Emotion Regulation

Ad J.J.M. Vingerhoets · Ivan Nyklíček
Johan Denollet
Editors

Emotion Regulation

Conceptual and Clinical Issues

Springer

Chapter 1
Introduction: Emotions, Emotion Regulation, and Health

Johan Denollet, Ivan Nyklíček, and Ad J.J.M. Vingerhoets

Emotions may be considered as the spices of our lives. They enable us to enjoy life to the fullest, but they also have other important functions. There is the interpersonal, communicative function aimed to signal to others information about our internal state and behavioral intentions (Frijda, 1986). In addition, specific intrapersonal functions of emotional expression have been demonstrated. For example, emotions make us aware of what really is important in our lives. As such, they are important for adequate decision making (Bechara, Damasio, & Damasio, 2000). In addition, they help and prepare us to better deal with environmental demands.

Emotions manifest themselves in specific cognitive, behavioral, and physiologic reactions and they are crucial for adaptation to new situations. Emotions result from the outcome of the evaluation of environmental stimuli. When attended to and appraised in certain ways, a coordinated set of responses involving behavioral and physiologic systems is triggered (John & Gross, 2004). As such, emotions provide the necessary physiologic support for emotion-specific action tendencies, thereby facilitating overt action. A clear example of this process is the fight-flight reaction, which implies increased heart rate and blood pressure, dilation of the bronchi, and increased blood flow to the muscles, preparing the body for action. Depressed affect and grief, as another example, are characterized by a quite different physiologic reaction pattern, aimed at the conservation of energy. There is apathy and often a reduced muscle tone with the head directed downward—there is no intention for action. Passivity prevails, and sexual and maternal drives are strongly reduced (Henry & Stephens, 1977; Vingerhoets & Perski, 2000). The idea is that this passive condition may reduce aggression and instead may act as a manifest signal to indicate that the person is in dire need of emotional or instrumental support from others (Nesse, 2000; Thornhill & Thornhill, 1989).

In light of their adaptive function, it is plausible that emotions have played an essential role for survival in the course of human evolution. It is important to note, however, that this does not mean that emotions should be regarded as outdated adaptation systems that were only advantageous for the human species in the very past. In fact, they still are crucial for proper psychologic functioning in the current modern society. For example, emotions are essential for adequate decision making. The notion that emotions should be considered as the opposite of the ratio and not important for cognition has to be qualified as obsolete and incorrect

A. Vingerhoets et al., (eds.), *Emotion Regulation.*

(Bechara, Damasio, & Damasio, 2000). But perhaps most important for this volume, the health-promoting effect of emotions in the social world depends on our ability to regulate these emotions in an adaptive way.

Adaptive Regulation of Emotions

As pointed out by John and Gross (2004), emotions are often helpful, but sometimes destructive. With reference to this issue, two important aspects of emotions need to be disentangled: (i) the subjective experience of emotions per se and (ii) the regulation of these emotions. Among other things, a major challenge is to find ways of regulating one's emotions so that one retains their helpful features while limiting their potentially destructive aspects. The things we do before an emotion response has become fully activated determine our physiologic and behavioral reactions. Cognitive reappraisal, or changing the way we perceive a potentially emotion-eliciting event, is one way of modifying the emotional impact of a situation (John & Gross, 2004). If one thinks that another person plans to do harm, this may induce anger; if an unpleasant situation is considered as being caused by one's own behavior, this will probably result in remorse, shame, or guilt. If a situation is appraised as involving danger, fear is a likely emotional outcome, whereas loss experiences generally evoke sadness.

Emotion regulation not only depends on our appraisal of the emotion-eliciting event. The things we do once the emotion process is already under way and response tendencies have already been generated, are of equal importance (John & Gross, 2004). For instance, in addition to cognitive reappraisal, emotion suppression is another emotion regulation strategy that is used commonly in everyday life. Emotion suppression is a form of emotion regulation that involves consciously inhibiting ongoing expression of emotion-related behavior. As such, nonexpression changes the way we respond behaviorally once we are already in an emotional state (Gross & Levenson, 1993).

When focusing on the effects of emotions on well-being and health, it should be kept in mind that this possible influence may not be the mere direct physiologic consequence of the expression of emotions. The many interpersonal aspects, including the nature of the relationship with the individual to whom one expresses and his or her reaction, are also important. For example, crying has been shown to very likely elicit emotional support. It may be this social support or the fact that an opponent becomes less aggressive that makes one feel better rather than the shedding of tears per se (see Hendriks et al., this volume).

In addition, the causal direction may also be the other way around: Using emotion suppression makes individuals feel inauthentic and bad about themselves and thus more prone to experience negative emotions and depressive symptoms (John & Gross, 2004). Suppression decreases the behavioral expression of negative emotions but not their subjective experience. In social contexts, suppressors may fail to respond appropriately to others and may avoid interpersonal interaction (John & Gross, 2004). Importantly, there is increasing evidence that emotion regulation styles aimed at not expressing emotion, either consciously or unconsciously—in the latter case often called repression—may have adverse effects on physical health (Myers et al., this volume; Nyklíček, Vingerhoets, & Denollet, 2002).

Nonexpression of Emotions and Health

Given the fact that suppression modifies the behavioral aspect of the emotion response tendencies without reducing the experience of negative emotion, these negative emotions may continue to linger and accumulate unresolved (John & Gross, 2004). There is little doubt that emotions may have an immediate impact on our physiologic functioning. Among the most dramatic examples is emotional fainting. Individuals suffering from blood phobia may lose their consciousness at the mere sight of blood or when undergoing rather innocent procedures such as taking blood samples (Vingerhoets & Schomaker, 1989). This is caused by a strong decrease in heart rate and a widening of the blood vessels. However, there is also evidence to suggest that chronic unresolved negative emotions can trigger acute, life-threatening cardiac events. Emotionally stressful events may trigger the onset of acute myocardial infarction. An outburst of anger, for example, may trigger the incidence of an acute myocardial infarction during the first 2 hours after the anger-evoking incident (Mittleman et al., 1995; Moller et al., 1999). But the risk of a myocardial infarction may also be increased during vacation travel; for example, adverse driving conditions or changes in climate may increase the risk for acute myocardial infarction during the first 2 days of vacation (Kop, Vingerhoets, Kruithof, & Gottdiener, 2003).

Sudden and profound emotional stress (e.g., death of relatives, domestic abuse, severe arguments, medical diagnoses, devastating financial loss) can also trigger acute heart failure in individuals who are free from cardiac disease (Engel, 1971). Reports of acute heart failure triggered by psychological stress thus are not confined to Japan, where this syndrome was labeled *Tako-tsubo cardiomyopathy*. Recent studies have also identified emotional stress as a trigger of acute heart failure in individuals from Western societies (Sharkey et al., 2005; Wedekind, Moller, & Scholz, 2006; Wittstein et al., 2005). This condition is characterized by a distinctive form of acute left ventricular dysfunction and is reversible with appropriate medical therapy. Exaggerated sympathetic stimulation is probably central to the cause of this syndrome of acute heart failure due to emotional stress (Wittstein et al., 2005).

In conclusion, there is ample evidence that experiencing intense negative emotions may have an acute effect on bodily functioning. However, chronic emotional distress is also a powerful determinant of adverse cardiovascular outcomes. Various psychological factors have been associated with the incidence and progression of heart disease, like chronic life stress (Rozanski, Blumenthal, & Kaplan, 1999), depression (Barth, Schumacher, & Herrmann-Lingen, 2004), anxiety (Moser et al., 2007), low social support (Orth-Gomer et al., 1998), and personality (Denollet et al., 1996; Denollet, Vaes, & Brutsaert, 2000). These factors often cluster together, and this clustering elevates the risk for cardiac events even more (Albus, Jordan, & Herrmann-Lingen, 2004).

However, it is important to consider the notion that—apart from the mere experience of negative emotions—the failure to use adaptive emotion regulation strategies might be detrimental to health as well. The popular literature is replete with warnings that it may be damaging for one's health to inhibit one's emotions and the expression of them. Anger must be released and tears must flow, because otherwise these emotions may seriously affect one's physical functioning (Cornelius, 2001; Bushman, 2002). In particular, when these behaviors are the consequence of specific stable personality traits, the person is said to be at increased risk of several somatic problems.

In contrast with this popular belief that nonexpression of emotions may be detrimental to health, the medical community has frequently qualified this notion as folklore and scientifically ungrounded. Despite this skepticism, there is empirical evidence to suggest that nonexpression of emotions increases the risk of somatic disease. Experimental research has shown that emotional inhibition is associated with increased cardiovascular reactivity (Gross & Levenson, 1997) and decreased cardiovascular recovery and heart rate variability (Brosschot & Thayer, 1998). Epidemiologic research has shown that anger inhibition is associated with high blood pressure (Steffen, McNeilly, Anderson, & Sherwood, 2003) and cardiovascular death (Graves, Mead, Wang, Liang, & Klag, 1994; Harburg, Julius, Kaciroti, Gleiberman, & Schork, 2003). Emotional inhibition has also been linked to immune dysregulation in patients with human immunodeficiency virus (Cole, Kemeny, Fahey, Zack, & Naliboff, 2003).

Undoubtedly, many issues concerning the health impact of emotion regulation strategies remain to be answered. Among other things, it is unclear to what extent and why some forms of emotion regulation may be healthier than others. It has been suggested that using cognitive reappraisal to regulate emotions is associated with healthier patterns of psychological functioning than applying suppression (John & Gross, 2004), but more experimental and epidemiologic research is needed to examine the validity of this notion. Another important issue relates to the determinants of individual differences in emotion regulation styles.

Individual Differences

The expectation that significant others will not be available appears to fuel the suppression of emotions (Dozier & Kobak, 1992). In addition, more temperamental precursors for suppression have been identified, including introversion (John & Gross, 2004) and shyness (Melchior & Cheek, 1990). The past decades have witnessed the description of several psychological constructs and personality features to describe more or less stable individual differences in emotion regulation strategies. Well-known examples include alexithymia (Lumley, Gustavson, Partridge, & Labouvie-Vief, 2005), the repressive coping style (Myers, Brewin,

& Power, 1998), Type C coping style (Temoshok, 1987), and lack of emotional intelligence (Salovey & Mayer, 1990).

Unfortunately, the clinical implications of this research are still far from clear and certain. The cross-sectional nature of many studies prevents drawing definitive conclusions about the nature of the relationship between nonexpression and health outcomes, and there is also a lack of insight into the underlying mechanisms that may explain this relationship. Some recent studies have tried to address these issues in research on the health implications of social inhibition in patients with human immunodeficiency virus infection (Cole, Kemeny, Fahey, Zack, & Naliboff, 2003) and coronary heart disease (Denollet et al., 2006).

With reference to this issue, research on the health effect of Type D personality in cardiac patients indicates that social inhibition may modulate the impact of negative emotions on long-term prognosis (Denollet et al., 2006). Type D personality refers to individuals who have an elevated score on negative affectivity (or the tendency to experience negative emotions across time and situations) and social inhibition (or the tendency to inhibit the expression of emotion and behavior during social interaction). This personality type has been shown to reliably predict mortality, morbidity, and poor quality of life in several groups of patients suffering from cardiovascular disease (e.g., Al-Ruzzeh et al., 2005; Aquarius, Denollet, Hamming, & De Vries, 2005; Denollet et al., 1996; Denollet, Vaes, & Brutsaert, 2000). Importantly, only those individuals who score high on *both* negative affectivity *and* social inhibition are at increased risk for poor health outcomes (Denollet et al., 1996). Recently, we have specifically examined the interaction between social inhibition and negative affectivity as a determinant of prognosis after balloon angioplasty treatment (Denollet et al., 2006). This study showed that the combined effect of social inhibition and negative affectivity, rather than negative emotions alone, was an independent predictor of poor prognosis. Interestingly, individuals with high negative affectivity but low social inhibition were not at increased risk for a major adverse cardiac event. Hence, more research is needed to test the hypothesis that inhibition or other emotion regulation strategies may modify the effect of negative emotions on physical health.

About This Book

In the past decade, we have organized three conferences focused on these issues at Tilburg University. During these conferences, international experts present their latest findings and discuss them with fellow researchers.

This book contains a selection of the updated body of knowledge based on the key contributions of the 2003 meeting. The contributions provide the latest insights into a wide array of topics such as the writing paradigm, alexithymia, crying, repression, and so forth. We included both fundamental and basic research on emotion regulation as well as more clinically oriented contributions in order to cover a wide range of relevant research. The contributions can be classified into two broad categories. In the first category, the focus is on conceptual and developmental issues. In the second category, clinical perspectives and interventions are the main issues.

The first part of this volume, on the fundamental, conceptual, and neurobiologic bases of emotion regulation, starts with a chapter by Koolhaas and de Boer. In their contribution, some intriguing findings from animal studies are summarized. The distinction between proactive (being also more expressive) and reactive (less expressive) coping styles among rodents has proved to be differently associated with overt behavior as well as with neuroendocrine responses to laboratory challenges. Interestingly, these differential reactions putatively make the two types of animals also differently susceptible to diseases and are additionally associated with different effects of pharmacologic agents.

In Chapter 3, the focus is on the personality aspects of different alexithymia types. Moormann and colleagues have developed a model containing five alexithymia types. Their different personality features, coping approaches, and vulnerability to stress-related mental and physical problems are discussed. Lumley and colleagues present in Chapter 4 their critical considerations concerning the relationship between alexithymia and the development of health problems. They show that various pathways may be responsible for research findings, ranging from direct physiologic effects of alexithymia to third-variable explanations. In addition, they put forth important challenges for future research on this topic. In Chapter 5, Myers and colleagues review the studies of the past three decades on repressive coping. They summarize the available evidence for a link between this style and various health problems and discuss the critique as well as the possible cognitive and psychophysiologic mechanisms explaining the link. The latter issue is just starting to be investigated systematically.

Chapter 6 is devoted to adult crying. Hendriks and colleagues put forth some challenging ideas about the potential mechanism of the effect of crying on well-being. From an attachment-theory perspective, they provide preliminary evidence for the view that the positive effects of crying may be brought about by positive responses from the social environment as a result of this potent signal of a need for caring, help, and support. Emotional intelligence is the topic of Chapter 7, written by Van Heck and Den Oudsten. In this comprehensive contribution, the authors critically discuss the concept of emotional intelligence and examine its relation with the standard intelligence concept. In addition, they address the important issue of its assessment and summarize the scarce research results regarding its impact on health.

The second part of this volume, on clinical perspectives and interventions, begins with Chapter 8, a contribution by Rottenberg and Vaughan on emotion expression in depression. Both naturalistic and experimental studies are reviewed, concluding that depression may be accompanied by emotion context insensitivity, which is characterized by rather stereotypical emotional response patterns without much variation across situations. Rodebaugh and Heimberg (Chapter 9) argue that many affective problems involve dysfunctional emotion regulation. In their view, treatment should more explicitly aim at enhancing self-regulation and emotion regulation. Van Dijke (Chapter 10) provides the readers with an example of how disturbances with emotion regulation are treated with a comprehensive, multidisciplinary approach in a psychiatric hospital setting. Emotional inhibition as a factor in eating disorders is discussed by Bekker and Spoor in Chapter 11. They argue that especially anger inhibition may be an important maladaptive response style highly prevalent among eating-disordered women displaying oversensitivity to others. In Chapter 12, Rieffe and colleagues present empirical findings relating to the relevance of emotional competence for somatic complaints in children. They present data supporting their view that maladaptive coping strategies, such as an attentional overemphasis on internal bodily symptoms, may be key factors promoting somatic complaints. In Chapter 13, Nelson describes various types of crying behavior, especially in the clinical context, which can be used to identify attachment styles of the patient.

The last two chapters of this volume are devoted to Pennebaker's renowned writing disclosure intervention. First, Smyth and colleagues provide an in-depth discussion of the writing paradigm in the clinical context. They consider issues such as the effects on physiologic systems, the mechanisms that may be responsible for the effects found, and the role of feedback that may be provided to the writer. In the final contribution (Chapter 15), Solano and colleagues present a critique on the emphasis on simple direct (main) effects when evaluating the writing paradigm. They argue and provide examples of studies showing that the effectiveness of this paradigm in the clinical context strongly depends on some specific characteristics of the patients and their situation, such as their personality, their primary disorder, and the recency of an adverse event they may have experienced.

Taken together, this volume provides the reader with a comprehensive and up-to-date overview of the state of the art with respect to emotion regulation in relation to mental and somatic health. The emphasis on clinically oriented papers makes it interesting reading for both researchers and clinicians. Those working in the fields of psychiatry, psychosomatics, behavioral medicine, health psychology, clinical psychology, and medical psychology all can benefit from this unique collection of papers written by internationally leading researchers. We hope that readers will enjoy this volume and that it will stimulate and inspire them.

References

Albus, C., Jordan, J., & Herrmann-Lingen, C. (2004). Screening for psychosocial risk factors in patients with coronary heart disease-recommendations for clinical practice. *European Journal of Cardiovascular Prevention and Rehabilitation, 11*, 75–79.

Al-Ruzzeh, S., Athanasiou, T., Mangoush, O., Wray, J., Modine, T., George, S., & Amrani, M. (2005). Predictors of poor mid-term health related quality of life after primary isolated coronary artery bypass grafting surgery. *Heart, 91*, 1557–1562.

Aquarius, A. E., Denollet, J., Hamming, J. F., & De Vries, J. (2005). Role of disease status and type D personality in outcomes in patients with peripheral arterial disease. *American Journal of Cardiology, 96*, 996–1001.

Barth, J., Schumacher, M., & Herrmann-Lingen, C. (2004). Depression as a risk factor for mortality in patients with coronary heart disease: a meta-analysis. *Psychosomatic Medicine, 66*, 802–813.

Bechara, A., Damasio, H., & Damasio, A. R. (2000). Emotion, decision making and the orbitofrontal cortex. *Cerebral Cortex, 10*, 295–307.

Brosschot, J. F., & Thayer, J .F. (1998). Anger inhibition, cardiovascular recovery, and vagal function: a model of the links between hostility and cardiovascular disease. *Annals of Behavioral Medicine, 20*, 326–332.

Bushman, B. (2002). Does venting anger feed or extinguish the flame? Catharsis, rumination, distraction, anger, and aggressive responding. *Personality and Social Psychology Bulletin, 28*, 724–731.

Cole, S. W., Kemeny, M. E., Fahey, J. L., Zack, J. A., & Naliboff, B. D. (2003). Psychological risk factors for HIV pathogenesis: mediation by the autonomic nervous system. *Biological Psychiatry, 54*, 1444–1456.

Cornelius, R. R. (2001). Crying and catharsis. In A. J. J. M. Vingerhoets & R. R. Cornelius (Eds.), *Adult crying: a biopsychosocial approach* (pp. 199–211). Hove, United Kingdom: Brunner-Routledge.

Denollet, J., Pedersen, S. S., Ong, A. T., Erdman, R. A., Serruys, P. W., & van Domburg, R. T. (2006). Social inhibition modulates the effect of negative emotions on cardiac prognosis following percutaneous coronary intervention in the drug-eluting stent era. *European Heart Journal, 27*, 171–177.

Denollet, J., Sys, S. U., Stroobant, N., Rombouts, H., Gillebert, T. C., & Brutsaert, D. L. (1996). Personality as independent predictor of long-term mortality in patients with coronary heart disease. *Lancet, 347*, 417–421.

Denollet, J., Vaes, J., & Brutsaert, D. L. (2000). Inadequate response to treatment in coronary heart disease: adverse effects of type D personality and younger age on 5-year prognosis and quality of life. *Circulation, 102*, 630–635.

Dozier, M., & Kobak, R. R. (1992). Psychophysiology in attachment interviews: converging evidence for deactivating strategies. *Child Development, 63*, 1473–1480.

Engel, G. L. (1971). Sudden and rapid death during psychological stress: folklore or folk wisdom? *Annals of Internal Medicine, 74*, 771–782.

Frijda, N. H. (1986). *The emotions*. New York: Cambridge University Press.

Graves, P. L., Mead, L. A., Wang, N. Y., Liang, K., & Klag, M. J. (1994). Temperament as a potential predictor of mortality: evidence from a 41year prospective study. *Journal of Behavioral Medicine, 17*, 111–126.

Gross, J. J., & Levenson, R. W. (1993). Emotional suppression: physiology, self-report, and expressive behavior. *Journal of Personality and Social Psychology, 64*, 970–986.

Gross J. J., & Levenson, R. W. (1997). Hiding feelings: the acute effects of inhibiting positive and negative emotions. *Journal of Abnormal Psychology, 106*, 95–103.

Harburg, E., Julius, M., Kaciroti, N., Gleiberman, L., & Schork, M.A. (2003). Expressive/suppressive anger-coping responses, gender, and types of mortality: a 17-year follow-up (Tecumseh, Michigan, 1971-1988). *Psychosomatic Medicine, 65*, 588–597.

Henry, J. P., & Stephens, P. M. (1977). *Stress, health and the social environment: a sociobiological approach to medicine*. Berlin: Springer.

John, O. P., & Gross, J. J. (2004). Healthy and unhealthy emotion regulation: personality processes, individual differences, and life span development. *Journal of Personality, 72*, 1301–1333.

Kop, W. J., Vingerhoets, A., Kruithof, G. J., & Gottdiener, J. S. (2003). Risk factors for myocardial infarction during vacation travel. *Psychosomatic Medicine, 65*, 396–401.

Lumley, M. A., Gustavson, B. J., Partridge, R. T., & Labouvie-Vief, G. (2005). Assessing alexithymia and related emotional ability constructs using multiple methods: interrelationships among measures. *Emotion, 5*, 329–342.

Melchior, L. A., & Cheek, J. M. (1990). Shyness and anxious self-preoccupation during a social interaction. *Journal of Social Behavior and Personality, 5*, 117–130.

Mittleman, M. A., Maclure, M., Sherwood, J. B., Mulry, R. P., Tofler, G. H., Jacobs, S. C., Friedman, R., Benson, H., & Muller, J. E. (1995). Triggering of acute myocardial infarction onset by episodes of anger. *Circulation, 92*, 1720–1725.

Moller, J., Hallqvist, J., Diderichsen, F., Theorell, T., Reuterwall, C., & Ahlbom, A. (1999). Do episodes of anger trigger myocardial infarction? A case-crossover analysis in the Stockholm

Heart Epidemiology Program (SHEEP). *Psychosomatic Medicine*, *61*, 842–849.
Moser, D. K., Riegel, B., McKinley, S., Doering, L. V., An, K., & Sheahan, S. (2007). Impact of anxiety and perceived control on in-hospital complications after acute myocardial infarction. *Psychosomatic Medicine*, *69*, 10–16.
Myers, L. B., Brewin, C. R., & Power, M. J. (1998). Repressive coping and the directed forgetting of emotional material. *Journal of Abnormal Psychology*, *107*, 141–148.
Nesse, R. M. (2000). Is depression an adaptation? *Archives of General Psychiatry, 57,* 14–20.
Nyklíček, I., Vingerhoets, A., & Denollet, J. (2002). Emotional non-expression and health: data, questions, and challenges. *Psychology & Health*, *17*, 517–528.
Orth-Gomer, K., Horsten, M., Wamala, S. P., Mittleman, M. A., Kirkeeide, R., Svane, B., Ryden, L., & Schenck-Gustafsson, K. (1998). Social relations and extent and severity of coronary artery disease. The Stockholm female coronary risk study. *European Heart Journal, 19,* 1648–1656.
Rozanski, A., Blumenthal, J. A., & Kaplan, J. (1999). Impact of psychological factors on the pathogenesis of cardiovascular disease and implications for therapy. *Circulation, 99,* 2192–2217.
Salovey, P., & Mayer, J. D. (1990). Emotional intelligence. *Imagination, Cognition & Personality, 9,* 185–211.
Sharkey, S. W., Lesser, J. R., Zenovich, A. G., Maron, M. S., Lindberg, J., Longe, T. F., & Maron, B. J. (2005). Acute and reversible cardiomyopathy provoked by stress in women from the United States. *Circulation*, *111*, 472–479.
Steffen, P. R., McNeilly, M., Anderson, N., & Sherwood, A. (2003). Effects of perceived racism and anger inhibition on ambulatory blood pressure in African Americans. *Psychosomatic Medicine, 65,* 746–750.
Temoshok, L. (1987). Personality, coping style, emotion and cancer: towards an integrative model. *Cancer Surveys*, *6*, 545–567.
Thornhill, R., & Thornhill, N. W. (1989). The evolution of psychological pain. In R. Bell & N. Bell (Eds.), *Sociobiology and the social sciences* (pp. 73–103). Lubbock, TX: Texas Technical University.
Vingerhoets, A. J. J. M., & Perski, A. (2000). The psychobiology of stress. In A. Kaptein, A. Appels, & K. Orth-Gomer (Eds.), *Psychology in medicine* (pp. 34–49). Houten, The Netherlands: Bohn, Stafleu Van Loghum.
Vingerhoets, A. J. J. M., & Schomaker, L. R .B. (1989). Emotional fainting: its physiological and psychological aspects. In C. D. Spielberger, I. G. Sarason, & J. Strelau (Eds.), *Stress and anxiety*, Vol. XII (pp. 181–198). New York: Hemisphere Publishing Corporation.
Wedekind, H., Moller, K., & Scholz, K. H. (2006). Tako-tsubo cardiomyopathy: incidence in patients with acute coronary syndrome. *Herz, 31*, 339–346.
Wittstein, I. S., Thiemann, D. R., Lima, J. A., Baughman, K. L., Schulman, S. P., Gerstenblith, G., Wu, K. C., Rade, J. J., Bivalacqua, T. J., & Champion, H. C. (2005). Neurohumoral features of myocardial stunning due to sudden emotional stress. *New England Journal of Medicine*, *352*, 539–548.

Chapter 2
Coping Styles and Aggression: A Biobehavioral Approach

Jaap M. Koolhaas and Sietse F. de Boer

Introduction

Health and stress-related disease are generally considered to be influenced by a complex interplay between the actual environmental demands and the individual's capacity to cope with these demands. A wide variety of medical, psychological, and biological studies both in humans and in animals demonstrate that individuals may differ in their capacities to cope with such environmental demands. Factors that have been shown to affect the individual coping capacity include genotype, ontogeny, adult experience, age, social support, and so forth. For ages, researchers have tried to determine the individual vulnerability to stress-related diseases using estimates of the individual coping capacity. These attempts date back to the times of Hippocrates who distinguished the following four temperaments: choleric, sanguine, phlegmatic and melancholic. Each of these temperaments was supposed to reflect a general attitude in dealing with everyday problems. More recent approaches use the concept of coping and try to classify coping responses into distinct coping strategies. Psychologists define coping in humans as the cognitive, behavioral, and emotional ways of managing stressful situations. According to Lazarus (1966), coping responses are determined by the appraisal of the degree of control over important resources available to the individual. In their conceptualization, psychologists divide coping responses into emotion-focused coping and problem-focused coping strategies. The concept of coping is also used by biologists to understand the behavioral and physiologic ways animals manage stressful conditions. A coping strategy can therefore be defined as a coherent set of behavioral and physiologic stress responses that is consistent over time and context and that is characteristic of a certain group of individuals. Most studies describe individual differences in behavior and physiology as trait characteristics that may determine the individual's vulnerability to stress-related diseases.

These studies are in the realm of biomedical sciences, yet there is a growing interest in individual differentiation in behavior and physiology in the science of ecology and evolutionary biology (Sih, Bell, Johnson, & Ziemba, 2004). Individual variation in coping with challenges in the natural habitat is not only considered as the origin of speciation but may be an important factor in the regulation of populations as well. It seems that coping strategies have been shaped by evolution and

A. Vingerhoets et al., (eds.), *Emotion Regulation.*

form general adaptive response patterns in reaction to everyday challenges in the natural habitat. The aim of this chapter is to describe coping strategies in animals as they might be observed in nature and to summarize the available evidence of their possible function. We will focus on aggressive behavior as an important indicator and component of coping strategy. It will be argued that the individual variation in aggressive behavior is related to a differentiation in behavioral flexibility. This differential degree of flexibility seems to be one of the major factors involved in the differential fitness of individuals under various environmental conditions in nature.

Aggression and Coping Strategies

Much of our current thinking on coping strategies is based on the work of Jim Henry (Henry & Stephens, 1977). He suggested, on the basis of social stress research in animals and man, that two different stress response patterns may be distinguished. The first type, the active response, was originally described by Cannon (1915) as the fight-flight response. Behaviorally, territorial control and aggression characterize this active response. Engel and Schmale (1972) originally described the second type of stress response as the conservation-withdrawal response. This response pattern is characterized behaviorally by immobility and low levels of aggression. These authors consider the degree in which animals react with an aggressive response to a stressor as an important discriminating factor of the two coping strategies. These ideas led to the expectation that the individual level of aggressive behavior (i.e., the tendency to defend the home territory) is related to the way individual male mice react to environmental challenges in general. This hypothesis was tested by Benus, Bohus, Koolhaas, and Van Oortmerssen (1991a) using male house mice that were genetically selected for either short attack latency (SAL) or a long attack latency (LAL). These selection lines of wild house mice were derived from a completely different line of research aimed at investigating the genetic basis of aggression. Also, when other indices of aggressive behavior are taken into account, the SAL males are considered extremely aggressive, whereas the LAL males have very low levels of intermale aggressive behavior. The results of a series of experiments in mice and rats, which are summarized in Table 2.1, demonstrate that the individual tendency to initiate aggressive behavior is indeed predictive of the individual reactions to other, nonsocial environmental challenges. This pattern of behavioral responses is consistent with the concept of stable coping strategies.

Table 2.1 shows that the individual level of aggressive behavior is related to the way in which the animals react to a wide variety of environmental challenges. It seems that aggressive males have a strong tendency to take the initiative (i.e., attack, active avoidance, or nest building). Nonaggressive males seem to accept the situation more easily as it is, responding only when absolutely necessary. This difference in response initiation forms the basis of the terminology we currently use for the different coping strategies. In our view, high levels of aggression are a reflection of

Table 2.1 Summary of the behavioral differences between high-aggressive and low-aggressive male rats and mice

Behavioral characteristics	High aggressive	Low aggressive
Tests for proactivity		
Attack latency	Low	High
Active avoidance	High	Low
Defensive burying	High	Low
Nest building	High	Low
Behavioral flexibility tests		
Routine formation	High	Low
Cue dependency	Low	High

Source: Koolhaas, J. M., Korte, S. M., De Boer, S. F., Van Der Vegt, B. J., Van Reenen, C. G., Hopster, H., et al. (1999). Coping styles in animals: current status in behavior and stress-physiology. *Neuroscience & Biobehavioral Reviews, 23,* 925–935.

a more general proactive coping strategy, whereas a low level of aggression reflects a reactive coping strategy.

An important fundamental question is whether the two types of behavior patterns can be considered to represent strategies of coping in the sense that they are both aimed at successful environmental control. Several experiments indicate that the different behavior patterns can indeed be considered as coping strategies. An illustrative example is the shock prod defensive burying test. In this test, the animal is confronted with a small, electrified prod in its home cage. Because this prod is a novel object, the experimental animal will explore it by sniffing at the object. Consequently, the animal receives a mild but aversive shock. As soon as it has experienced the shock, the animal has two options to avoid further shocks. It may either hide in a corner of the cage to avoid further contact with the shock prod or it may actively bury the shock prod with the bedding material of the cage. Under these free-choice conditions, aggressive males spend most of the 10 minutes of test-time burying, whereas nonaggressive males show immobility behavior. Notice, however, that the two types of responding are equally successful in avoiding further shocks (De Boer & Koolhaas, 2003). In this particular test, successful coping can be defined operationally as avoidance of further shocks. In that sense, both response types in the defensive burying test can be considered as successful coping. However, Treit, Pinel, and Fibiger, (1981) described the defensive burying test originally as an anxiety test. High levels of burying behavior would indicate a high level of anxiety. Therefore, one may argue that the differences in burying behavior reflect a difference in baseline emotional state such as anxiety. We think that this interpretation is not correct. When high and low aggressive males (rats and mice) are tested in a well-validated anxiety test, the elevated plus maze, no differences are observed. The difference between both anxiety tests is that the elevated plus maze is more a test for baseline anxiety, whereas the burying test is a test for fear induced by the electric shock. In line with the concept of proactive and reactive coping, this fear can be expressed either as burying behavior or as immobility behavior (De Boer, Van Der Vegt, & Koolhaas, 2003).

It is important to emphasize that the differentiation in coping strategies may not be expressed equally clearly in all challenging situations. In particular, tests that measure aspects of initiative or proactivity seem to be most discriminative. This holds, for example, for latency measures such as the attack latency test in males or the defensive burying test, which allow the animal a choice between proactive and reactive coping. Although female mice usually do not show territorial aggression, females of the short attack latency selection line show much more defensive burying than female mice of the long attack latency selection line. This supports our view that aggression is only one of a larger set of behavioral characteristics that make up the proactive coping strategy.

Behavioral Flexibility

The concept of coping strategies is basically descriptive; that is, it describes the correlations and consistencies of the behavior of individual animals under different environmental conditions. The question is to what extent these differences might be causally related to differential cognitive abilities? Several experiments indicate that proactive and reactive coping strategies differ in the degree to which behavior is guided by environmental cues (Koolhaas et al., 1999). Aggressive males easily develop routines (i.e., a rather intrinsically driven rigid type of behavior). Nonaggressive males are more flexible and react to environmental stimuli all the time. This can be demonstrated for example by the way in which aggressive and nonaggressive males react to a small change in an otherwise stable environment. Animals can be trained to run a maze for a food reward. Rats and mice can learn such a task easily. When they reached a stable task performance, the reaction to a small change in the maze was studied. In one experiment, a small piece of tape was put on the floor in one of the alleys of the maze, while in another experiment, the maze was turned 90 degrees with respect to the extra maze cues. In both experiments, aggressive males paid little or no attention to the change (i.e., there was no increase in time to complete the task and no increase in the number of errors made in the maze). Nonaggressive males, on the other hand, started exploring the maze again and hence took much more time to get to the goal box and made more errors in the task. This suggests that the behavior of the nonaggressive male may be much more guided by environmental stimuli, whereas aggressive males seem to develop routines. A similar difference in behavioral plasticity can be demonstrated in the response to a 12-hour shift in light-dark cycle. Aggressive male mice stay in their original day-night rhythm for a few days after which their rhythm gradually shifts to the new cycle. Nonaggressive males on the other hand shift their rhythm immediately; they are twice as fast in adapting to the new light-dark cycle as the aggressive males (Benus, Koolhaas, & Van Oortmerssen, 1988).

These experiments show that the two coping strategies differ more generally in the use of feedback and feed-forward behavioral control. The proactive animal acts primarily on the basis of previous experience (i.e., feed-forward control). The reactive coping animal seems to rely on feedback information. This fundamental difference in behavioral control may causally explain why the animals differ in such a wide variety of behavioral tests. One may conclude that the concept of coping strategies can be reduced to an underlying difference in a limited number of behavioral control mechanisms. Moreover, this differential use of behavioral control mechanisms also relates to the adaptive character of the two coping strategies. A proactive coping animal may be adapted to stable environmental conditions. After all, a feed-forward behavioral control works best under highly predictable conditions. The reactive coping strategy may do better under variable and unpredictable environmental conditions. Indeed, field studies on feral mouse populations indicate that aggressive males are more successful under stable colony conditions, whereas nonaggressive males do better during migration (see below).

Neuroendocrinology of Coping Strategies

Coping strategies are not only characterized by differences in behavior but also by differences in physiology and neuroendocrinology. As mentioned earlier, tests that measure aspects of initiative or proactivity seem to be most discriminative. The defensive burying test in rodents is such a test, which allows the animal a choice between proactive and reactive coping. In general, high plasma noradrenalin and relatively low plasma adrenaline and corticosterone accompany defensive burying, whereas freezing behavior is associated with relatively low plasma noradrenalin and high plasma corticosterone levels. In a strain of wild-type rats, the more aggressive males showed the highest levels of burying behavior and showed a larger catecholaminergic (both plasma noradrenalin and adrenaline) reactivity after electrified prod exposure than did the nonaggressive rats (Sgoifo, De Boer, Haller, & Koolhaas, 1996). Also, during social defeat, the more competitive proactive male rats react with higher responses of blood pressure and catecholamines than the more reactive rats. In addition, these competitive males had higher baseline levels of noradrenalin (Fokkema, Smit, Van der Gugten, & Koolhaas, 1988). The same can be observed in a comparison between strains. The aggressive wild-type rats responded to social defeat with larger sympathetic (plasma noradrenalin levels) reactivity and concomitantly lower parasympathetic reactivity (as measured by increased heart rate response and decreased heart rate variability) than the less aggressive Wistar rats (Sgoifo et al., 1997). Thus, proactive coping rodents show in response to stressful stimulation a low Hypothalamus-Pituitary-Adrenocortical (HPA) axis reactivity (low plasma corticosterone response) but high sympathetic reactivity (high levels of catecholamines). In contrast, reactive coping rodents show higher HPA-axis reactivity and higher parasympathetic reactivity (Table 2.2). Differences in endocrine activity have also been observed for HPA axis and gonadal axis activity under baseline conditions. In aggressive mice, reduced circadian peak plasma corticosterone levels have been observed compared with nonaggressive mice (Korte et al., 1996). In mice of the short attack latency selection line and in wild-type male rats, high baseline levels of testosterone have been observed, while the proactive coping male

Table 2.2 Summary of the physiologic and neuroendocrine differences between proactive and reactive animals

Physiologic and neuroendocrine characteristics	Proactive	Reactive
HPA-axis activity	Low	Normal
HPA-axis reactivity	Low	High
Neurosympathetic reactivity	High	Low
Adrenomedullary reactivity	High	Medium
Parasympathetic reactivity	Low	High
Testosterone production	High	Low
Testosterone sensitivity	High	Low

is also more sensitive to the behavioral effects of testosterone (Ruiter, Koolhaas, Keijser, Van Oortmerssen, & Bohus, 1992).

Neurobiology of Coping Strategies

Several studies in our rats and mice show a widespread central nervous differentiation between the two coping strategies. This takes place, for example, at the level of the peptidergic modulation of the central nucleus of the amygdala (Roozendaal, Wiersma, Driscoll, Koolhaas, & Bohus, 1992), the vasopressinergic neurons in the bed nucleus of the stria terminalis and its innervation of the lateral septum (Compaan, Buijs, Pool, De Ruiter, & Koolhaas, 1992), the suprachiasmatic nucleus (Bult, Hiestand, Van der Zee, & Lynch, 1993), postsynaptic 5-HT1a receptor sensitivity, the hippocampal mossy fiber system (Sluyter, Jamot, Van Oortmerssen, & Crusio, 1994), and striatal dopaminergic mechanisms (Benus, Bohus, Koolhaas, & Van Oortmerssen, 1991b). These differences reflect differences in the state of brain mechanisms in terms of number of neurons, degree of arborization of neurons, hormonal and neurotransmitter receptor binding capacity, and so forth, which in concert may determine the tendency to cope either proactively or reactively with environmental challenges.

It is interesting to notice that the vasopressinergic system of the lateral septal area is well-known to be sexually dimorphic and testosterone dependent. Males are characterized by a considerably higher density of Lateral Septum Arginine Vasopressin (LS-AVP) fibers than females. However, the differences in density of LS-AVP fibers as observed in the proactive and reactive coping strategies within the male gender turn out to be as large as the differences between the sexes. This indicates that the differentiation in coping strategies is somehow related to the differentiation between the sexes. Indeed, there is some evidence that the perinatal processes involved in the sexual differentiation are also involved in the development of the two coping strategies within the male gender (Koolhaas, Everts, de Ruiter, De Boer, & Bohus, 1998).

An intriguing recent observation in mice indicates that the nonaggressive, reactive coping mouse shows the strongest hippocampal neuronal plasticity in terms of stress-induced changes in hippocampal neurogenesis. This is correlated with a

Table 2.3 Summary of the central nervous differences between proactive and reactive male rats and mice

Neurochemical characteristics	Proactive	Reactive
Septum AVP-ir fibers	Low density	High density
SCN AVP-ir fibers	Low density	High density
AVP infusion in ACE	Insensitive	Immobility
AVP infusion in ACE	Insensitive	Bradycardia
CRH infusion in ACE	Behavioral activity	Insensitive
CRH infusion in ACE	Tachycardia	Insensitive
Hippocampal mossy fibers	Small	Large
Striatal dopamine	Sensitive	Insensitive
5-HT turnover	High	Low
5-HT1a binding	High	Low
5-HT1a receptor mRNA	High	Low
5-HT1a receptor sensitivity	High	Low

AVP-ir, Arginine Vasopressin Immunoreactivity; SCN, Suprachiasmatic Nucleus; ACE, Central Amygdala; CRH, Corticotropin Releasing Hormone; 5-HT, 5-hydroxytryptamine.

significantly higher hippocampal expression of genes coding for cytoskeleton proteins (Feldker, De Kloet, Kruk, & Datson, 2003).

Stress Vulnerability

The concept of coping styles implies that animals have a differential capacity to adapt to various environmental conditions. Negative health consequences might arise if an animal cannot cope with the stressor or needs very demanding coping efforts. In view of the differential neuroendocrine reactivity and neurobiological makeup, one may expect different types of stress pathology to develop under conditions in which a particular coping style fails. Although there are only a limited number of studies performed concerning pathology in relation to the type of coping style adopted, there are some indications that the two coping styles differ in susceptibility to develop cardiovascular pathology, ulcer formation, stereotypies, and infectious disease.

Cardiovascular Pathology

Various studies emphasize the differences between the two coping styles in autonomic balance. Because of the role of the two branches of the autonomic nervous system in cardiovascular control, one may expect a differential vulnerability for various types of cardiovascular pathology as well. Indeed, a number of experiments found evidence that the proactive coping animal is more vulnerable to develop hypertension, atherosclerosis, and tachyarrhythmia due to the high sympathetic reactivity (Fokkema, Koolhaas, & Gugten, 1995; Fokkema, Smit, Van der

Gugten, & Koolhaas, 1988; Manuck, Kaplan, & Clarkson, 1983; Sgoifo, De Boer, Haller, & Koolhaas, 1996; Sgoifo et al., 1997). However, it seems that these types of cardiovascular pathology only develop under conditions of threat to control rather than loss of control (Koolhaas & Bohus, 1991). The reactive coping style is characterized by a higher parasympathetic reactivity as can be observed by a strong bradycardia response in reaction to a sudden unexpected stressor. Although there have been no systematic studies of the cardiovascular consequences of this response, one may suggest that these types of animals are more vulnerable to sudden cardiac death.

Gastric Ulceration

The classical studies of Weiss, (1972) showed that the development of ulcers was high when the number of active coping attempts was high in the absence of informational feedback or with negative informational feedback present. In the experimental animal that could actively control the aversive shock by either pressing a lever during the warning signal or during the shock itself, the total length of stomach wall erosions was much smaller than in the yoked partner, which received exactly the same amount of shocks, but could not control them. Moreover, in the absence of informational feedback, a positive correlation was observed between the number of active coping attempts and the amount of gastric ulceration. In line with these results is an observation in the Roman high avoidance (RHA) and Roman low avoidance (RLA) rats, which can be considered to represent the proactive and reactive coping styles, respectively. It was shown that RHA rats, after stress of food deprivation for 5 days, had more stomach lesions than RLA rats (Driscoll, Martin, Kugler, & Baettig, 1983). A negative correlation between attack latency in the intruder test and gastric ulceration induced by restraint-in-water stress (Murison & Skjerve, 1992) also suggests that animals that prefer a proactive coping style are more vulnerable for the formation of ulcers during uncontrollable stress. In rat colonies, dominant animals that are usually representatives of the proactive coping style are reported to develop stomach wall erosions when they have lost their leading position (social outcast) after frequent attacks by other colony members. These studies suggest that the proactive individual is most vulnerable to stomach ulcers under conditions of loss of control. This observation is supported by studies in cattle (Wiepkema & Adrichem, 1987; Wiepkema & Schuiten, 1992).

Immunologic Defense

Contemporary psychoneuroimmunology emphasizes the role of the HPA axis and the sympathetic branch of the autonomic nervous system in the communication between the brain and the immune system (Felten et al., 1987). In view of the differential reactivity of these two systems in the two coping styles, one may expect to see differences in the immune system as well. Indeed, several studies in rats and mice demonstrate that individual differentiation in coping is an important factor in stress and immunity. In particular in the social stress models, the individual level of social activity seems to be an important explanatory variable in some studies (Bohus & Koolhaas, 1990; Raab et al., 1986). Although these studies do not specifically address the issue of coping styles, it is tempting to consider the possibility that these socially active animals represent the proactive coping style. Sandi, Castanon, Vitiello, Neveu, and Mormede (1991) specifically addressed the question of the significance of individual differentiation in emotional responsiveness to the differentiation in immunology. They used the RHA and RLA rats that have been genetically selected on the basis of their active avoidance behavior (Driscoll, Demek, D'Angio, Claustre, & Scatton, 1990). These selection lines have been shown to differ in a number of behavioral and neuroendocrine stress responses in a similar way as the proactive and reactive coping styles as mentioned above. It was shown that the Natural Killer (NK) cell activity and the proliferation response of splenocytes to mitogenic stimulation was lowest in the RLA males, a difference that was even more pronounced after the stress of active shock avoidance learning. In a study of pigs, Hessing (1994) demonstrated that aggressive, resistant pigs had a higher in vivo and in vitro cell-mediated immune response to specific and nonspecific antigens than nonaggressive, nonresistant pigs. After stress, the aggressive, resistant pigs showed the strongest immunosuppression. This difference in immunologic reactivity in relation to coping style may explain the differential disease susceptibility in relation to social rank in group-housed pigs after a challenge with Aujeszky virus. These observations in pigs are consistent with similar data obtained in colony-housed male rats (Bohus & Koolhaas, 1990). Finally, it was demonstrated that proactive coping male rats are more vulnerable for the experimental induction of the autoimmune disease experimental allergic encephalomyelitis (EAE), which is considered to be an animal model for multiple sclerosis in humans. This high vulnerability seems to be due to the high sympathetic reactivity in the proactive coping males (Kavelaars, Heijnen, Tennekes, Bruggink, & Koolhaas, 1999).

Evolutionary Significance

Most of the data mentioned so far have been obtained using males under rather limited experimental conditions in the laboratory. To allow conclusions about the adaptive significance of coping strategies, one needs data from more complex natural populations as well. There are several examples in mammals, birds, and fish showing that phenotypic variation is somehow maintained within a single natural population. These field studies support the general view as outlined above on the adaptive significance of individual variation in behavior and physiology of animals. On the basis of extensive ecology studies in a sunfish species (*Lepomis gibbosus*), Coleman and Wilson (1998) found evidence that two morphologically different phenotypes occupy different habitats while both seem to have an advantage over morphologically intermediate individuals. Subsequently, they considered the possibility that the same might be true for the individual differentiation in behavior, in particular for the differentiation in shy and bold animals. The way in which the distinction between shy and bold is described in a number of species, including monkeys, octopus, and fish, suggests that the shy individual might be similar to the reactive coping male, and the bold individual might be similar to the proactive coper. This leads to the question whether there is any evidence from rodent field studies that the proactive and reactive coping strategy have a differential adaptive significance. In feral mouse populations, there is some evidence that different behavioral phenotypes may have a differential fitness depending on the environmental conditions. In nature, mouse populations are known to go through phases of growth and decline. Such population cycles may cover a period from 4 to 7 years and can be so extreme that the population suddenly collapses at the end of a cycle and becomes extinct. Chitty (1967) hypothesized that the cyclic nature of rodent populations might be due to a disruptive selection for aggressive behavior in the course of the population cycle. Evidence that this might be the case was obtained in a study by Van Oortmerssen and Busser (1989) in seminatural populations of house mice consisting of both males and females. Phenotypic characterization of the laboratory-bred male offspring (F1) of fathers caught from these colonies revealed a bimodal distribution of attack latencies as measured in a standardized resident intruder paradigm. Subsequent selective breeding for high and low attack latencies resulted within five generations in a stable short attack latency (SAL) selection line. After a number of failures due to infertility of the offspring, we managed to obtain a long attack latency (LAL) selection line as well. Cross-fostering and back-cross experiments show that the phenotypic differentiation in aggressive behavior as observed in the colonies has a strong genetic basis.

An analysis of the mortality reveals a strong increase in females, juveniles, and preweanling juveniles just before the crash of the population (Fig. 2.1). The idea that this increase in mortality is due to enhanced levels of aggression in the males is supported by an index of territoriality. Figure 2.2 shows the number of males present in the nests. In the growth phase of the population, on average four males were found together in each nest. Toward the crash, however, males were generally found alone, indicating a reduced tolerance for additional males in the nest. During the whole population cycle, animals are migrating from the population. It seems that the nonaggressive phenotype is more successful in establishing a new colony than the highly aggressive phenotype. This leads to the more general view that the two phenotypes observed in seminatural populations of house mice might have a differential fitness depending on the phase of the population cycle.

Recent studies in the great tit (*Parus major*), a small song bird, show a similar differentiation of phenotypes like in our rodent studies. Bold animals are relatively aggressive, superficial explorers and more prone to develop behavioral routines than shy birds. In a field study, Verbeek, Drent, and Wiepkema, (1994) observed a bimodal distribution of aggressive behavior of individual birds. Subsequent experiments showed that this differentiation has a genetic basis and can be considered behaviorally as a differentiation in proactive and reactive coping strategy.

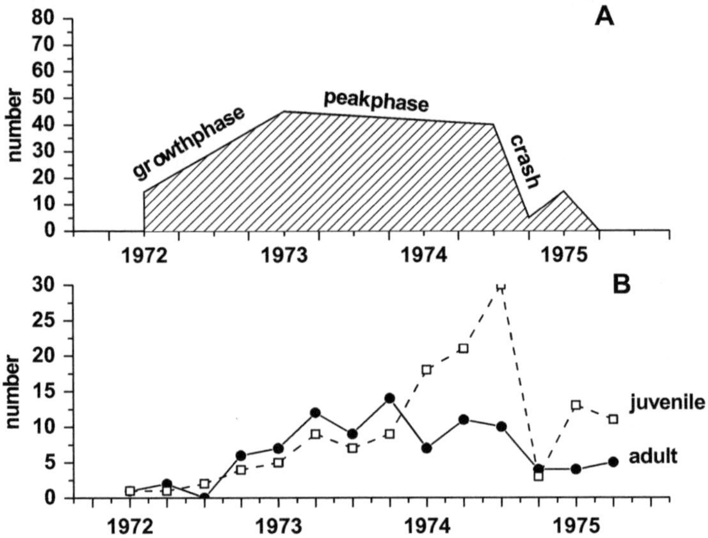

Fig. 2.1 (**A**) Change in population density of a feral population of house mice. (**B**) Mortality of adult and juvenile house mice during the various phase of the population cycle.

Observations in natural bird populations support the idea that the individual variation in coping strategy buffers the species against the negative effects of environmental variation such as food availability (Dingemanse, Both, Van Noordwijk, Rutten, & Drent, 2003). In this sense, the concept of coping strategies addresses a fundamental issue in evolutionary biology.

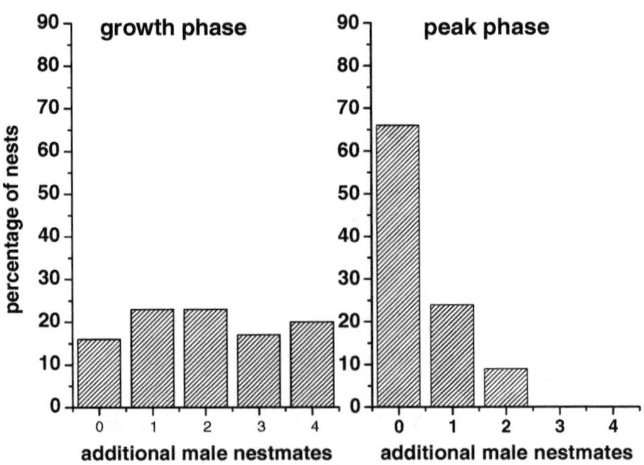

Fig. 2.2 Number of males found together in one nest during the growth phase and at the end of the peak phase of a colony of wild house mice.

Conclusion

Individual differentiation in behavior and physiology is a well-known phenomenon in many animal species. Unfortunately, there are relatively few studies using a more systematic approach to characterize individual response patterns across various environmental conditions. However, the scarce literature suggests that the dimension of proactive and reactive coping strategies can be distinguished in a wide variety of animal species (Koolhaas et al., 1999). Authors may use different terms to characterize phenotypes, such as shyness and boldness or proactive and reactive, but they all seem to share the same basic characteristics. Detailed analysis of coping strategies in rats and mice indicates that the most fundamental difference between proactive and reactive coping is the degree to which behavior is guided by feedback and feed-forward control. This results in a differential degree of behavioral flexibility. This degree of flexibility may have its origin in a differential survival value in nature. The challenge for the future is to integrate ethologic, stress physiologic, and ecologic approaches in the study of coping strategies.

From a biomedical point of view, the concept of coping strategies implies that different animals have a differential capacity to adapt to the same environmental conditions. Negative health consequences might arise if an animal cannot cope with the stressor or needs very demanding coping efforts. In view of the differential neuroendocrine reactivity and neurobiological makeup, one may expect different types of stress pathology to develop under conditions in which a particular coping strategy fails. Although there are only a limited number of studies performed concerning pathology in relation to the type of coping strategy adopted, there are some indications that the two coping strategies differ in susceptibility to develop cardiovascular pathology, ulcer formation, stereotypes, and infectious disease (Koolhaas et al., 1999).

If we accept the idea that nature somehow favors the existence of different phenotypes within one species, one may wonder how this relates to animals bred by humans in laboratory or animal husbandry conditions. Both in wild house mice and in a small bird, the great tit (*Parus major*), latency measures seem to have a bimodal distribution (Verbeek et al., 1994). Many studies use heavily domesticated animals that are usually selected for specific traits as well. In general, individual behavioral scores are normally distributed in these animals. Moreover, it is hard to tell how a certain inbred or domesticated strain relates to the original and presumably functional distribution of its wild ancestors. Nevertheless, it is intriguing that the extremes of this normal distribution often still fulfill the criteria for proactive and reactive coping strategies, both behaviorally and physiologically (De Boer, Van Der Vegt, & Koolhaas, 2003). Although the discussion on the shape of the distribution curve is important from an evolutionary point of view, it does not seem to matter much when the individual vulnerability to stress-related diseases is concerned. After all, it has been repeatedly shown that the extremes in a population, irrespective of the detailed distribution curve, may differ not only quantitatively but also qualitatively in their behavioral and physiologic response pattern to stress.

References

Benus, R. F., Bohus, B., Koolhaas J. M., & Van Oortmerssen, G. A. (1991a). Heritable variation in aggression as a reflection of individual coping strategies. *Experientia, 47,* 1008–1019.

Benus, R. F., Bohus, B., Koolhaas J. M., & Van Oortmerssen, G. A. (1991b). Behavioural differences between artificially selected aggressive and non-aggressive mice: response to apomorphine. *Behavioural Brain Research, 43,* 203–208.

Benus, R. F., Koolhaas J. M., & Van Oortmerssen, G. A. (1988). Aggression and adaptation to the light-dark cycle: role of intrinsic and extrinsic control. *Physiology & Behavior, 43,* 131–137.

Bohus, B., & Koolhaas J. M. (1990). Psychoimmunology of social factors in rodents and other subprimate vertebrates. In R.Ader, D. L. Felten, & N. Cohen (Eds.), *Psychoneuroimmunology* (2nd ed., pp. 807–830). San Diego, New York: Academic Press Inc.

Bult, A., Hiestand, L., Van der Zee, E. A., & Lynch, C. B. (1993). Circadian rhythms differ between selected mouse lines: a model to study the role of vasopressin neurons in the suprachiasmatic nuclei. *Brain Research Bulletin, 32,* 623–627.

Cannon, W. B. (1915). *Bodily changes in pain, hunger, fear and rage.* New York: Appleton.

Chitty, D. (1967). The natural selection of self-regulatory behaviour in animal populations. *Proceedings of the Ecological Society of Australia 2,* 51–78.

Coleman, K., & Wilson, D. (1998). Shyness and boldness in pumpkinseed sunfish: individual differences are context-specific. *Animal Behaviour, 56,* 927–936.

Compaan, J. C., Buijs, R. M., Pool, C. W., De Ruiter, A. J. H., & Koolhaas J. M. (1992). Differential lateral septal vasopressin innervation in aggressive and nonaggressie male mice. *Brain Research Bulletin, 30,* 1–6.

De Boer, S. F., & Koolhaas J. M. (2003). Defensive burying in rodents: ethology, neurobiology and psychopharmacology. *European Journal of Pharmacology, 463,* 145–161.

De Boer, S. F., Van Der Vegt, B. J., & Koolhaas J. M. (2003). Individual variation in aggression of feral rodent strains: a standard for the genetics of aggression and violence? *Behavior Genetics, 33,* 485–501.

De Ruiter, A. J. H., Koolhaas J.M., Keijser, J. N., Van Oortmerssen, G. A., & Bohus, B. (1992). Differential testosterone secretory capacity of the testes of aggressive and non-aggressive house mice during ontogeny. *Aggressive Behavior, 18,* 149–157.

Dingemanse, N. J., Both, C., Van Noordwijk, A. J., Rutten, A. L., & Drent, P. J. (2003). Natal dispersal and personalities in great tits (Parus major). *Proceedings of the Royal Society of London. Series B: Biological Sciences, 270,* 741–747.

Driscoll, P., Demek, J., D'Angio, M., Claustre, Y., & Scatton, B. (1990). A genetically-based model for divergent stress responses: behavioral, neurochemical and hormonal aspects. In V. Pliska & G. Stranzinger (Eds.), *Farm animals in biomedical research* (5th ed., pp. 97–107). Hamburg: Verlag Paul Parey.

Driscoll, P., Martin, J. R., Kugler, P., & Baettig, K. (1983). Environmental and genetic effects on food-deprivation induced stomach lesions in male rats. *Physiology & Behavior, 31,* 225–228.

Engel, G. L. & Schmale, A. H. (1972). Conservation withdrawal: a primary regulatory process for organic homeostasis. In R. Porter & J. Knight (Eds.), *Physiology, emotions and psychosomatic illness. CIBA Foundation Symposium* (pp. 57–95). Amsterdam: Elsevier.

Feldker, D. E., De Kloet, E. R., Kruk, M. R., & Datson, N. A. (2003). Large-scale gene expression profiling of discrete brain regions: potential, limitations, and application in genetics of aggressive behavior. *Behavior Genetics, 33,* 537–548.

Felten, D. L., Felten, S. Y., Bellinger, D. L., Carlson, S. L., Ackerman, K. D., Madden, K. S., et al. (1987). Noradrenergic sympathetic neural interactions with the immune system: structure and function. *Immunology Review, 100,* 225–260.

Fokkema, D. S., Koolhaas J. M., & Van der Gugten, J. (1995). Individual characteristics of behavior, blood pressure, and adrenal hormones in colony rats. *Physiology & Behavior, 57,* 857–862.

Fokkema, D., Smit, K., Van der Gugten, J., & Koolhaas J. M. (1988). A coherent pattern among social behavior, blood pressure, corticosterone, and catecholamines measures in individual male rats. *Physiology & Behavior, 42,* 485–489.

Henry, J. P., & Stephens, P. M. (1977). *Stress, health and the social environment: a sociobiological approach to medicine*. Berlin: Springer.

Hessing, M. (1994). *Individual behavioural characteristics in pigs and their consequences for pig husbandry*. Ph.D. thesis. Wageningen: Agricultural University.

Kavelaars, A., Heijnen, C. J., Tennekes, R., Bruggink, J. E., & Koolhaas J. M. (1999). Individual behavioral characteristics of wild-type rats predict susceptibility to experimental autoimmune encephalomyelitis. *Brain Behavior Immunology, 13,* 279–286.

Koolhaas J. M., & Bohus, B. (1991). Coping strategies and cardiovascular risk: a study of rats and mice. In A. Appels (Ed.), *Behavioral observations in cardiovascular research* (pp. 45–58). Amsterdam: Swets & Zeitlinger.

Koolhaas, J. M., Everts, H., de Ruiter, A. J., De Boer, S. F., & Bohus, B. (1998). Coping with stress in rats and mice: differential peptidergic modulation of the amygdala-lateral septum complex. *Progress in Brain Research, 119,* 437–448.

Koolhaas, J. M., Korte, S. M., De Boer, S. F., Van Der Vegt, B. J., Van Reenen, C. G., Hopster, H., et al. (1999). Coping styles in animals: current status in behavior and stress-physiology. *Neuroscience & Biobehavioral Reviews, 23,* 925–935.

Korte, S. M., Meijer, O. C., De Kloet, E. R., Buwalda, B., Keijser, J., Sluyter, F., et al. (1996). Enhanced 5-HT1a receptor expression in forebrain regions of aggressive house mice. *Brain Research, 736,* 338–343.

Lazarus, R. (1966). *Psychosocial stress and the coping process*. New York: McGraw-Hill.

Manuck, S. B., Kaplan, J. R., & Clarkson, T. B. (1983). Behaviorally induced heart rate reactivity and atherosclerosis in cynomolgous monkeys. *Psychosomatic Medicine, 45,* 95–108.

Murison, R., & Skjerve, A. (1992). Individual behavioral characteristics and extent of stress-induced gastric ulceration in rats. *Acta Physiologica Hungarica, 80,* 127–133.

Raab, A., Dantzer, R., Michaud, B., Mormede, P., Taghzouti, K., & Simon, H. (1986). Behavioral, physiological and immunological consequences of social status and aggression in chronically coexisting resident-intruder dyads of male rats. *Physiology & Behavior, 36,* 223–228.

Roozendaal, B., Wiersma, A., Driscoll, P., Koolhaas J. M., & Bohus, B. (1992). Vasopressinergic modulation of stress responses in the central amygdala of the Roman high-avoidance and low-avoidance rat. *Brain Research, 596,* 35–40.

Sandi, C., Castanon, N., Vitiello, S., Neveu, P. J., & Mormede, P. (1991). Different responsiveness of spleen lymphocytes from two lines of psychogenetically selected rats (Roman high and low avoidance). *Journal of Neuroimmunology, 31,* 27–33.

Sgoifo, A., De Boer, S. F., Haller, J., & Koolhaas J. M. (1996). Individual differences in plasma catecholamine and corticosterone stress responses of wild type rats: relationship with aggression. *Physiology & Behavior, 60,* 1403–1407.

Sgoifo, A., De Boer, S. F., Westenbroek, C., Maes, F. W., Beldhuis, H., Suzuki, T., et al. (1997). Incidence of arrhythmias and heart rate variability in wild type rats exposed to social stress. *American Journal of Physiology, 273,* H1754–H1760.

Sih, A., Bell, A. M., Johnson, J. C., & Ziemba, R. E. (2004). Behavioral syndromes: an integrative overview. *The Quarterly Review of Biology, 79,* 241–277.

Sluyter, F., Jamot, L., Van Oortmerssen, G. A., & Crusio, W. E. (1994). Hippocampal mossy fiber distribution in mice selected for aggression. *Brain Research, 646,* 145–148.

Treit, D., Pinel, J. P. J., & Fibiger, H. C. (1981). Conditioned defensive burying: a new paradigm for the study of anxiolytic agents. *Pharmacology, Biochemistry, and Behavior, 15,* 619–626.

Van Oortmerssen, G. A., & Busser, J. (1989). Studies in wild house mice III: disruptive selection on aggression as a possible force in evolution. In P. F. Brain, D. Mainardi, & S. Parmigiani (Eds.), *House mouse aggression: a model for understanding the evolution of social behavior* (pp. 87–117). Chur Switzerland: Harwood.

Verbeek, M. E. M., Drent, P. J., & Wiepkema, P. R. (1994). Consistent individual differences in early exploratory behavior of male great tits. *Animal Behavior, 48,* 1113–1121.

Weiss, J. M. (1972). Influence of psychological variables on stress-induced pathology. In R. Porter & J. Knight (Eds.), *Physiology, emotion and psychosomatic illness. CIBA Foundation Symposium* (pp. 253–265). Amsterdam: Elsevier.

Wiepkema, P. R., & Van Adrichem, P. W. M. (1987). *Biology of stress in farm animals.* Dordrecht: Nijhoff.

Wiepkema, P. R., & Schuiten, W. G. P. (1992). Stereotypes in sows during chronic stress. *Psychotherapy and Psychosomatics, 57,* 194–199.

Chapter 3
New Avenues in Alexithymia Research: The Creation of Alexithymia Types

Peter Paul Moormann, Bob Bermond, Harry C.M. Vorst, Anthony F.T. Bloemendaal, Stefan M. Teijn, and Lea Rood

Introduction

In this chapter, a new approach to alexithymia is launched by the introduction of five alexithymia types, each being characterized by its own specific psychological makeup. This idea is inspired by the results of several studies, two of which will be discussed in greater detail. In the first study (Bloemendaal & Teijn, 1998; Bloemendaal, Teijn, & Moormann, 1999; Janssons 2004), the relation between alexithymia types and personality disorders has been explored among psychiatric patients. The other study (see Rood, 2003; and Moormann, Bermond, & Albach, 2004) concerns university psychology students and athletes. Here the relation between alexithymia types and personality traits has been investigated. The chapter concludes with a graphic representation of each alexithymia type with its corresponding personality profile (Fig. 3.1). The meaning of alexithymia types will be discussed with regard to both theoretical implications (the development of a biologically based personality theory) and practical implications (psychological health, stress resistance,
psychotherapy, interpersonal relationships, vocational interests, and creativity).

Construction of Alexithymia Types

The following features of alexithymia are discerned by Vorst and Bermond (2001) in the Bermond Vorst Alexithymia Questionnaire (BVAQ): (a) reduced ability to differentiate between emotional feelings, (b) reduced ability to fantasize, (c) reduced ability to verbalize emotional experiences, (d) reduced ability to experience emotional feelings, and (e) "pensée opératoire" (Marty & M'Uzan, 1963), or a reduced tendency to reflect upon emotions.

The alexithymia types can be created by using the second order factor structure, representing a cognitive (a, c, e) and an affective (b, d) dimension of the BVAQ. Percentile scores can be computed for both the affective (A) and the cognitive (C) components of the BVAQ. Only subjects with scores above percentile 70 (reduced ability to experience emotions) and below percentile 30 (augmented ability to experience emotions) are selected to form the following four alexithymia subtypes: (1) Type I or full-blown alexithymia (A > 70, C>70); (2) lexithymia (A < 30, C < 30); (3) Type II alexithymia (A < 30, C > 70); and (4) Type III alexithymia (A > 70, C < 30). The fifth group, "modals," consists of individuals in the scoring range of percentiles 30–70. Persons who do not meet the criteria of any of the five types can be labeled as having a "mixed profile."

- *Type I alexithymia* is characterized by low emotionality and a poor fantasy life in combination with poorly developed cognitions accompanying the emotions.
- The opposite of Type I alexithymia is *lexithymia*, characterized by both high emotionality and an enriched fantasy-life in combination with well-developed cognitions accompanying the emotions.
- *Type II alexithymia* is characterized by high emotionality and a rich fantasy-life in combination with poorly developed cognitions accompanying the emotions.
- The opposite of Type II alexithymia is *Type III alexithymia*, characterized by a low emotionality and a poor fantasy-life, but with well-developed cognitions accompanying emotions.
- The fifth group is called *modals* with average scores on both the emotion and cognitive dimension of alexithymia.
- Individuals who fail to meet the criteria belonging to these five types have *mixed profiles*.

Alexithymia Types and Personality Disorders

The sample in the first study consisted of a mixed group of 105 *psychiatric patients* (28 males and 75 females, 19 to 77 years of age; two missing values regarding age). All patients were volunteers who had signed an informed consent. The following six groups could be distinguished: (1) chronic psychiatric patients in an open ward with a complex pathology who were under 24 hours attendance; (2) patients in an open ward receiving short-term psychotherapy for mixed psychiatric disorders; (3) patients recovering from Axis-1 disorders after a serious negative life event; (4) patients receiving long-term psychotherapy of neurotic and/or depressive symptoms, life-span problems, and personality disorders; (5) patients with a serious character neurosis with a prognosis of fundamental changes in personality; and (6) patients receiving part-time treatment for personality problems, life-span problems, or mood disorders with an average treatment duration of 9 months. Patients with a psychosis, dementia, suicidality, and analphabetism were excluded.

The results of this research confirmed the notion that both Type I and Type II alexithymia are disorders of affect regulation, supposedly linked to psychiatric illness, because 61.0% of the psychiatric patients could be classified as either Type I (42.9%) or Type II (18.1%). Only 16.2% of the psychiatric patients seemed to fit the three other types, which are supposed to have a healthy form of affect regulation; more precisely Type III (3.8%), lexithymia (2.9%), and modals (9.5%). No statements can be made concerning the remaining 22.8% with a mixed profile of alexithymia scores.

Type I individuals can be characterized as being concrete and rational, as lacking emotional warmth, as being distant in interpersonal relationships and socially clumsy, and as having a poor fantasy life. It is therefore not surprising that Type I turned out to be positively related to the Schizoid Personality Disorder and negatively to the Theatrical or Histrionic Personality Disorder. According to Millon and Davis (2000), the schizoid individual is someone who lacks a personality. Schizoids prefer isolation, as relationships seem to hold no rewards for them. They are often described as detached and emotionally flat, but in general they are rarely noticed by anyone, because they are so quiet and unobtrusive. In many respects, they are the opposite of the Histrionic or Theatrical Personalities, who are always eager to make themselves the center of attention. They are perpetually "on stage to impress, if not to control and to become angry, jealous, or depressed if not acknowledged" (Millon & Davis, 2000).

Type II individuals are emotionally unstable, which is in line with the established strong association with the Borderline Personality Disorder. Borderliners are notably emotionally unstable, and especially angry. Their relationships are stormy and intense, with so many breakups and reconciliations that life becomes a crossing between a soap opera and a roller coaster (Millon & Davis, 2000).

The Relationships Between Alexithymia Types and Personality

In the second study, 354 second-year *psychology students* (267 females, 86 males; one missing value) participated. Their ages ranged between 18 and 56 years (mean, 23 years). One hundred forty-three (40%) of them did fit the criteria of any of the five (a)lexithymia types and were selected for further analyses. The remaining respondents had mixed profiles on the emotion and cognitive dimension of alexithymia and were therefore excluded from further analyses.

First, the prevalence of the alexithymia types was examined. A comparison between the healthy and unhealthy alexithymia types revealed the following: A total of 20.4% belonged to Type I (11.6%) and Type II (8.8%), which are considered to be "unhealthy" types. Considerably more of them (33%) could be classified as lexithymics (13%), Type III (9.0%), and modal (11.0%), which are considered to be "healthy" types. The remaining 46.6% had mixed profiles.

The comparison between psychiatric patients and psychology students demonstrates that in the psychiatric patients, the majority (61.0%) is classified as either Type I or Type II (the "unhealthy" types) compared with 20.4% in the students. In contrast, the "healthy" types (lexithymia, Type III, and modals) and mixed profiles are more prevalent among the students (33.0% and 46.6% vs. 16.2% and 22.8%).

Regarding sex differences, it was found that significantly more men could be classified as Type I and significantly more women as Type II. This confirms the stereotype that men are more rational, whereas women tend to be more emotionally unstable (see also Carpenter & Addis, 2000).

The relation between personality features and alexithymia types was investigated by administering a large test battery. For the investigation of the different personality profiles associated with each alexithymia type, a distinction was made between *determinants* and *behavioral manifestations* of alexithymia types.

Determinants include both personality traits with possible hereditary components and parental styles. Binary logistic regression analyses were used to test which factors measured with the three instruments below could predict which alexithymia type.

- The Leiden Parent-Child Interaction Questionnaire-Revised (LPCIQ-R/LOK-R; Moormann et al., 1997). Scales: Emotional Neglect and Control, both for father and mother separately.
- The Dutch Personality Questionnaire (DPQ/NPV; Luteijn et al., 1985). Scales: Inadequacy, Social Inadequacy, Rigidity, Aggrievedness, Self-sufficiency, Dominance, and Self-esteem.
- The Shortened Dutch adaptation of the Minnesota Multiphasic Personality Inventory (MMPI-S/NVM; Luteijn et al., 1980). Scales: Negativism, Somatization, Shyness, Psychopathology, and Extraversion.

Behavioral manifestations refer to psychological constructs supposed to be the consequence of a particular alexithymia type; for example, poor self concept, poor well-being and complaints (state measure of psychoneuroticism), achievement motivation, debilitating and facilitating anxiety, coping styles, and defenses. Analyses of variance (ANOVAs) with post hoc comparisons were used to examine on which constructs the alexithymia types differed from each other.

- The Leiden Self Concept Questionnaire (LSQ/LZL; Moormann et al., 1997). Scales: Past Self, Present Self, and Future Self. Subscales: Relatedness, Competence, Coping, and Self-esteem.
- The Dutch adaptation of Derogatis' Symptom Checklist (SCL-90; Arrindell & Ettema, 1981). Scales: Agoraphobia, Anxiety, Depression, Somatization, Insufficiency of Thinking and Acting (obsessive compulsiveness), Interpersonal Sensitivity & Mistrust (paranoid ideation and psychoticism), Hostility, and Sleeping problems.
- The Achievement Motivation test (AMT/PMT; Hermans, 1967). Scales: Achievement motivation, Debilitating Anxiety, and Facilitating Anxiety.
- The Utrecht Coping List (UCL; Schreurs et al., 1988) Scales: Active coping, Palliative reactions, Avoidant reactions, Social support seeking, Depressive reactions, Expression of emotions/anger, and Comforting thoughts.
- The Dutch adaptation of the Defense Mechanism Inventory (DMI; Passchier & Verhage, 1986). Scales: Turning Against Object, Projection, Principalization, Turning Against Self, Reversal.
- The Perceptual Defense Test (PDT; Brand et al., 1991; Moormann et al., 2003). A visual half-field task. Scales: Perceptual Defense (Repression) and a Right-Left Index for lateral dominance.

The results can be summarized as described in the following sections.

Type I Alexithymia

Determinants

Self-sufficiency (satisfaction with oneself and a disinterest in others and their problems) of the DPQ and shyness (feeling shy and having difficulties in relating with others) of the MMPI-S predicted Type I alexithymia. The core features of Type I alexithymia include being detached from social relationships and a restricted range of expression of emotions in interpersonal settings, caused by a lack of empathy and sociability.

Behavioral Manifestations

Type I alexithymia is neither related to complaints nor to symptoms of psychological disease (SCL-90). It is also not associated with a debilitating or facilitating anxiety (AMT) or to low self-esteem (LSQ). However, Type I individuals are defensive (DMI). Unacceptable emotions (as far as they are felt) or personal qualities are disowned by attributing them to others (*Projection*). When experiencing setbacks, they turn to others and blame them for their own problems (*Turning Against Object*). This might be a reaction against the intrusiveness and overcontrol of others who might try to socialize them through forced participation (McWilliams, 1994). Type I persons share with schizoid persons aversion of engulfment; the notion that others will enmesh them in relationships, thereby obliterating their individuality and identity. Autism in this way becomes a form of opposition or defiance against a "devouring external world" that would digest and assimilate them. When having problems, these individuals will not seek social support with others as a way of coping (UCL).

Profile

Type I persons are emotionally cold and socially/emotionally clumsy or incompetent. However, they are not plagued by thoughts of failure. Type I has the characteristic features of the *Einzelgänger*, a loner with a defect social antenna. They possess a rational inclination to life, which can be an advantage in many professions where rational thinking devoid of emotional interference is an advantage. However, in personal and intimate relations, the emotionally cold and distant behavior may cause interpersonal problems. Because of the lack of emotionality, Type I alexithymics are not likely to suffer from emotional exhaustion. The reduced emotionality and fantasy make Type I individuals less suited for professions in the performing arts or professions in which creativity and expressivity are required. The Type I alexithymia profile shows a remarkable resemblance with features of the schizoid personality style. According to Millon and Davis (2000), several normal-range variants of the schizoid personality can be distinguished. Oldham and Morris (1995) describe the *solitary style*, individuals with a limited need for companionship and social support: "As dispassionate observers of life, these solitary individuals rarely get excited about anything" (p. 314). In work they function efficiently but not as team players. Millon, Weiss, Millon, and Davis (1994) describe a similar pattern of characteristics within the normal range, referred to as the *retiring style*. Those individuals are unobtrusive and work quietly and methodically behind the scenes, content to remain in the background. Others often perceive them as lacking spontaneity and vitality.

Type II Alexithymia

Determinants

Inadequacy and Social Inadequacy of the DPQ predicted Type II alexithymia. Inadequacy means that one feels tense, depressive, or unstable. Type II alexithymics suffer from a lack of emotional stability (neuroticism). Social Inadequacy means that one considers oneself incompetent in comparison with others and one feels shy and inhibited.

Behavioral Manifestations

Type II individuals report a high level of complaints (SCL-90). Type II individuals are anxious, agoraphobic (one suffers from anxiety and panic attacks when left alone), and depressive. These persons report vague somatic complaints and sleeping problems. In addition, they adopt a suspicious, somewhat paranoid attitude toward other people, implying that they are difficult to handle, and they feel insufficient in thinking and acting (compulsiveness, an inclination to exaggerated precision, and afraid to make mistakes). In stress situations, they experience debilitating anxiety, whereas levels of facilitating anxiety stay low (AMT). When a Type II person is in a situation in which s/he is put under pressure, s/he will massively underachieve due to thoughts of failure (AMT). As for defense (DMI), Type II uses *Turning Against Self* (TAS). These individuals turn against or blame themselves when experiencing problems or setbacks. As for coping (UCL), they are inclined to avoid problems or to react in a depressive manner to problems or setbacks. Type II individuals have a low past, present, and future self. Their LSQ subscale scores reveal that they are not capable of feeling very related to others (their own problems seems to consume all the energy). Their sense of self-esteem is weak and they feel incompetent. The Type II individuals have a poor coping style and they expect to have little control over situations.

Profile

Type II alexithymics are the least stress resistant of all types and they suffer from psychiatric problems and psychosomatic complaints. Predominately, they manifest a psychoneurotic personality structure, a character neurosis. They lose balance quickly and easily become victims of debilitating anxiety. They have little self-confidence, possess a negative self-image, suffer from a lot of psychological complaints, and have somewhat compulsive traits. Type II individuals are tense and afraid of making mistakes. They blame themselves for inadequacies and show maladjusted coping. Depressive signs are not uncommon. In stress situations, the uncontrolled emotion regulation makes them vulnerable to splitting of consciousness (dissociation), such as blackouts, depersonalizations, derealizations, and anesthesias (see Moormann, Bermond, & Albach, 2004; Moormann, Bermond, & Albach, 2004). Experiencing emotions but lacking the cognitions that belong to them indeed is a highly unpleasant and confusing mental state. There is a correspondence between the Type II alexithymic profile and the Borderline Personality Style. The *mercurial style* for instance (see Oldham and Morris, 1995) is described as living on a roller-coaster life. Frequent ups and downs are the rule and attachment is the central theme in all relationships, with frantic attempts to avoid abandonment (separation anxiety) and a desire always to be involved in a romantic relationship. The more adapted borderline style tends to be spontaneous and emotionally intense but occasionally overreacts and dramatizes (see Millon & Davis, 2000, who refer to Sperry, 1995). According to Millon and Davis (2000), the adult borderline represents what happens when "the difficult temperament" (see Thomas & Chess, 1977) meets an "invalidating environment." The consequences of this developmental pattern should not be neglected. Without adequate mirroring and validation, individuals cannot learn to label their private and emotional experiences accurately (e.g., it leads to problems with verbalizing, identifying, and analyzing emotions), they are not able to develop realistic life goals, fail to develop normal expectations concerning what normal interactions might be like, and they cannot trust their own reactions as valid (e.g., it induces feelings of inadequacy and social inadequacy). Other factors that indirectly contribute to the development of the borderline personality include sexual abuse and the role of cultural ideas, in particular in the case of women (Linehan, 1993). This notion is in agreement with our finding that Type II alexithymia was often found in women with childhood sexual abuse (Albach, Moormann, & Bermond, 1996; Moormann et al., 1997; Moormann et al., 2004). In addition, Type II alexithymia was common among female psychology students. In other studies among athletes, Type II alexithymia was associated with a debilitating anxiety. This specific subgroup therefore was in need of mental training (Moormann, Bermond, & Albach, 2004). Among psychology students, a strong tendency to handle conflicts by directing aggressive behavior toward the self was characteristic (Moormann et al., 2003).

Lexithymia

Determinants

Emotional warmth of the mother (LPCIQ-R) predicts lexithymia. This result confirms the notion that early childhood experiences determine personality later in life.

Both Freud and Erikson (see Carver & Scheier, 2000) emphasize that a mother-child interaction characterized by basic trust is likely to contribute to the development of a healthy personality. In our research, it is confirmed that the role of a warm, caring, and loving mother is associated with an optimal affect regulation later in life.

Behavioral Manifestations

Lexithymia is neither related to psychological complaints (SCL-90) nor to defense (DMI). In contrast, lexithymics score high on facilitating anxiety (AMT) which means that they can excel in challenging situations. As for coping (UCL), lexithymic individuals are inclined to work actively on problems instead of denying or avoiding them. Sometimes they will try to alleviate problems by searching for distraction (palliative reaction), or by seeking support in comforting thoughts. They also seek social support in hard times. Lexithymic individuals have a high present and future self (LSQ). They report a high self-esteem, relate to others very well, and consider themselves as competent.

Profile

The core element of lexithymia is a well-developed affective organism. Both the emotional and the cognitive component of affect regulation are well tuned. Our findings also indicate that lexithymic individuals are "emotionally intelligent" and possess a healthy personality structure. They have the capacity to rise above their own standards in demanding situations. This notion is in line with Goleman's (1995) statement about the relation between flow and emotional intelligence, derived from an interview he had with Csikszentmihalyi, the "father of flow." Lexithymics additionally report adequate coping mechanisms. They are also high on self-confidence, and their well-developed affect regulation is a sound base for the realization of their creative and expressive potential. The profile of lexithymics shows resemblances with features of the well-adapted histrionic personality. The *dramatic style*, described by Oldham Morris (1990), emphasizes feeling, color, and attention. These persons deal with their world effectively, value the impact of emotion, and display their emotions easily and openly. This notion is supported by the results from a study by Niessen (2001), where lexithymics were found to score significantly higher than modals on the subscales Emotional Perception and Emotional Expression of the Social Intelligence Scale (Riggio, 1986; Uterwijk, 1998). According to Oldham and Morris, persons with a dramatic style are also highly intuitive and quickly sense what to talk about and how others wish to be regarded. The *outgoing style* (Millon et al., 1994) focuses more on sociability than on theatrics. With their great confidence in their influence and charm, such persons just naturally know how to manipulate others and make others to like them. Usually, they are described as warm, lively, dramatic, energizing, or provocative. Most are open to new possibilities and find tremendous joy in new experiences. Their joy in life is infectious, stimulating others to equal exuberance (see Millon & Davis, 2000). However, just like narcissists, histrionics can also be exhibitionists and manipulators. Niessen's (2001) findings demonstrate that lexithymic individuals have a tendency to manipulate. They score significantly higher than modals on emotional manipulation. Regarding exhibitionism, histrionics demonstrate their wares and read the desires of others to create intense interest and attraction. They become engaging, charming, or even seductive when "on stage." Daily life examples of such behavior can be seen when watching the numerous attention-seeking performances in talk shows on television, for instance in the provocative Jerry Springer show with displays of overt, sexually seducing behavior or in the less brutal Oprah Winfrey Show with a more sophisticated formula. Nowadays, with the introduction of emotion television, it seems as if the dramatic style has become a worldwide success in the entertainment business and has become a hallmark of modern Western culture, the culture of exhibitionism. It has become a trend for being successful, being in the picture.

Type III Alexithymia

Determinants

Adequacy and Social Adequacy (DPQ) predict Type III alexithymia. Adequacy relates to emotional stability. Social adequacy means that one reports to get along with others very well. One speaks easily, feels open, and is easy-going and sociable. Hence, Type III individuals possess good social skills and do not show signs of neuroticism

Behavioral Manifestations

Type III individuals show a healthy profile. Type III is a negative predictor of depressive complaints (SCL-90), debilitating anxiety (AMT), palliative coping, avoidant coping, seeking relief in comforting thoughts, depressive coping (all UCL), and Turning Against Self (DMI). The last result means that, as a mechanism of defense, they are not likely to blame themselves when frustrated. Type III individuals also have a high past, present, and future self. They feel related to other people, think of themselves as being competent, and have high self-appreciation. They consider themselves as being able to handle problems, and they expect to have sufficient control over situations. Interestingly, Type III predicts Perceptual Defense (for the Perceptual Defense Test, see Brand et al., 1991; Moormann et al., 2003). Only Type III individuals demonstrate a significantly higher preference for neutral pictures as opposed to threatening pictures on the visual half-field task. From a psychodynamic point of view, this may mean that threatening events are repressed or banned from conscious awareness (supposedly as a compensation for self-inflation; see Horney, 1939). It is striking that Type III individuals score less favorably only on this ambiguous test, where it is difficult for naive subjects to deduct what it is really measuring. As it is hard to fake on this kind of test, our result strongly suggests that Type III individuals are repressors.

Profile

Type III individuals are characterized by low scores on the emotion and high scores on the cognitive dimension of alexithymia. On pure intuitive grounds and from a theoretical point of view, this combination of scores seems odd (Moormann, 2004). It is not easy to understand how persons exhibiting reduced emotion arousability can have well-developed cognitions accompanying this reduced ability to experience emotions. In a recent publication on the cognitive neuropsychology of alexithymia, an explanation for this paradox has been put forward (Bermond et al., 2006). From a behavioral point of view, the combination of low scores on the emotion dimension and high scores on the cognitive dimension suggests a well-adapted person, who is neither overwhelmed by emotions, nor fantasy-prone, but who still has the ability to react upon the emotions of others in a socially coherent way. The questionnaire results seem to confirm this notion. Type III persons report an extremely healthy, almost suspect personality profile. However, there is one dissonant. Type III individuals may be repressors. Negative, threatening experiences are not allowed to enter their conscious awareness. Moreover, Niessen's (2001) results reveal that Type III individuals have a tendency to manipulate. They score significantly higher on SIS emotional and social manipulation. In conclusion, the whole cluster of personality features strongly suggests that the profile of Type III alexithymics shows resemblances with the narcissistic personality.

Modals

Determinants

Neither personality nor parent-child relationship were significantly associated with modal scores on alexithymia.

Behavioral Manifestations

Mean scores on the Affective and Cognitive dimensions of alexithymia were not systematically related to psychological complaints (SCL-90), to a debilitating or facilitating anxiety (AMT), nor to defense (DMI). Negative associations were found with the use of comforting thoughts as coping strategy (UCL). In addition, a relation with a negative future self-image has been found, which means that modals fail to regard their future in an optimistic way.

Profile

Not much remarkable is to be noted concerning the modals, although the somewhat pessimistic view of the future suggests a *normal-range variant of the depressive personality* (see Millon & Davis, 2000).

Discussion and Conclusion

The creation of five alexithymia types opens new avenues in alexithymia research. The personality profiles associated with each alexithymia type have been graphically represented in Figure 3.1, which can be used as a working model for psychological health and stress resistance. The neurobiological basis of each alexithymia type has recently been outlined elsewhere (Bermond et al., 2006). It is outside the scope of this chapter to expand in full detail the putative neurologic structures associated with each alexithymia type. Rather, we want to emphasize that insight into the neurobiological substrates, underlying alexithymia types with their corresponding personality profiles, can be seen as an important first step toward the development of a biologically based personality theory. The finding that Type II alexithymics are the most vulnerable to stress of all alexithymia types fits well within the diathesis-stress model (Davison & Neale, 1997), according to which people are predisposed (by the very nature of their specific neurobiological makeup) to react adversely to environmental stressors.

In addition to new theoretical perspectives discussed above, the creation of alexithymia types may have some practical applications as well, notably in the pathology area of personality disorders and psychotherapy. Now, with the information about the relation between alexithymia types and personality disorders or styles, psychotherapy for Type I shall be primarily directed at the schizoid, for Type II at the borderline, for Type III at the narcissistic, and for lexithymics at the histrionic personality (for treatment specifications, we refer to Beck, 1976; Beck, Freeman, & Associates, 1990; Linehan, 1993; Millon & Davis, 2000). However, it should be noted that both alexithymia and personality disorders have a reputation of being difficult to treat.

When looking in the normal score range, knowledge of alexithymia types can be applied in the domain of vocational interests, the arts, and sports. For instance, Type I individuals are not suited for teamwork, Type II individuals have affinities with the arts, Type III individuals may become good managers or professors, and lexithymics possess the characteristics of excellent performing artists or entertainers. Type II athletes are not stress resistant and often suffer from performance anxiety, motivation dips, and a negative self-image. Cognitive Behavioral (CBT) or Rational Emotive Therapy (RET) can be applied in teaching the athlete how to cope with performance anxiety, as in both CBT and RET the relation between cognition, emotion, and conation is the major focus (see Moormann, Bermond, & Albach, 2004).

Figure 3.1 is helpful for highlighting some broad lines in our research findings. It supplies us with a helicopter view of the current findings on alexithymia types, described in the following text.

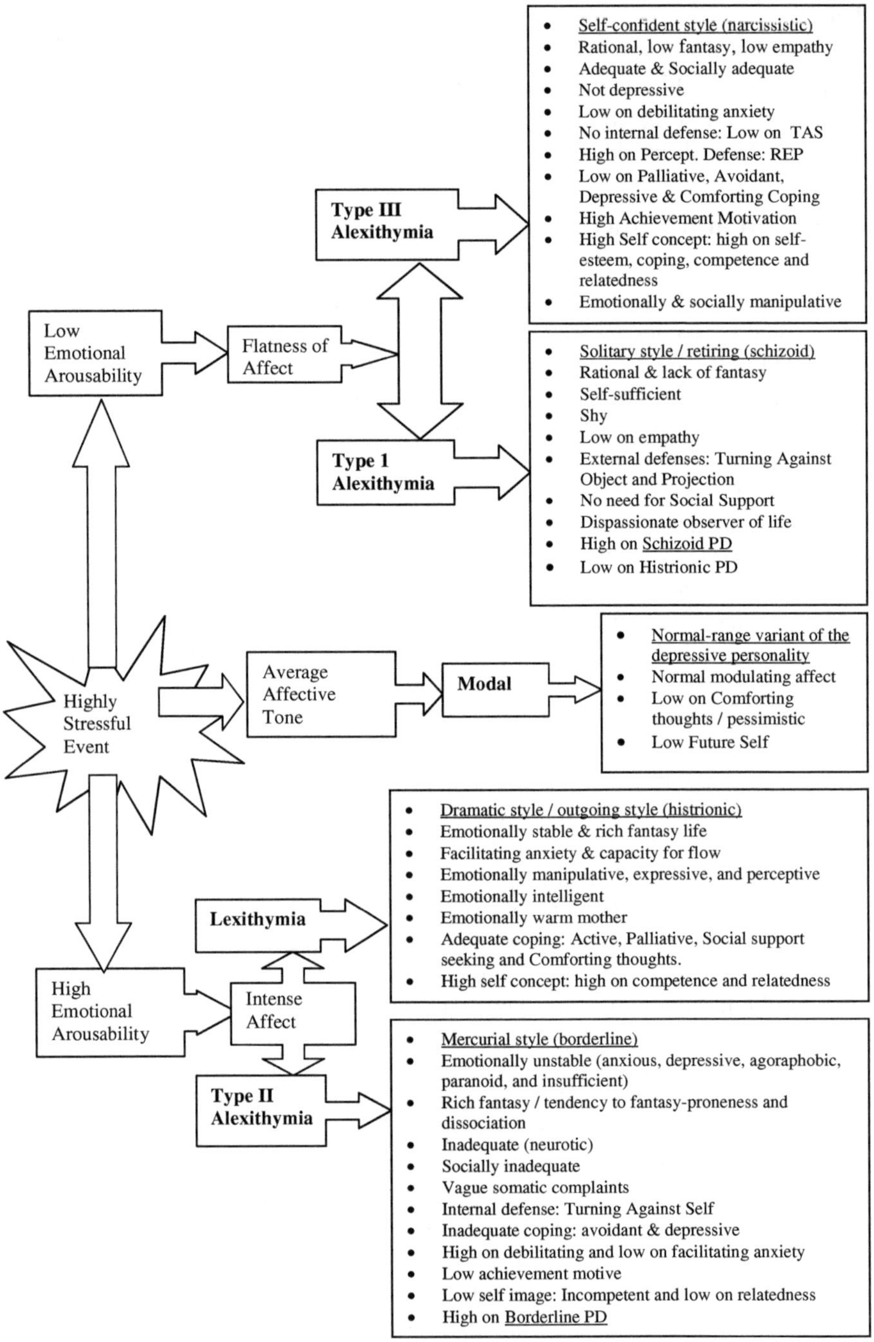

Fig. 3.1 Personality profiles of alexithymia types.

The Cognitive Component of Alexithymia Is Crucial for Psychological Health

Persons who experience problems with the cognitive components of alexithymia display a more pathologic personality profile (Type I and Type II), whereas more healthy personality profiles can be seen in persons where the cognitions accompanying the emotions are highly articulated (lexithymia and Type III).

The Emotion Component of Alexithymia Is Crucial for Stress Resistance, Interpersonal Relationships, and Creativity

Persons with low scores on the emotion component (e.g., low on emotionality and poor on fantasy) are stress resistant (Type I and Type III). They are not easily overwhelmed by emotions, but their lack of empathy may cause problems in interpersonal relationships and in psychotherapy. Type I alexithymics withdraw, whereas Type III alexithymics (who can rely on their cognitions) may become manipulative. Furthermore, the poorly developed emotion component in Type I and Type III may hamper creativity (see Moormann et al., 2004). In contrast, highly emotional persons may either outperform themselves, if the cognitions accompanying the emotions are well-matched (lexithymics report facilitating anxiety under stress and are more open for flow experiences), or may perform far below their standards in stress situations if the cognitions accompanying the emotions are nearly absent (Type II alexithymics report debilitating anxiety and are vulnerable to dissociative states that can lead to blackouts). In fact, Type II persons are the least stress resistant, but it should be noted as well that they might be artistic-creative (painters, composers, choreographers, etc.). The discrepancy between intense feeling and at the same time not being able to say what one feels fuels other modes of expression. According to Bell (1919/1975), this discrepancy acts as the artistic impulse. It is the drive behind artistic-creativity. Hence, although Type II alexithymics do possess neurotic features, which may be regarded as pathologic, it is just this character neurosis, this pathologic part among Type II alexithymics that functions as the drive behind artistic-creative endeavors. Marcel Proust, the famous French novelist, a notorious neurotic himself, once claimed "All great things come from neurotics." Becker (1978), in *The Mad Genius Controversy*, shares this point of view. He refers to Freud's theorizing on the sublimation of libidinal energies on behalf of higher intellectual and aesthetic concerns that allows the genius to escape the fate of neurosis; it is the failure to successfully sublimate fixated infantile desires that creates a nearly insurmountable disposition to "obsessional neurosis." In this context, Becker refers to Stekel (1912), who considers the struggle inherent in the sublimation of libidinal impulses as leading to an inevitable disposition to neurosis: as such, all men of genius are judged neurotic. Indeed, Stekel argued that the neurotic condition constitutes the germ of creation and source of all progress.

Strictly Speaking, Only Type I and Type II Are Part of the Construct of Alexithymia

Alexithymia is a disorder of affect regulation, and therefore only Type I and Type II should be related to psychological illness. In contrast, lexithymia and Type III are associated with psychological well-being. Although it may be a bit misleading to speak of alexithymia types when dealing with lexithymia, Type III, and modals, representing normal manifestations of affect regulation, for matters of convenience we leave it that way. Furthermore, our data also show that, although alexithymia is defined as a disorder of affect regulation, in the normal range both Type I and Type II individuals can be well adjusted, even gifted, thereby questioning the notion that alexithymia should be considered as a disorder.

References

Albach, F., Moormann, P. P., & Bermond, B. (1996). Memory recovery of childhood sexual abuse. *Dissociation, 9,* 258–269.

Arrindell, W. A., & Ettema, J. H. M. (1986). *Handleiding SCL-90. Nederlandse bewerking van de Symptom Checklist van L.R. Derogatis* [Manual SCL-90. Dutch adaptation of L.R. Derogatis' Symptom Checklist]. Lisse, The Netherlands: Swets & Zeitlinger.

Beck, A. T. (1976). *Cognitive therapy and the emotional disorders.* New York: International Universities Press.

Beck, A. T., Freeman, A., & Associates (1990). *Cognitive therapy of personality disorders.* New York: Guilford Press.

Becker, G. (1978). *The mad genius controversy.* Beverly Hills, CA: Sage.

Bell, C. (1975). The artistic problem In W. G. Bywater (Ed.), *Clive Bell's eye.* Detroit, MI: Wayne State University Press. [First published in 1919 by Athenaeum.]

Bermond, B., Vorst, H. C. M., & Moormann, P .P. (2006). Cognitive neuropsychology of alexithymia: Implications for personality typology.*Cognitive Neuropsychiatry, 11,* 332–360.

Bloemendaal, A. F. T., & Teijn, S. M. (1998). *Alexithymie in de psychiatrie* [Alexithymia in psychiatry]. Master's thesis. Leiden, The Netherlands: Department of Clinical & Health Psychology, Leiden University.

Bloemendaal, A. F. T., Teijn, S. M., & Moormann, P. P. (1999). Alexithymia and personality disorders in a psychiatric population. In A. J. J. M. Vingerhoets & I. Nyklíhek (Eds.), *Abstracts 1999 of the Second International Conference on The (Non)Expression of Emotions in Health and Disease* (pp. 77–78). Tilburg, The Netherlands: Tilburg University.

Brand, A. N., Olff, M., Hulsman, R., & Slagman, C. (1991). Perceptual defense: the use of digitized pictures. In M. Olff, G. Godaert, & H. Ursin (Eds.), *Quantification of human defense* (pp. 293–301). Heidelberg, Germany: Springer-Verlag.

Carpenter, K. M., & Addis, M. E. (2000). Alexithymia, gender and responses to depressive symptoms. *Sex Roles, 43*, 629–644.

Carver, C. S., & Scheier, M. F. (2000). *Perspectives on personality* (4th ed.). Needham Heights, MA: Allyn & Bacon.

Davison, G. C., & Neale, J. M. (1997). *Abnormal psychology* (7th ed.). New York: Wiley.

Goleman, D. (1995).*Emotional intelligence.* New York: Bantam Books.

Hermans, H. J. M. (1967). *Prestatie Motivatie Test: Handleiding* [Achievement Motivation Test: Manual]. Amsterdam, The Netherlands: Swets & Zeitlinger.

Horney, K. (1939). *New ways in psychoanalysis.* New York: Norton.

Janssons, M. S. (2004). *Typen alexithymie en persoonlijkheidsstoornissen onder psychiatrische patiënten* [Alexithymia types and personality disorders among psychiatric patients]. Master's thesis. Leiden, The Netherlands: Depatment of Clinical & Health Psychology, Leiden University.

Linehan, M. M. (1993). *Cognitive-behavioral therapy of borderline personality disorder.* New York: Guilford Press.

Luteijn, F., Kok, A. R., & Van der Ploeg, F. A. E. (1980). *Handleiding bij de NVM* [Manual NVM]. Lisse, The Netherlands: Swets & Zeitlinger.

Luteijn, F., Starren, J., & Van Dijk, H. (1985). *Handleiding bij de NPV* [Manual NPV]. Lisse, The Netherlands: Swets & Zeitlinger.

Marty, P., & M'Uzan, M. (1963). La pensé opératoire. *Revue Française de psychanalyse, 27* (suppl. XXIIIe Congrès des psychanalystes de langues romanes, Barcelone, June 1962), 345–356.

McWilliams, N. (1994). *Psychoanalytic diagnosis.* New York: Guilford Press.

Millon, T., & Davis, R. (2000). *Personality disorders in modern life.* New York: Wiley.

Millon, T., Weiss, L., Millon, C., & Davis, R. (1994). *MIPS: Millon index of personality styles manual.* San Antonio, TX: Psychological Corporation.

Moormann, P. P., & Pijpers R. (2004). *Scoren tussen de oren: De theorie en praktijk van individuele mentale training* [Believing is achieving: theory and practice of individual mental training]. Lisse, The Netherlands: Harcourt International.

Moormann, P. P., Bermond, B., & Albach, F. (2004). The Reality Escape Model: the intricate relation between alexithymia, dissociation, and anesthesia in victims of child sexual abuse. In I. Nyklíhek, A. J. J. M. Vingerhoets, & L. Temoshok (Eds.), *Emotional expression and health* (pp. 82–89). Hove, UK: Brunner Routledge.

Moormann, P. P., Bermond, B., Albach, F., & Van Dorp, I. (1997). The etiology of alexithymia from the perspective of childhood sexual abuse. In A. J. J. M. Vingerhoets, F. J. Van Bussel, & A. J. W. Boelhouwer (Eds.), *The (non)expression of emotions in health and disease* (pp. 139–153). Tilburg, The Netherlands: Tilburg University Press.

Moormann, P. P., Brand, N., Behrendt, E., & Massink, J. (2003). A conceptualization of alexithymia and defense mechanisms in relation to lateral brain dominance. In F. J Maarse, A. E. Akkerman, A. N. Brand, & L. J. M. Mulder (Eds.), *Clinical assessment, computerized methods, and instrumentation* (pp. 71–91). Lisse, The Netherlands: Swets & Zeitlinger.

Niessen, M. A. J. (2001). *Emotionaliteit en cognitieve gevoelscontrole als invloedrijke factoren in persoonlijkheid: Het alexithymie construct nader onderzocht* [Emotionality and cognitive feeling control as influential factors in personality: Further investigation on the alexithymia construct]. Master's thesis. Amsterdam, The Netherlands: Department of Psychology, University of Amsterdam.

Oldham, J. M., & Morris, L. B. (1990). *The personality self-portrait.* New York: Bantam Books.

Oldham, J. M., & Morris, L. B. (1995). *The new personality self-portrait: why you think, work, love, and act the way you do.* New York: Bantam Books.

Passchier, J., & Verhage, F. (1986). The Defense Mechanism Inventory. Preliminary findings on reliability and validity of the Dutch translation. *Gedrag & Gezondheid, 14*, 119–124.

Riggio, E. R. (1986). Assessment of basic social skills. *Journal of Personality and Social Psychology, 51*, 649–660.

Rood, L. (2003). *Typen van affectregulatie: ontstaansfactoren en psychisch welzijn* [Types of affect regulation: origins and psychological well-being]. Master's thesis. Leiden, The Netherlands: Department of Clinical & Health Psychology, Leiden University.

Schreurs, P. J. G., Van de Willige, G., Tellegen, B., & Brosschot, J. F. (1988). *Handleiding Utrechtse Copinglijst: UCL* [Manual Utrecht Coping List: UCL]. Lisse, The Netherlands: Swets & Zeitlinger.

Sperry, L. (1995). *Handbook of diagnosis and treatment of the DSM-IV personality disorders.* New York: Brunner/Mazel.

Stekel, W. (1912). *Träume der Dichter: Eine vergleichende Untersuchung der unbewussten Triebkrafte bei Dichtern, Neurotikern und Verbrechern* [Poet's dreams: a comparative study of unconscious urges among poets, neurtics, and offenders]. Wiesbaden, Germany: Verlag J. F. Bergmann.

Thomas, A., & Chess, S. (1977). The behavioral study of temperament. In J. Strelau, F. H. Farley, & A. Gale (Eds.), *The biological basis of personality and behavior: theories, measurement techniques, and development* (Vol. 1, pp. 213–255). Washington, DC: Hemisphere.

Uterwijk, J. (1998). *Constructie en validering van een Sociale Intelligentie Schaal* [Constructionand validation of a Social Intelligence Scale]. Unpublished intern report. Psychologische Methodenleer. Amsterdam, The Netherlands: University of Amsterdam.

Vorst, H. C. M., & Bermond, B. (2001). Validity and reliability of the Bermond-Vorst Alexithymia Questionnaire. *Personality and Individual Differences, 30*, 413–434.

Chapter 4
Alexithymia and Physical Health Problems: A Critique of Potential Pathways and a Research Agenda

Mark A. Lumley, Jonathan Beyer, and Alison Radcliffe

Early Observations on Alexithymia and Physical Health

In the late 1960s and early 1970s, there were reports that patients with various physical illnesses had relatively poor outcomes with psychodynamic psychotherapy (Nemiah & Sifneos, 1970; Sifneos, 1967). Many of these physically ill patients had difficulty reflecting upon, describing, and expressing their emotions; and they struggled to identify connections between psychological or mental processes and their physical symptoms or disease exacerbations. They were described as unproductive, unimaginative, boring, and stiff; and therapists often had difficulty establishing close working alliances with them. The word *alexithymia* was coined to describe these patients and their primary difficulty—putting feelings into words.

These initial observations of alexithymia in patients with health problems undergoing psychotherapy indicated the need for research. But what direction should such research take? In retrospect, at least two research directions could have ensued during the subsequent decades. First, research could have examined the *treatment implications of alexithymia*, addressing questions such as, "Why do alexithymic patients have difficulty with insight-oriented therapy?" "What alternative treatments might be useful for them?" "Can alexithymia be reduced, and will this lead to improved health?" However, this first research direction was almost completely ignored. Instead, a second direction, based on the observation of elevated alexithymia in physically ill patients, has been diligently pursued—what are the *health implications of alexithymia*? This second line of research has been dominant in subsequent years as researchers have sought to demonstrate that alexithymia is indeed a risk factor for physical illness.

Although research on alexithymia was sporadic during the 1970s and early 1980s, the literature has flourished during the past 20 years. This has been due, in large part, to the development, validation, and promotion of the Toronto Alexithymia Scale (Taylor, Ryan, & Bagby, 1985) and its 20-item revision (Bagby, Parker, & Taylor, 1994; Bagby, Taylor, & Parker, 1994). The TAS-20 provides not only a global alexithymia score but also scores on three dimensions or facets of alexithymia: (a) difficulty identifying one's feelings, (b) difficulty describing one's feelings, and (c) an externally oriented mode of cognition.

A computer literature search (Medline) revealed that by mid-2003, more than 1,300 research articles had been published on alexithymia. To provide a sense for

A. Vingerhoets et al., (eds.), *Emotion Regulation.*

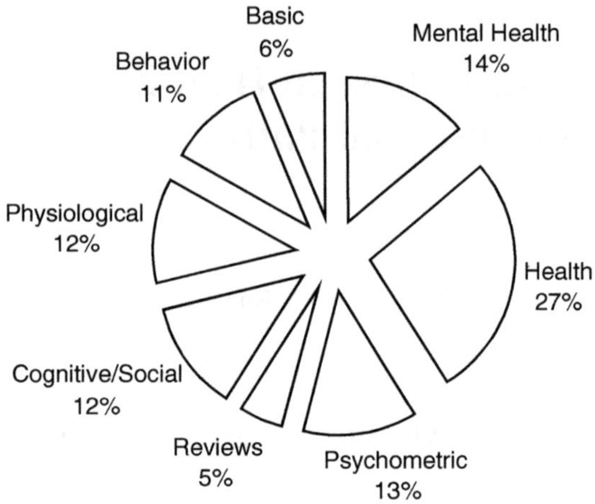

Fig. 4.1 Distribution of research studies on alexithymia, published in 2001 and 2002 ($n = 164$).

the types of alexithymia research being conducted, we reviewed all 164 alexithymia articles published in 2001 and 2002. We classified the content of the articles into one of eight categories that appeared to be exhaustive and mutually exclusive. Figure 4.1 presents the percentage of the 164 articles falling into each of these eight categories. As can be seen, small percentages (5% or 6%) of the articles were review articles or basic laboratory studies of alexithymia. Slightly larger percentages (11% to 14%) of the articles examined the relationship of alexithymia to health behaviors, cognitive and social factors, physiologic measures, or mental health; or the articles were psychometric, dealing with the development of assessment approaches, factor-analytic studies, or translations of measures to other languages. Noteworthy, however, is that more than one quarter of the articles examined the relationship of alexithymia to some aspect of physical illness or medical status. If one includes studies of physiology and health behaviors—domains related to physical health that we discuss below—it can be seen that more than one-half of the papers are related to physical health and illness. Notably missing from these eight categories is one pertaining to treatment; indeed, no alexithymia studies were published during these 2 years that examined issues of intervention. Clearly, the research path most taken has been the health implications of alexithymia.

Is Alexithymia a Risk Factor for Physical Health Problems? Possible Pathways

A leading view of alexithymia is that it is a risk factor not only for psychiatric and behavioral problems but also for the development, maintenance, or exacerbation of those medical or physical health problems that are influenced by disordered affect regulation (Taylor, Bagby, & Parker, 1997). Indeed, many studies have assessed alexithymia in people with various physical illnesses and diseases, typically by comparing patients to healthy controls. We have found at least one study that has been published in the past two decades that has shown elevated levels of alexithymia in patients who have a wide range of health problems: rheumatoid arthritis, hypertension, irritable bowel syndrome, inflammatory bowel disease, cardiac disease, noncardiac chest pain, breast cancer, diabetes, headaches, morbid obesity, chronic pain, eating disorders, kidney failure, peptic ulcer, HIV infection, fibromyalgia, low sperm counts, panic disorder, sexual dysfunction, and more. Clearly, the list is long and is likely to grow, and it certainly gives the impression that alexithymia must be a robust and pervasive risk factor for many physical health problems. Yet, is this conclusion reasonable from these findings?

In this chapter, we critically evaluate the research evidence, methods, and conclusions drawn regarding the hypothesis that alexithymia is a risk factor for physical illness. To do so, we investigate several possible alternative explanations for the recurrent finding that alexithymia is elevated in patients with various health problems. In Figure 4.2, we present a model delineating the various pathways linking alexithymia and physical illness. Some years ago, we presented a similar model and a comprehensive literature review (Lumley Stettner, & Wehmer, 1996), but because the literature has grown so large, our examination of studies in this chapter will not be exhaustive. Rather, we will try to faithfully represent the state of alexithymia research by identifying studies that examine various linkages between alexithymia and health, and we will focus on recent studies (published since our 1996 review). Our primary goal, however, is to advance the quality of the research and sophistication of interpretations made, so that the risk factor question can be more clearly answered. At the end of the chapter, we revisit the research direction not taken—the treatment implications of alexithymia—and also examine several current controversies and challenges in alexithymia research.

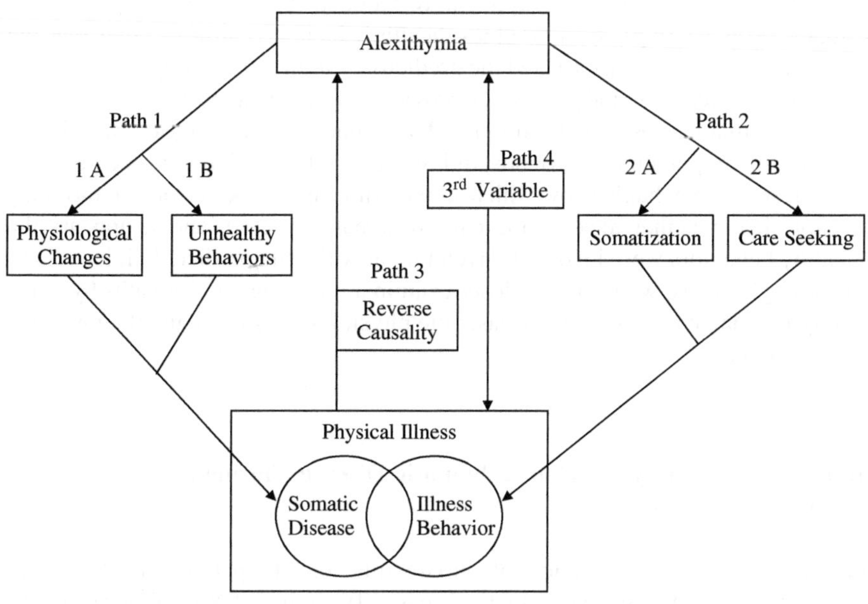

Fig. 4.2 Model of the various pathways linking alexithymia to physical illness.

As illustrated in Figure 4.2, there are at least four explanations for the observed relationships between alexithymia and physical illness. The first path shows that alexithymia may *cause or exacerbate somatic disease*. If so, it should do so via one of two possible mechanisms (or subpaths): alexithymia may induce *physiologic changes* that lead to disease, or alexithymia may prompt *unhealthy behaviors* that support disease processes. The second path suggests that alexithymia causes or prompts *illness behavior*, but not necessarily somatic disease. This pathway also has two subpaths: alexithymia leads to *somatization* (increased reporting of symptoms), or alexithymia prompts *health care seeking*, resulting in higher levels of alexithymia in patient or clinic populations. The third path shown in Figure 4.2 indicates that alexithymia may result from, rather than contribute to, physical illness; that is, alexithymia is *secondary to illness*. The fourth path is that some *third variable* leads to both alexithymia and physical illness. In the following sections of the chapter, we discuss the rationale for each pathway, briefly present and critique evidence for or against it, and suggest methodological and interpretive advances that are needed to more fully test each path.

Path 1: Alexithymia Causes (or Exacerbates) Somatic Disease

The first path in the model presents the traditional psychosomatic view, that alexithymia causes or exacerbates somatic disease. As this chapter will show, there is little solid evidence for this proposal. However, one study that we find to be quite convincing is the longitudinal study of 2,297 middle-aged men, which found that baseline alexithymia predicted an increased risk of death over a 5.5-year follow-up (Kauhanen, Kaplan, Cohen, Julkunen, & Salonen, 1996). The study controlled for many variables (e.g., demographics, health behaviors, cardiovascular risk factors, social factors, depression), and the predictive validity of alexithymia remained. Yet even this excellent study does not provide definitive support for the proposal that alexithymia causes somatic disease. Unfortunately, the analyses, which controlled for many potential confounds, did not reveal the mediating processes, leaving unclear the mechanism by which alexithymia is a risk factor for mortality. It is not clear whether alexithymia caused somatic disease, and it appears that unhealthy behaviors were involved, given that alexithymia predicted violent deaths quite strongly. Thus, we turn to a closer examination of the two subpaths by which alexithymia may cause somatic disease: the physiologic subpath and the unhealthy behavior subpath.

Subpath 1A: Alexithymia Causes Somatic Disease Through Physiologic Changes

Does the poor affect regulation of alexithymia lead to pathologic physiologic changes that could eventuate in somatic disease? Two types of physiologic processes have been examined: immune function and psychophysiologic activity (Guilbaud, Corcos, Hjalmarsson, Loas, & Jeammet, 2003). Only a handful of studies have examined immune functioning and alexithymia, and all suggest that alexithymia is related to poorer immune functioning. Two excellent studies by one research team found that alexithymia was related to reduced lymphocyte levels and to the presence of precancerous cervical lesions among women who were undergoing diagnostic testing (Todarello, Casamassima, Daniele, et al., 1997; Todarello, Casamassima, Marinaccio, et al., 1994). These studies are quite convincing because they demonstrated that alexithymia was linked to both a potential physiologic mediating pathway as well as to a clinical disease end point—something that no other studies have done. Two other studies also support a link between alexithymia and immune impairments. Alexithymic men had lower cytotoxic lymphocyte counts (subsets of natural killer cells and killer effector T cells) than nonalexithymic men, even after controlling for smoking and alcohol intake (Dewaraja et al., 1997), and alexithymia was related to lower levels of interleukin-4 in a small sample of young women even after controlling for depression (Corcos et al., 2004). Thus, although there is need of more studies of alexithymia and immune functioning, the available evidence supports this pathway.

More than a dozen studies have examined alexithymia and psychophysiology, particularly cardiovascular and sympathetic nervous system activity before and during laboratory-based stressors. A number of studies have found that alexithymia is related to higher resting or tonic sympathetic activity (Friedlander et al., 1997; Fukunishi, Sei et al., 1999; Gundel, Greiner, Ceballos-Baumann, Von Rad, Forstl, & Jahn, 2002; Henry et al., 1992; Infrasca, 1997; Stone & Nielson, 2001; Wehmer, Brejnak, Lumley, & Stetner, 1995), although other studies have found no alexithymia effect on resting measures (Luminet, Rimé, Bagby, & Taylor 2004; Newton & Contrada, 1994; Roedema & Simons, 1999; Waldstein, Kauhanen, Neumann, & Katzel, 2002). No studies, however, have shown that alexithymia is associated with lower resting physiologic activity. Most of these studies also have examined physiologic reactivity to various laboratory stressors. Although two studies have found that alexithymia, or at least some facet of it, predicts greater heart rate or blood pressure reactivity to stressors controlling for any baseline differences (Luminet et al., 2004; Waldstein et al., 2002), most studies suggest that there is either no effect of alexithymia on stressor reactivity beyond baseline (Friedlander et al., 1997; Fukunishi, Sei et al., 1999; Martinez-Sanchez et al., 2001), or that alexithymia predicts reduced stressor reactivity (Hyer, Woods, Summers, Boudewyns, & Harrison, 1990; Linden, Lenz, & Stossel, 1996; Neumann, Sollers, Thayer, & Waldstein, 2004; Newton & Contrada, 1994; Roedema & Simons, 1999; Wehmer et al., 1995; Zonnevylle-Bender et al., 2005). Thus, there is some evidence for elevated resting sympathetic arousal among people with alexithymia, which could, if frequent or prolonged, alter physiology and lead to somatic disease. In contrast, there is little evidence that alexithymia leads to hyperreactivity to stressors but more evidence for alexithymic hyporeactivity to various stressors. The latter finding does not support a link between alexithymia and somatic disease.

Yet, most of these psychophysiology studies have additional limitations. The primary finding of no acute stressor hyperreactivity related to alexithymia may be due to the use of stressors that are not appropriate. Emotion or imagery-based stressors (e.g., viewing a supposedly disturbing video or using autobiographical emotional memories) may fail to elicit physiologic activity because the deficits of alexithymia render these "stressors" less vivid or less powerful. We would like to see the simultaneous use of multiple stressors, including behavioral (e.g., exercise), cognitive (e.g., math), emotional, as well as interpersonal (e.g., dyadic conflict) stressors. It is possible that interpersonal conflict—which we suspect is the most common and important type of stressor in people's lives—activates the alexithymic person's affective and physiologic systems in ways that isolated, interpersonally irrelevant stressors do not. In addition, more attention should be paid to the physiologic measures and underlying processes. The measures that have been used in alexithymia studies have been fairly narrow in range—we would like to see research on alexithymia and parasympathetic activity (e.g., as assessed by vagal tone). Also, laboratory assessments may not capture real-world, ecologically valid physiologic activity, such as can be obtained with ambulatory monitoring. We know of no studies of alexithymia and naturalistic assessment of physiologic activity. Such studies would reveal the frequency and duration of physiologic activation and test whether the elevated baseline sympathetic activity seen in laboratory studies is due to novelty effects—new people, procedures, and experiences—that alexithymic people modulate poorly. Finally, we find that most researchers conducting studies on physiology and alexithymia—including ourselves—have been relatively naïve about the construct validity of the physiologic measures, typically viewing them simply as measures of "arousal." There is a sophisticated body of literature on the psychobehavioral processes underlying these measures, and this literature needs to be incorporated into studies of alexithymia and psychophysiology.

Subpath 1B: Alexithymia Causes Somatic Disease Through Unhealthy Behaviors

Alexithymia may also lead to somatic disease, not through the failure of affect regulation to regulate one's physiology, but through behavioral processes—unhealthy actions that have somatic consequences. There is a long list of potentially unhealthy behaviors, and alexithymia—by leading to the failure to regulate affect—may prompt people to engage in behaviors that are risky for health. The longitudinal study of alexithymia and mortality noted above (Kauhanen et al., 1996) found increased violent deaths among alexithymic participants, suggesting the presence of behavioral mechanisms, but that study did not indicate what behavioral processes might be involved. What evidence is there that alexithymia influences unhealthy behavior?

There is consistent evidence that alexithymia is elevated in people with eating disorders (Beales & Dolton, 2000; Carano et al., 2006; De Panfilis, Salvatore, Avanzini, Gariboldi, & Maggini, 2001; Kessler, Schwarze, Filipic, Traue, & von Wietersheim, 2006; Mazzeo & Espelage, 2002; Pinaquy, Chabrol, Simon, Louvet, &

Barbe, 2003; Zonnevylle-Bender, Van Goozen, Cohen-Kettenis, Van Elburg, & Van Engeland, 2002; Zonnevylle-Bender et al., 2004), and alcohol or drug abuse or dependence (El Rasheed, 2001; Haviland, Hendryx, Shaw, & Henry, 1994; Kauhanen, Julkunen, & Salonen, 1992). There also is some evidence that alexithymic people are more likely to engage in problematic gambling (Lumley & Roby, 1995; Parker, Wood, Bond, & Shaughnessy, 2005), have poorer nutrition and a sedentary lifestyle (Helmers & Mente, 1999), and a greater body mass index (Neumann et al., 2004). In contrast, at least one study indicated that cigarette smoking and the degree of nicotine dependence among smokers was unrelated to alexithymia (Lumley, Downey, Stettner, Wehmer, & Pomerleau, 1994), and another study suggested that alexithymia is related to less frequent sexual intercourse among women (Brody, 2003), which suggests a decreased risk for sexually transmitted diseases, although perhaps an increased risk of relationship difficulties.

Another health behavior is compliance (adherence) to medical recommendations. Alexithymia was unrelated to compliance with psychotherapy recommendations (Aarela, Saarijarvi, Salminen, & Toikka, 1997) and unrelated to compliance in diabetes treatment (Friedman et al., 2003). Interestingly, one study found that alexithymic patients were more likely to remain in cognitive behavioral therapy for smoking cessation (Lumley et al., 1994) but more likely to drop from group psychotherapy that focused on feelings (Beresnevaite, 2000). Thus, currently, there is no clear relationship between alexithymia and medical adherence.

In general, we know little about the relationship of alexithymia with many health behaviors, ranging from daily hygiene to diet to preventive medical care to risky driving. This void in the literature is noteworthy, given how straightforward such research is to conduct. The simplest approach is to conduct surveys of both alexithymia and various health behaviors. Better methodology, such as diary research or ecologic momentary assessment, can examine health behaviors in the natural environment and reduce recall and reporting biases that accompany retrospective reports. Studies also could track patients for compliance while they are in physical rehabilitation or a clinical trial of medication. Ideally, this research should go beyond simply documenting a relationship between alexithymia and health behavior; it should address the motivation or reasons for the behaviors. Alexithymia may prompt unhealthy behavior as a way to regulate negative affect, but this has not been verified, so research should examine whether health behaviors are engaged in (or avoided) for affect regulation purposes.

Path 2: Alexithymia Causes Illness Behavior but Not Somatic Disease

Somatic disease usually co-occurs with illness behavior, which is the subjective experience of symptoms (e.g., pain, fatigue) as well behavioral manifestations such as functional disability and the seeking of health care. Because of the overlap between somatic disease and illness behavior, a reasonable hypothesis is that alexithymia is a risk factor for illness behavior but not for somatic disease, per se. As noted in Figure 4.2, we suggest that there are two potential illness behavior pathways accounting for the elevated levels of alexithymia in patients with various physical illnesses.

Subpath 2A: Alexithymia Causes Somatization

Alexithymia may lead to somatization, or the experience and reporting of somatic symptoms, rather than to somatic disease, per se. There is substantial evidence that alexithymia is associated with the report of somatic symptoms. A review of 18 samples found a mean correlation of $r = .23$ between alexithymia scores and somatic symptoms and also found that alexithymia was more prevalent in people with somatoform disorders than in healthy controls (De Gucht & Heiser, 2003). This review is supported by more recent studies (De Gucht, Fischler, & Heiser, 2004a, 2004b; Wearden, Lamberton, Crook, & Walsh, 2005).

Yet, most studies of alexithymia and symptoms lack objective measures, such as clinical or laboratory indices. A few studies have included both, and these studies can test directly whether alexithymia is related to both subjective symptoms and objective markers in the same sample. For example, alexithymia is positively associated with reports of pain but not the presence of clinically verified tissue dysfunction (Glaros & Lumley, 2005; Miranda, Viikari-Juntura, Heistaro, Heliövaara, & Riihimäki, 2005). Similarly, alexithymia is related to subjective but not objective measures of health during blood donation (Byrne & Ditto, 2005), during testing for coronary artery disease (Kauhanen, Kaplan, Cohen, Salonen, & Salonen, 1994; Valkamo et al., 2001), and among HIV-positive patients (Lumley, Tomakowsky, & Torosian, 1997).

Thus, alexithymia is clearly linked with physical symptoms, but it is not typically related to objective disease or somatic pathology. Yet, we do not know the direction of the relationship between alexithymia and symptoms. It is unclear whether alexithymia prompts the reporting of symptoms, whether symptoms creates alexithymia, or whether both the report of symptoms and alexithymia are manifestations of some third variable; the latter two alternatives are discussed below in Paths 3 and 4.

Subpath 2B: Alexithymia Causes Health Care Seeking

Alexithymia may be elevated in patients because alexithymia prompts health care utilization rather than somatic disease. Elevated health care use could result in higher levels of alexithymia in samples recruited from health care settings, especially when such samples are compared with nonpatient healthy controls. Several studies shed light on the relationship of alexithymia and health care utilization. Alexithymic men were more likely to report having been diagnosed with coronary heart disease (specifically, angina pectoris) but had less atherosclerosis, suggesting that alexithymic men were more likely to seek evaluations than to have diseased arteries (Kauhanen et al., 1994). Another study found that alexithymia was related to greater health utilization, at least among depressed patients (Joukamaa, Karlsson, Sholman, & Lehtinen, 1996). Several studies from our laboratory make the picture more complicated, however, because different facets of the TAS-20 predicted health care use differently. Difficulty identifying feelings predicted more outpatient medical seeking, whereas externally oriented thinking predicted less utilization (Lumley & Norman, 1996). We also found that externally oriented thinking—but not global alexithymia—predicted unawareness of symptoms in coronary artery disease, which implies that this facet leads to less health care seeking (Torosian, Lumley, Pickard, & Ketterer, 1997).

The proposal that alexithymia, or at least the difficulty identifying and communicating feelings facets, drives care seeking rather than somatic disease may explain the "negative" findings of some alexithymia studies that compared samples of patients with different disorders—such as "explained" versus "unexplained" symptoms, or epilepsy versus psychogenic nonepileptic events (Kooiman, Bolk, Brand, Trijsburg, & Rooijmans, 2000; Posse & Haellstroem, 1998; Tojek, Lumley, Barkley, Mahr, & Thomas, 2000). Although not all studies have shown similar levels of alexithymia among patient groups (Porcelli, Taylor, Bagby, & De Carne, 1999), this "care-seeking" perspective may explain why clinic-recruited patients with "medically explained" problems may be similar in alexithymia to those with unexplained disorders—alexithymia may drive care seeking rather than disorders.

Yet, different facets of alexithymia may predict different outcomes. For example, difficulty identifying and describing one's feelings may prompt complaints or symptoms and increased health care use, but externally oriented thinking may actually decrease bodily awareness, resulting in decreased health care use. Clearly, studies of health care use need to examine the facets of alexithymia separately. It might be useful to study the motives and decision-making processes that lead to care seeking to better understand how alexithymia influences treatment seeking. In addition, there is a useful research design that should be employed in studies of care seeking. The traditional design compares clinic patients with healthy nonpatient controls, but this confounds the presence of disorder with the status of being a patient. Several novel studies have compared clinic patients with nonpatients who have the same disorder but who are recruited from the community. Studies using this design have found that stress and related constructs (e.g., depression) are elevated only in the clinic patients, but not in nonpatients with the same disorder, suggesting that stress drives care seeking rather than disorder (Aaron et al., 1996). We know of no alexithymia studies that have used this design, but future research should try to determine whether alexithymia drives care seeking rather than disorder.

Path 3: Alexithymia Is Caused by Physical Illness

Correlations between alexithymia and physical illness are often interpreted as alexithymia causing illness. We suspect that this interpretive bias is due to the long-standing emphasis in the field of psychosomatics–where the literature on alexithymia developed and has primarily been published—to view psychological factors as causal. Yet, such correlations could mean that alexithymia results from illness or disease. Is such "secondary alexithymia" possible?

An examination of other theoretical literatures suggests that alexithymic characteristics may be consequence of stressors. The Dynamic Model of Affect (Reich, Zautra, & Davis, 2003) proposes that stressors, including pain, lead to poorer differentiation of positive from negative affect. The "levels of thinking" model has demonstrated that elevated stress can lead to lower thinking levels; that is, simplistic, dichotomous, and concrete thought (Pennebaker et al., 1990). The Dynamic Integration Theory suggests that stress can shift individuals away from complex, integrated thought that tolerates ambiguity, toward attempts to maintain positive affect through the use of simplistic thinking, such as occurs with stereotypes (Labouvie-Vief, 2003). All three of these concepts—poor affect differentiation, low levels of thinking, and low complexity—appear to be components of alexithymia, and these theories support the proposal that stressful illness or disease may lead to alexithymic characteristics. Yet, it is not clear whether chronic stress, pain, or health problems can result in full presentation of alexithymia.

Some studies suggest that alexithymia is secondary to illness or stressors. Alexithymia is increased in people who have experienced sexual violence (Zeitlin, McNally, & Cassiday, 1993), head injury (Williams et al., 2001), or severe burns (Fukunishi, Chishima, & Anze, 1994), or who have posttraumatic stress disorder (Badura, 2003; Fukunishi, Sasaki, Chishima, Anze, & Saijo, 1996; Zlotnick, Mattia, & Zimmerman, 2001). Patients with stressful health conditions that appear less "psychosomatic," such as HIV infection (Fukunishi, Hirabayashi, Matsumoto, Yamanaka, & Fukutake, 1999) or kidney failure (Jin, Mai, & Ding, 2001), also have elevated levels of alexithymia, which may result from these life-threatening illnesses.

Yet, these studies do not confirm that alexithymia is a consequence of a stressor; rather, they indicate only that alexithymia is a correlate of some stressor. Traumatic events or stressful medical conditions are not randomly distributed in the population; thus, alexithymia could have been a risk factor for exposure to the traumatic event or for developing the health problem in the first place, or for generating posttraumatic symptoms. Other studies also do not support the secondary alexithymia hypothesis. In theory, more severe pain or stress should lead to greater secondary alexithymia, but this has not typically been found (Cox, Kuch, Parker, Shulman, & Evans, 1994). Also, it is difficult to conceptualize alexithymia as being secondary to asymptomatic disorders, such as hypertension, which has been repeatedly associated with elevated alexithymia (Jula, Salminen, & Saarijarvi, 1999; Lu, Yue, & Shu, 2001; Todarello, Taylor, Parker, & Fanelli, 1995).

With respect to the temporal stability of alexithymia, some longitudinal studies have suggested that alexithymia is a stable trait (e.g., Martinez-Sanchez, Ato-Garcia, & Ortiz-Soria, 2003), whereas the frequently observed association between alexithymia and depression or anxiety has suggested a state-dependent phenomenon (Honkalampi, Hintikka, Laukkanen, Lehtonen, & Viinamaki, 2001; Honkalampi et al., 2004; Marchesi, Fontò, Balista, Cimmino, & Maggini, 2005).

Recent studies appear to have reached a consensus on this issue, however, by distinguishing absolute from relative stability. A test of absolute stability refers to changes in mean alexithymia scores and is typically tested with paired *t*-tests; a test of relative stability examines the ranking of scores over time, as indicated by correlations. A number of studies have reported that alexithymia scores have relative stability—similar rank orders over time—but not absolute stability, in that mean alexithymia scores often change, in part due to changes in negative affect or other symptoms (Luminet, Bagby, & Taylor, 2001; Mikolajczak & Luminet, 2006; Posse, Hällström, & Backenroth-Ohsako, 2004; Saarijarvi, Salminen, & Toikka, 2006).

What conclusions can be drawn about secondary alexithymia? It appears likely that stress, pain, and threatening disease can result in cognitive/affective changes—such as simple and undifferentiated emotion and environmentally or bodily-focused cognition—that might be viewed as alexithymia. We suspect that there are cases in which adults develop alexithymia after some illness or stressor. Clearly, however, we need longitudinal rather than cross-sectional studies that start prior to the onset of the stressor or disease. Such studies might assess alexithymia prior to diagnostic testing, after the diagnosis, when the illness or disease has become manifest, and when recovery has occurred. Similarly, studies of soldiers or other healthy people who are at risk for stress or injury could assess alexithymia before and then again after some have experienced a stressor. Tracking of alexithymia levels over the entire course of a person's experience with illness or stress will clarify the cause and effect relationship between alexithymia and stress or health problems.

Path 4: Alexithymia and Illness Are Both Due to a Third Variable

Relationships between two variables such as alexithymia and physical illness might be due to a third factor that is correlated with both. Genetic vulnerabilities or temperamental variables (e.g., shyness) may result in various health problems as well as elevated alexithymia scores. Unfortunately, little research has examined these possibilities. Sociodemographic factors are also potential third variables. Lower socioeconomic status is a risk for health problems (Adler et al., 1994), as is older age. Although some studies indicate that alexithymia is elevated among older people and those of lower socioeconomic status (Lane, Sechrest, & Riedel, 1998; Salminen, Saarijarvi, Aarela, Toikka, & Kauhanen, 1999; Sayar, Ebrinc, & Ak, 2001), these findings are not consistent (Parker, Taylor, & Bagby, 1989) and do not appear robust enough to account for the consistent relationship between alexithymia and poor health.

By far, the most commonly considered third variable in alexithymia research is negative affect or neuroticism, including depression, anxiety, and distress. We have seen two types of these "third variable" arguments. First, it is sometimes suggested that negative affect causes both alexithymia and illness. This argument hinges partly on Path 3 described above ("secondary alexithymia") with the additional consideration that negative affect or stress causes illness behavior—a link that has substantial support from a range of studies. Yet this type of third variable explanation has received little attention. A second argument is that the generalized response disposition of negative affect—being excessively self-critical and reporting negative emotions and other self-states—confounds the assessment of both alexithymia and health status, particularly when both of these are self-reported (Watson & Pennebaker, 1989). This second concern rears its head in many studies, particularly because alexithymia is typically self-reported with the TAS-20, which is consistently related to negative affect. Many authors statistically control for negative affect, and this has met with mixed results, with some studies concluding that negative affect accounts for the effects of alexithymia (Bydlowski et al., 2005; Eizaguirre, Saenz de Cabezón, Alda, Olariaga, & Juaniz, 2004; Lumley, Smith, & Longo, 2002), and others reporting that alexithymia remains uniquely predictive (e.g., Luminet, Rimé, Bagby, & Taylor 2004; Vermeulen, Luminet, & Corneille, 2006). We have not observed a consistent conclusion about the independence of alexithymia from negative affect, and this is due, in part, to methodological and statistical variation.

First, whether alexithymia remains a significant predictor of health beyond the effects of a competing construct (e.g., negative affect) is due both to the magnitude of correlation of each variable with the other two and to the sample size. The size of the independent effect of alexithymia can easily become nonsignificant in relatively small samples but remain significant in larger samples—even if the unique alexithymia effect is smaller in the second sample. Thus, sample sizes need to be considered when comparing studies that conclude either the uniqueness or redundancy of alexithymia. Furthermore, many authors appear to focus on statistical significance to the exclusion of effect sizes when examining the independent or redundant effects of alexithymia. Imagine the following hypothetical results:

"In this study, alexithymia correlated with illness ($p = .03$), and depression correlated significantly with both alexithymia ($p = .001$) and illness ($p = .01$). Controlling for depression, we found that alexithymia was no longer significantly related to illness ($p = .11$), but depression was still related to illness ($p = .04$)."

From such data, we have seen authors make two conclusions: (a) that alexithymia is redundant with depression, and there is nothing unique about alexithymia; (b) that depression mediates the relationship between alexithymia and health because this relationship becomes nonsignificant when depression is in the model. However, neither of these two conclusions is justified from these data. We need to know more than p-values; we need to examine the magnitude of direct and indirect effects of alexithymia on health (Holmbeck, 1997). Furthermore, conclusions about mediation need to be based not only on patterns of correlations but also on theoretically based mechanisms, and the cross-sectional nature of the data limits conclusions about mediation.

Is there support for the "third variable" pathway in the alexithymia/health relationship? In the current state of the literature, we find no consistent evidence for this. Genetic or temperamental variables are rarely tested, and the literature on both socioeconomic factors and negative affect as potential confounds is not clear. Furthermore, we caution that correlating self-rated alexithymia with self-reported health status—which is very common—is likely confounded by general response dispositions, and researchers need to consider alternate methods of assessing both alexithymia and health. This is a theme we return to at the end of the chapter.

Summary

What can be concluded from the research on alexithymia and physical illness? It appears that there is some support for each of the pathways that we have described. Alexithymia appears to be related to altered physiology—there is growing evidence that alexithymia is related to impaired immune function, and there is rather consistent evidence that alexithymia is related to elevated resting sympathetic activity—although not to stressor reactivity. In addition, alexithymia probably prompts several unhealthy behaviors, such as substance abuse, disordered eating, and perhaps life-threatening behavior. Unfortunately, most of these studies have not related the physiologic or behavioral changes to clinical disease states. We also believe that alexithymia is associated with—and probably contributes to—somatization, although alexithymia has no consistent relationship to care seeking or medical adherence. It also appears that alexithymia—or at least cognitive and affective reactions that appear like alexithymia—can be secondary to some stressors, particularly threatening or painful ones. Finally, it appears likely that a third variable—particularly negative affect and related constructs—contributes to some of the overlap between self-reported alexithymia and self-reported health, although it does not account fully for this relationship.

Yet, interpretations of the links between alexithymia and physical illness will remain limited as long as researchers continue in the same vein. Fully 81% of all alexithymia studies published in 2001 and 2002 (excluding literature reviews and psychometric articles) were cross-sectional and correlational, whereas only 10% were longitudinal, and 9% were experimental. Cross-sectional, correlational studies, especially those relating self-reported alexithymia to self-reported criterion measures, will only generate results with multiple possible interpretations. We believe that new directions are needed. Alternative research designs such as longitudinal and experimental approaches, non–self-report measures of alexithymia, and objective health indices are needed to answer the pathway questions. Perhaps more fundamentally, we suggest that the questions that researchers ask should be expanded, and we suggest that it is time to explore the research direction not taken—the treatment implications of alexithymia.

Treatment Implications of Alexithymia

The early observations that alexithymic, physically ill patients had difficulty with psychodynamic psychotherapy stimulated the field of alexithymia research, but that research focused on health rather than intervention. Indeed, we know almost nothing about the treatment implications of alexithymia. We envision several potential approaches to such research.

Alexithymia as a Predictor or Moderator of Treatment Outcomes

The most straightforward study is to evaluate whether pretreatment alexithymia predicts the prognosis of patients in medical, psychiatric, or behavioral treatments. Alexithymia has been found to predict poorer outcomes of treatment for depression (Ogrodniczuk, Piper, & Joyce, 2004), alcoholism (Cleland, Magura, Foote, Rosenblum, & Kosanke, 2005; Loas, Fremaux, Otmani, Lecercle, & Delahousse, 1997), functional gastrointestinal disorders (Porcelli, Bagby, Taylor, De Carne, Leandro, & Todarello, 2003; Porcelli, De Carne, & Todarello, 2004), and mixed psychiatric disorders (McCallum, Piper, Ogrodniczuk, & Joyce, 2003). Alexithymia predicted poorer outcomes of group psychotherapy for complicated grief, and this effect was mediated by the therapists' negative responses to alexithymic patients (Ogrodniczuk, Piper, & Joyce, 2005).

In contrast with the generally negative outcomes of alexithymic people in these treatments, there may be no influence, or perhaps even a positive influence, of alexithymia on cognitive-behavioral treatments (CBT). Baseline alexithymia was unrelated to outcomes of CBT for obsessive-compulsive disorder (Rufer, Hand, Braatz, Alsleben, Fricke, & Peter, 2004), a behavioral management program for psoriasis symptoms (Fortune, Richards, Griffiths, & Main, 2004), and relaxation training (Friedlander et al., 1997). Alexithymic patients were somewhat more likely to remain in group CBT for smoking cessation (Lumley et al., 1994), and alexithymia predicted better success in group CBT for substance use (Rosenblum et al., 2005). A study of women undergoing in vitro fertilization found that alexithymia predicted better outcomes of this treatment (Kakatsaki et al., 2004).

These studies, however, have many limitations. The treatments themselves were often heterogeneous or poorly specified, and these studies lacked control conditions with which to compare alexithymia's effect. As a result, correlations between alexithymia and treatment response could be due to a host of other uncontrolled variables often associated with alexithymia, such as being unhealthier, less educated, more distressed, and so forth.

Ideally, alexithymia should be tested as a moderator of treatment effects by determining how alexithymia predicts outcomes of one treatment compared with either a control condition or very different type of treatment. Very few studies have done this, but alexithymia has been tested as a moderator of emotional disclosure or expressive writing. In this paradigm, participants are randomized to write (or in some studies, talk) for 15–30 minutes daily for several days about either personal stressful experiences or emotionally neutral control topics (Pennebaker & Beall, 1986). Health is assessed at baseline and follow-up, and potential moderators, such as alexithymia, can be assessed at baseline and tested to determine whether they predict health outcomes of the disclosure group differently than the control group.

Do alexithymic people respond better, worse, or no differently than nonalexithymic people to emotional disclosure? Two studies have been published and our group also has conducted several of these studies. Unfortunately, these studies are not consistent regarding alexithymia's role in emotional disclosure. One study found that greater difficulty describing feelings (a facet of the TAS-20) predicted improved affect several months after expressive writing among college students compared with control writing (Paez, Velasco, & Gonzalez, 1999), and another study found that the greater alexithymia (TAS-20 total), and specifically the difficulty describing feelings facet, predicted less postsurgical distress and quicker hospital discharge among patients undergoing bladder papilloma resection (Solano, Donati, Pecci, Persichetti, & Colaci, 2003). These two studies suggest that alexithymia, particularly the difficulty describing feelings facet, predicts better responses to disclosure writing.

In contrast with these two studies, we have found that alexithymia predicts poorer responses to disclosure in three studies of people with chronic pain (Lumley, 2004). In 68 patients with rheumatoid arthritis, the difficulty identifying feelings facet of the TAS predicted less improvement in disability and joint impairment compared with controls. In 48 women with chronic pelvic pain, higher TAS-20 total scores predicted worse pain outcomes in the disclosure group but better outcomes in the control group, and there was a similar trend for the use of pain medications. Finally, in 82 young adults with migraine headaches, greater TAS-20 scores again predicted worse outcomes in the disclosure group (increased negative affect, sensory and affective pain, and headache frequency) compared with improvements in the control group on these variables. Thus, our research suggests that alexithymia interferes with the benefits of emotional disclosure—a finding that is consistent with the original observations of insight-oriented therapists, although the conclusion differs from that of the other two disclosure studies (Paez et al., 1999; Solano et al., 2003). Perhaps the different facets or subscales of the TAS-20 have different effects. Paez et al. and Solano et al. both found that difficulty describing feelings predicted better outcomes after disclosure, whereas we have found that difficulty identifying feelings and externally oriented thinking predicted worse outcomes. Perhaps difficulty describing feelings, which is closely linked to introversion, inhibition, and shame, predicts beneficial responses to emotional disclosure, because the private, solitary nature of the intervention allows introverted or ashamed patients to process emotionally difficult issues in a nonthreatening manner. In contrast, true alexithymia (including deficits in emotional awareness, differentiation, and a lack of introspection) should predict poorer outcomes to disclosure.

Thus, it appears that alexithymia is a negative prognostic indicator for many psychological treatments, particularly those focusing on insight, emotional awareness, and a close alliance with a therapist. In contrast, alexithymia may not affect more structured cognitive-behavioral treatments and may even be associated with better outcomes of such treatments. Perhaps the compulsive nature and external focus of people with alexithymia prompt greater adherence to structured exercises and behavioral recommendations.

In truth, however, we know little about how alexithymia influences most interventions. How might alexithymia influence people's engagement in and responses to classic behavioral interventions, such as relaxation training, classical conditioning-based interventions (e.g., systematic desensitization), or operant procedures (e.g., stimulus control)? We might expect that the externally focused, nonaffective orientation of alexithymic people would fit well with such interventions. How might alexithymia influence cognitive therapy? Would alexithymic people engage well in the logical, analytic aspects of such approaches, or would the requirement to monitor, verbalize, and evaluate one's beliefs challenge the alexithymic person's abilities? How about the experiential, interpersonal, and affect-oriented therapies? These approaches appear to require more attention to feelings, psychological processes, and nuances of relationships, and alexithymia should interfere with successful engagement in and outcomes of such therapies. What about pharmacologic interventions? We know of clinicians who preferentially prescribe serotonin reuptake inhibiting medications for alexithymic patients, because they believe that such patients see no relevance of most psychotherapeutic approaches and prefer "nonpsychological" interventions such as medication. We strongly suggest that researchers routinely assess alexithymia (and other individual difference measures of interest) prior to conducting intervention studies and then evaluate whether alexithymia predicts differential treatment effects. Ideally, such studies will have more than one condition, such as a treatment group and a placebo group or two contrasted treatment groups, to see whether alexithymia moderates the effects of groups. Yet, even when only a single intervention is used, assessing alexithymia can provide insight as to how alexithymia influences the course and outcomes of routine clinical practice.

Interventions to Change Alexithymia

Is it possible to directly reduce alexithymia; that is, "treat" it? Although alexithymia may be a fairly stable personality trait that is not easily changed, some studies show that alexithymia decreases over time during treatment, and that these decreases are related to improved symptoms (Becker-Stoll & Gerlinghoff, 2004; Clyne, & Blampied, 2004; de Groot, Rodin, & Olmsted, 1995). Yet, these studies were not designed to reduce alexithymia, and the change in alexithymia may have been a reflection of reduced symptoms. Clearly, a control group is needed.

We know of only one controlled study that attempted to reduce alexithymia and examine whether reduced alexithymia mediated the treatment's effect on health outcomes. Beresnevaite (2000) randomized 37 patients who had both a myocardial infarction and elevated TAS scores to either 4 months of weekly group therapy or two sessions of an education control. Group therapy involved relaxation training, identifying and communicating feelings, imagery, music, and nonverbal emotional expression. Significant decreases in the TAS scores were found in the treatment group but not in the control group. Furthermore, the decreases in TAS scores were linked to better cardiovascular disease outcomes 2 years later. In our view, this study provides some of the strongest support that alexithymia is a risk factor for health problems, because this methodology—using a randomized trial to reduce a risk factor and determine whether health improves—is the gold standard method of determining risk factor status in humans. (In actuality, research that creates or administers the risk factor and shows that it leads to poorer health is the ideal method, but this cannot ethically be done with humans, and we cannot envision an animal model of alexithymia.) Yet, even this study has interpretive limitations, because we do not know what else might have changed in addition to alexithymia, such as depression or social support. Other competing constructs would need to be assessed for their effects on outcome and statistically controlled to rule out alternative explanations.

Although there is little research on alexithymia interventions, clinicians have suggested approaches. Levant (2001) views alexithymia as a result of maladaptive social learning, especially in males, and he developed a cognitive-behavioral intervention in which men are taught to observe symptoms, learn emotion terms, label emotional situations, and link emotional labels with symptoms. Others have suggested variations of psychodynamic therapy—such as labeling feelings for patients rather than asking them how they feel (Taylor et al., 1997). Treatments that encourage greater attention to internal experience, such as mindfulness or the focusing technique of experiential psychotherapy, may result in greater emotional awareness and less alexithymia. We hope that the near future will witness treatment studies that directly target alexithymia, that track changes in alexithymia (and competing constructs), and that determine whether reduced alexithymia mediates health improvements.

Major Challenges Facing Alexithymia Research

There are a number of controversial issues and challenges facing alexithymia researchers. We close this chapter by briefly noting five issues that will need to be addressed in the future.

Challenge 1: Is the Reliance on Self-Reports a Problem?

It is noteworthy that just over 60% of the alexithymia articles published in 2001 and 2002 (excluding reviews and measure development articles) used only self-report measures of both alexithymia and the outcome variable of the study. Thus, a limitation of much of the literature on alexithymia is the presence of shared method variance between predictor and criterion, which spuriously inflates the magnitude of correlations. Yet, beyond this psychometric issue, there has been a long-standing concern over the ability of self-report measures to faithfully capture the construct of alexithymia. Although numerous studies show that the leading self-report alexithymia measure (TAS-20) has some validity, validity is not a dichotomy but a continuum, and more is better! We do not know the various reasons that any given person may obtain an elevated score, nor do we know whether very highly alexithymic people can accurately observe their alexithymia and report it. The common observation that negative affect is routinely associated with elevated TAS-20 scores is an ongoing cause of concern. Self-reported alexithymia measures have dominated the literature for nearly two decades. On the one hand, their ease of use is attractive, but other approaches to assessing alexithymia, such as the Observer Alexithymia Scale, the Beth Israel Hospital Scale as rated by an interviewer, the Levels of Emotional Awareness Scale, or emotional intelligence based on performance testing should be explored more seriously than they have been to date (Lumley, Gustavson, Partridge, & Labouvie-Vief, 2005). We encourage researchers to consider adding non–self-report measures of alexithymia and to include objective measures of health, so that we can reduce the problem inherent in correlating self-reports.

Challenge 2: Is Alexithymia a Single Construct or Separate Facets?

Is alexithymia one homogeneous construct or are the dimensions or facets distinct and more important? Although almost all of the early studies used only the TAS or TAS-20 total score, the occasional failure to find significant effects led to explorations of the facets. Many studies have found that the difficulty identifying feelings and describing feelings facets of the TAS-20 often predict criterion measures, whereas the externally oriented thinking facet often does not. Sometimes, the facets predict different criteria in one sample, such as different forms of health care use (Lumley & Norman, 1996) or asthma symptoms versus objective lung function (Feldman, Lehrer, & Hochron, 2002). We noted above how studies of the TAS-20 as a moderator of the effects of emotional disclosure appear to find different effects as a function of the facet. Perhaps this should not be surprising, given that different personality dimensions (e.g., neuroticism, introversion, low openness) relate differentially to the three TAS-20 facets. Yet this state of affairs is problematic for the full alexithymia construct. Researchers might consider defining a truly alexithymic person as scoring highly on all facets, not just obtaining an elevated total score, which can occur because of elevations on only one or two facets.

Challenge 3: Are There Different Subtypes of Alexithymia?

It has been suggested that there may be different types of alexithymia. The longstanding issue of primary versus secondary alexithymia was noted above, but there are recent arguments that alexithymia should be subtyped according to the level of affective and cognitive characteristics a person demonstrates (Larsen, Brand, Bermond, & Hijman, 2003; Moorman, Bermond, Albach, & van Dorp, 1997). According to these authors, Type 1 alexithymia refers to the prototypic or classic alexithymic person, who has low emotionality along with minimal emotional awareness and verbalization, and a pronounced external orientation. The Type 2 alexithymic, in contrast, experiences elevated levels of negative emotion, tends to be self-focused, but has difficulty identifying and labeling affects. Although there is as yet very little validation of these subtypes, and this conceptual scheme may confuse emotions with experienced feelings, such a scheme does account for some of our clinical observations. We have observed more of the proposed Type 1 alexithymia among men and those in "externally oriented" careers, such as engineering and accounting, and whom others describe as "unemotional." In contrast, we have observed more of the proposed Type 2 alexithymia among those with trauma histories, particularly women with posttraumatic stress disorder, bulimia, or borderline personality. We encourage research on the possibility of these subtypes, because if they do exist, then failing to distinguish between them will greatly limit knowledge. For example, the health and treatment implications of these two types of alexithymia may be quite different.

Challenge 4: Are There Gender Differences in the Correlates of Alexithymia?

A growing number of studies report gender differences in how alexithymia relates to outcomes. This has been observed in studies of hemispheric functioning, the anterior cingulate cortex, stroke, health care use, attention, somatosensory amplification, and childhood cancer (Grabe, Möller, Willert, Spitzer, Rizos, & Freyberger, 2004; Gundel, Lopez-Sala, Ceballos-Baumann, Deus, Cardoner, Marten-Mittag, 2004; Jyvasjarvi, Joukamaa, Vaisanen, Larivaara, Kivela, & Keinanen-Kiukaanniemi, 1999; Lumley & Sielky, 2000; Morrison & Pihl, 1990; Spalletta et al., 2001; van Dijk, Grootenhuis, de Boer, Bermond, & Last, 2002; Wise & Mann, 1994). Indeed, most of the early alexithymia studies did not specifically test for gender differences or it was just statistically controlled; the latter approach not only ignores possible gender differences in how alexithymia relates to criterion variables but also is statistically inappropriate if gender does interact with alexithymia. Therefore, we recommend that researchers not only analyze the entire group but also examine the genders separately and report how alexithymia relates to criterion measures for the two genders. Apparent gender differences in the correlates of alexithymia should be confirmed by direct statistical tests, such as testing gender by alexithymia interactions.

Challenge 5: Should Alexithymia Have Main Effects on Health or Only Interactions?

Most studies of alexithymia test for its main effect on some outcome measures. Yet, one should question whether alexithymia (or any emotion regulation process) is related to poorer health in general or whether it affects health only when emotions have been activated. It is quite possible that under low or no activation conditions, alexithymia does not matter. Yet, almost no studies of alexithymia and illness examine the interaction between life stress and alexithymia. We propose that a better paradigm would examine the effects of alexithymia when the person is under stress, particularly naturally experienced stressors. Alternatively, research might identify the subset of participants who have elevated life stress and determine the effects of alexithymia in these people. We predict that health problems will be most pronounced in alexithymic people whose emotion regulation systems have been challenged by stressful life events.

Acknowledgement Preparation of this chapter was supported, in part, by a Clinical Science Award from the Arthritis Foundation and by NIH grants AR049059 and AG009203.

References

Aarela, E., Saarijarvi, S., Salminen, J. K., & Toikka, T. (1997). Alexithymic features do not predict compliance with psychotherapy in consultation-liaison patients. *General Hospital Psychiatry, 19*, 229–233.

Aaron, L. A., Bradley, L. A., Alarcon, G. S., Alexander, R. W., Triana-Alexander, M., Martin, M. Y., et al. (1996). Psychiatric diagnoses in patients with fibromyalgia are related to health care-seeking behavior rather than to illness. *Arthritis & Rheumatism, 39*, 436–445.

Adler, N. E., Boyce, T., Chesney, M. A., Cohen, S., Folkman, S., Kahn, R. L., et al. (1994). Socioeconomic status and health: the challenge of the gradient. *American Psychologist, 49*, 15–24.

Badura, A. S. (2003). Theoretical and empirical exploration of the similarities between emotional numbing in posttraumatic stress disorder and alexithymia. *Journal of Anxiety Disorders, 17*, 349–360.

Bagby, R. M., Parker, J. D., & Taylor, G. J. (1994). The twenty-item Toronto Alexithymia Scale—I. Item selection and cross-validation of the factor structure. *Journal of Psychosomatic Research, 38*, 23–32.

Bagby, R. M., Taylor, G. J., & Parker, J. D. (1994). The Twenty-item Toronto Alexithymia Scale—II. Convergent, discriminant, and concurrent validity. *Journal of Psychosomatic Research, 38*, 33–40.

Beales, D. L., & Dolton, R. (2000). Eating disordered patients: personality, alexithymia, and implications for primary care. *British Journal of General Practice, 50*, 21–26.

Becker-Stoll, F., & Gerlinghoff, M. (2004). The impact of a four-month day treatment programme on alexithymia in eating disorders. *European Eating Disorders Review, 12*, 159–163.

Beresnevaite, M. (2000). Exploring the benefits of group psychotherapy in reducing alexithymia in coronary heart disease patients: a preliminary study. *Psychotherapy & Psychosomatics, 69*, 117–122.

Brody, S. (2003). Alexithymia is inversely associated with women's frequency of vaginal intercourse. *Archives of Sexual Behavior, 32*, 73–77.

Bydlowski, S., Corcos, M., Jeammet, P., Paterniti, S., Berthoz, S., Laurier, C., et al. (2005). Emotion-processing deficits in eating disorders. *International Journal of Eating Disorders, 37*, 321–329.

Byrne, N., & Ditto, B. (2005). Alexithymia, cardiovascular reactivity, and symptom reporting during blood donation. *Psychosomatic Medicine, 67*, 471–475.

Carano, A., De Berardis, D., Gambi, F., Di Paolo, C., Campanella, D., Pelusi, L., et al. (2006). Alexithymia and body image in adult outpatients with binge eating disorder. *International Journal of Eating Disorders, 39*, 332–340.

Cleland, C., Magura, S., Foote, J., Rosenblum, A., & Kosanke, N. (2005). Psychometric properties of the Toronto Alexithymia Scale (TAS-20) for substance users. *Journal of Psychosomatic Research, 58*, 299–306.

Clyne, C., & Blampied, N. M. (2004). Training in emotion regulation as a treatment for binge eating: a preliminary study. *Behaviour Change, 21*, 269–281.

Corcos, M., Guilbaud, O., Paterniti, S., Curt, F., Hjalmarsson, L., Moussa, M., et al. (2004). Correlation between serum levels of interleukin-4 and alexithymia scores in healthy female subjects: Preliminary findings. *Psychoneuroendocrinology, 29*, 557–562.

Cox, B. J., Kuch, K., Parker, J. D., Shulman, I. D., & Evans, R. J. (1994). Alexithymia in somatoform disorder patients with chronic pain. *Journal of Psychosomatic Research, 38*, 523–527.

De Groot, J. M., Rodin, G., & Olmsted, M. P. (1995). Alexithymia, depression, and treatment outcome in bulimia nervosa. *Comprehensive Psychiatry, 36*, 53–60.

De Gucht, V., & Heiser, W. (2003). Alexithymia and somatisation: A quantitative review of the literature. *Journal of Psychosomatic Research, 54*, 425–434.

De Gucht, V., Fischler, B., & Heiser, W. (2004a). Neuroticism, alexithymia, negative affect, and positive affect as determinants of medically unexplained symptoms. *Personality and Individual Differences, 36*, 1655–1667.

De Gucht, V., Fischler, B., & Heiser, W. (2004b). Personality and affect as determinants of medically unexplained symptoms in primary care: a follow-up study. *Journal of Psychosomatic Research, 56*, 279–285.

De Panfilis, C., Salvatore, P., Avanzini, M., Gariboldi, S., & Maggini, C. (2001). Alexithymia in eating disorders: a personality disturbance? *Psichiatria e Psicoterapia Analitica, 20*, 349–361.

Dewaraja, R., Tanigawa, T., Araki, S., Nakata, A., Kawamura, N., Ago, Y., et al. (1997). Decreased cytotoxic lymphocyte counts in alexithymia. *Psychotherapy & Psychosomatics, 66*, 83–86.

Eizaguirre, A. E., Saenz de Cabezón, A. O., Alda, I. O. d., Olariaga, L. J., & Juaniz, M. (2004). Alexithymia and its relationships with anxiety and depression in eating disorders. *Personality and Individual Differences, 36*, 321–331.

El Rasheed, A. H. (2001). Alexithymia in Egyptian substance abusers. *Substance Abuse, 22*, 11–21.

Feldman, J. M., Lehrer, P. M., & Hochron, S. M. (2002). The predictive value of the Toronto Alexithymia Scale among patients with asthma. *Journal of Psychosomatic Research, 53*, 1049–1052.

Fortune, D. G., Richards, H. L., Griffiths, C. E., & Main, C. J. (2004). Targeting cognitive-behaviour therapy to patients' implicit model of psoriasis: results from a patient preference controlled trial. *British Journal of Clinical Psychology, 43*, 65–82.

Friedlander, L., Lumley, M. A., Farchione, T., & Doyal, G. (1997). Testing the alexithymia hypothesis: Physiological and subjective responses during relaxation and stress. *Journal of Nervous & Mental Disease, 185*, 233–239.

Friedman, S., Vila, G., Even, C., Timsit, J., Boitard, C., Dardennes, R., et al. (2003). Alexithymia in insulin-dependent diabetes mellitus is related to depression and not to somatic variables or compliance. *Journal of Psychosomatic Research, 55*, 285–287.

Fukunishi, I., Chishima, Y., & Anze, M. (1994). Posttraumatic stress disorder and alexithymia in burn patients. *Psychological Reports, 75*, 1371–1376.

Fukunishi, I., Sasaki, K., Chishima, Y., Anze, M., & Saijo, M. (1996). Emotional disturbances in trauma patients during the rehabilitation phase: Studies of posttraumatic stress disorder and alexithymia. *General Hospital Psychiatry, 18*, 121–127.

Fukunishi, I., Hirabayashi, N., Matsumoto, T., Yamanaka, K., & Fukutake, K. (1999). Alexithymic characteristics of HIV-positive patients. *Psychological Reports, 85*, 963–970.

Fukunishi, I., Sei, H., Morita, Y., & Rahe, R. H. (1999). Sympathetic activity in alexithymics with mother's low care. *Journal of Psychosomatic Research, 46*, 579–589.

Glaros, A. G., & Lumley, M. A. (2005). Alexithymia and pain in temporomandibular disorder. *Journal of Psychosomatic Research, 59*, 85–88.

Grabe, H.-J., Möller, B., Willert, C., Spitzer, C., Rizos, T., & Freyberger, H.-J. (2004). Interhemispheric transfer in alexithymia: a transcallosal inhibition study. *Psychotherapy & Psychosomatics, 73*, 117–123.

Guilbaud, O., Corcos, M., Hjalmarsson, L., Loas, G., & Jeammet, P. (2003). Is there a psychoneuroimmunological pathway between alexithymia and immunity? Immune and physiological correlates of alexithymia. *Biomedicine & Pharmacotherapy, 57*, 292–295.

Gundel, H., Greiner, A., Ceballos-Baumann, A. O., Von Rad, M., Forstl, H., & Jahn, T. (2002). Increased level of tonic sympathetic arousal in high-vs. low-alexithymic cervical dystonia patients. *Psychotherapie, Psychosomatik, Medizinische Psychologie, 52*, 461–468.

Gundel, H., Lopez-Sala, A., Ceballos-Baumann, A. O., Deus, J., Cardoner, N., Marten-Mittag, B., et al. (2004). Alexithymia correlates with the size of the right anterior cingulate. *Psychosomatic Medicine, 66*, 132–140.

Haviland, M. G., Hendryx, M. S., Shaw, D. G., & Henry, J. P. (1994). Alexithymia in women and men hospitalized for psychoactive substance dependence. *Comprehensive Psychiatry, 35*, 124–128.

Helmers, K. F., & Mente, A. (1999). Alexithymia and health behaviors in healthy male volunteers. *Journal of Psychosomatic Research, 47*, 635–645.

Henry, J. P., Haviland, M. G., Cummings, M. A., Anderson, D. L., Nelson, J. C., MacMurray, J. P., et al. (1992). Shared neuroendocrine patterns of post-traumatic stress disorder and alexithymia. *Psychosomatic Medicine, 54*, 407–415.

Holmbeck, G. N. (1997). Toward terminological, conceptual, and statistical clarity in the study of mediators and moderators: examples from the child-clinical and pediatric psychology literatures. *Journal of Consulting and Clinical Psychology, 65*, 599–610.

Honkalampi, K., Hintikka, J., Laukkanen, E., Lehtonen, J., & Viinamaki, H. (2001). Alexithymia and depression: a prospective study of patients with major depressive disorder. *Psychosomatics, 42*, 229–234.

Honkalampi, K., Koivumaa-Honkanen, H., Hintikka, J., Antikainen, R., Haatainen, K., Tanskanen, A., et al. (2004). Do stressful life-events or sociodemographic variables associate with depression and alexithymia among a general population?—a 3-year follow-up study. *Comprehensive Psychiatry 45*, 254–260.

Hyer, L., Woods, M. G., Summers, M. N., Boudewyns, P., & Harrison, W. R. (1990). Alexithymia among Vietnam veterans with posttraumatic stress disorder. *Journal of Clinical Psychiatry, 51*, 243–247.

Infrasca, R. (1997). Alexithymia, neurovegetative arousal and neuroticism. An experimental study. *Psychotherapy & Psychosomatics, 66*, 276–280.

Jin, Y., Mai, C., & Ding, K. (2001). A study of alexithymia of hemodialysis patients. *Chinese Journal of Clinical Psychology, 9*, 226–227.

Joukamaa, M., Karlsson, H., Sholman, B., & Lehtinen, V. (1996). Alexithymia and psychological distress among frequent attendance patients in health care. *Psychotherapy & Psychosomatics, 65*, 199–202.

Jula, A., Salminen, J. K., & Saarijarvi, S. (1999). Alexithymia: a facet of essential hypertension. *Hypertension, 33*, 1057–1061.

Jyvasjarvi, S., Joukamaa, M., Vaisanen, E., Larivaara, P., Kivela, S. L., & Keinanen-Kiukaanniemi, S. (1999). Alexithymia, hypochondriacal beliefs, and psychological distress among frequent attenders in primary health care. *Comprehensive Psychiatry, 40*, 292–298.

Kakatsaki, D., Chatziandreou, M., Vaslamatzis, G., Daphnes, O., Loutrades, D. s., & Christodoulou, G. N. (2004). Anxiety, depression, alexithymia and personality traits: Are they related with the outcome of in vitro fertilization? *Psychiatriki, 15*, 27–36.

Kauhanen, J., Julkunen, J., & Salonen, J. T. (1992). Coping with inner feelings and stress: Heavy alcohol use in the context of alexithymia. *Behavioral Medicine, 18*, 121–126.

Kauhanen, J., Kaplan, G. A., Cohen, R. D., Salonen, R., & Salonen, J. T. (1994). Alexithymia may influence the diagnosis of coronary heart disease. *Psychosomatic Medicine, 56*, 237–244.

Kauhanen, J., Kaplan, G. A., Cohen, R. D., Julkunen, J., & Salonen, J. T. (1996). Alexithymia and risk of death in middle-aged men. *Journal of Psychosomatic Research, 41*, 541–549.

Kessler, H., Schwarze, M., Filipic, S., Traue, H. C., & von Wietersheim, J. (2006). Alexithymia and facial emotion recognition in patients with eating disorders. *International Journal of Eating Disorders, 39*, 245–251.

Kooiman, C. G., Bolk, J. H., Brand, R., Trijsburg, R. W., & Rooijmans, H. G. (2000). Is alexithymia a risk factor for unexplained physical symptoms in general medical outpatients? *Psychosomatic Medicine, 62*, 768–778.

Labouvie-Vief, G. (2003). Dynamic integration: affect, cognition, and the self in adulthood. *Current Directions in Psychological Science, 12*, 201–206.

Lane, R. D., Sechrest, L., & Riedel, R. (1998). Sociodemographic correlates of alexithymia. *Comprehensive Psychiatry, 39*, 377–385.

Larsen, J. K., Brand, N., Bermond, B., & Hijman, R. (2003). Cognitive and emotional characteristics of alexithymia: a review of neurobiological studies. *Journal of Psychosomatic Research, 54*, 533–541.

Levant, R. F. (2001). Desperately seeking language: Understanding, assessing, and treating normative male alexithymia. In G. R. Brooks & G. E. Good (Eds.), *The new handbook of psychotherapy and counseling with men: a comprehensive guide to settings, problems, and treatment approaches* (pp. 424–443). San Francisco, CA: Jossey-Bass/Pfeiffer.

Linden, W., Lenz, J. W., & Stossel, C. (1996). Alexithymia, defensiveness and cardiovascular reactivity to stress. *Journal of Psychosomatic Research, 41*, 575–583.

Loas, G., Fremaux, D., Otmani, O., Lecercle, C., & Delahousse, J. (1997). Is alexithymia a negative factor for maintaining abstinence? A follow-up study. *Comprehensive Psychiatry, 38*, 296–299.

Lu, N., Yue, Z., & Shu, F. (2001). Alexithymia of patients with essential hypertension or type II diabetes mellitus. *Chinese Mental Health Journal, 15*, 163–165.

Luminet, O., Bagby, R. M., & Taylor, G. J. (2001). An evaluation of the absolute and relative stability of alexithymia in patients with major depression. *Psychotherapy & Psychosomatics, 70*, 254–260.

Luminet, O., Rimé, B., Bagby, R. M., & Taylor, G. J. (2004). A multimodal investigation of emotional responding in alexithymia. *Cognition & Emotion, 18*, 741–766.

Lumley, M. A. (2004). Alexithymia, emotional disclosure, and health: a program of research. *Journal of Personality, 72*, 1271–1300.

Lumley, M. A., & Norman, S. (1996). Alexithymia and health care utilization. *Psychosomatic Medicine, 58*, 197–202.

Lumley, M. A., & Roby, K. J. (1995). Alexithymia and pathological gambling. *Psychotherapy & Psychosomatics, 63*, 201–206.

Lumley, M. A., & Sielky, K. (2000). Alexithymia, gender, and hemispheric functioning. *Comprehensive Psychiatry, 41*, 352–359.

Lumley, M. A., Downey, K., Stettner, L., Wehmer, F., & Pomerleau, O. F. (1994). Alexithymia and negative affect: relationship to cigarette smoking, nicotine dependence, and smoking cessation. *Psychotherapy & Psychosomatics, 61*, 156–162.

Lumley, M. A., Stettner, L., & Wehmer, F. (1996). How are alexithymia and physical illness linked? A review and critique of pathways. *Journal of Psychosomatic Research, 41*, 505–518.

Lumley, M. A., Tomakowsky, J., & Torosian, T. (1997). The relationship of alexithymia to subjective and biomedical measures of disease. *Psychosomatics, 38*, 497–502.

Lumley, M. A., Smith, J. A., & Longo, D. J. (2002). The relationship of alexithymia to pain severity and impairment among patients with chronic myofascial pain: Comparisons with self-efficacy, catastrophizing, and depression. *Journal of Psychosomatic Research, 53*, 823–830.

Lumley, M. A., Gustavson, B. J., Partridge, R. T., & Labouvie-Vief, G. (2005). Assessing alexithymia and related emotional ability constructs using multiple methods: interrelationships among measures. *Emotion, 5*, 329–342.

Marchesi, C., Fontò, S., Balista, C., Cimmino, C., & Maggini, C. (2005). Relationship between alexithymia and panic disorder: a longitudinal study to answer an open question. *Psychotherapy & Psychosomatics, 74*, 56–60.

Martinez-Sanchez, F., Ortiz-Soria, B., & Ato-Garcia, M. (2001). Subjective and autonomic stress responses in alexithymia. *Psicothema, 13*, 57–62.

Martinez-Sanchez, F., Ato-Garcia, M., & Ortiz-Soria, B. (2003). Alexithymia—state or trait? *Spanish Journal of Psychology, 6*, 51–59.

Mazzeo, S. E., & Espelage, D. L. (2002). Association between childhood physical and emotional abuse and disordered eating behaviors in female undergraduates: an investigation of the mediating role of alexithymia and depression. *Journal of Counseling Psychology, 49*, 86–100.

McCallum, M., Piper, W. E., Ogrodniczuk, J. S., & Joyce, A. S. (2003). Relationships among psychological mindedness, alexithymia and outcome in four forms of short-term psychotherapy. *Psychology & Psychotherapy, 76*, 133–144.

Mikolajczak, M., & Luminet, O. (2006). Is alexithymia affected by situational stress or is it a stable trait related to emotion regulation? *Personality and Individual Differences, 40*, 1399–1408.

Miranda, H., Viikari-Juntura, E., Heistaro, S., Heliövaara, M., & Riihimäki, H. (2005). A population study on differences in the determinants of a specific shoulder disorder versus nonspecific shoulder pain without clinical findings. *American Journal of Epidemiology, 161*, 847–855.

Moorman, P. P., Bermond, B., Albach, F., & van Dorp, I. (1997). The etiology of alexithymia from the perspective of childhood sexual abuse. In A. J. J. M. Vingerhoets, F. J. van Bussel, & A. J. W. Boelhouwer (Eds.), *The (non)expression of emotions in health and disease* (pp. 139–153). Tilburg, The Netherlands: Tilburg University Press.

Morrison, S. L., & Pihl, R. O. (1990). Alexithymia and stimulus augmenting/reducing. *Journal of Clinical Psychology, 46*, 730–736.

Nemiah, J. C., & Sifneos, P. E. (1970). Affect and fantasy in patients with psychosomatic disorders. In O. W. Hill (Ed.), *Modern trends in psychosomatic medicine* (Vol. 2, pp. 26–34). London: Butterworths.

Neumann, S. A., Sollers, J. J., 3rd, Thayer, J. F., & Waldstein, S. R. (2004). Alexithymia predicts attenuated autonomic reactivity, but prolonged recovery to anger recall in young women. *International Journal of Psychophysiology, 53*, 183–195.

Newton, T. L., & Contrada, R. J. (1994). Alexithymia and repression: contrasting emotion-focused coping styles. *Psychosomatic Medicine, 56*, 457–462.

Ogrodniczuk, J. S., Piper, W. E., & Joyce, A. S. (2004). Alexithymia as a predictor of residual symptoms in depressed patients who respond to short-term psychotherapy. *American Journal of Psychotherapy, 58*, 150–161.

Ogrodniczuk, J. S., Piper, W. E., & Joyce, A. S. (2005). The negative effect of alexithymia on the outcome of group therapy for complicated grief: What role might the therapist play? *Comprehensive Psychiatry*, *46*, 206–213.

Paez, D., Velasco, C., & Gonzalez, J. L. (1999). Expressive writing and the role of alexythimia as a dispositional deficit in self-disclosure and psychological health. *Journal of Personality & Social Psychology, 77*, 630–641.

Parker, J. D., Taylor, G. J., & Bagby, R. M. (1989). The alexithymia construct: Relationship with sociodemographic variables and intelligence. *Comprehensive Psychiatry, 30*, 434–441.

Parker, J. D., Wood, L. M., Bond, B. J., & Shaughnessy, P. (2005). Alexithymia in young adulthood: a risk factor for pathological gambling. *Psychotherapy & Psychosomatics, 74*, 51–55.

Pennebaker, J. W., & Beall, S. K. (1986). Confronting a traumatic event: toward an understanding of inhibition and disease. *Journal of Abnormal Psychology, 95*, 274–281.

Pennebaker, J. W., Czajka, J. A., Cropanzano, R., Richards, B. C., Brumbelow, S., Ferrara, K., et al. (1990). Levels of thinking. *Personality & Social Psychology Bulletin, 16*, 743–757.

Pinaquy, S., Chabrol, H., Simon, C., Louvet, J. P., & Barbe, P. (2003). Emotional eating, alexithymia, and binge-eating disorder in obese women. *Obesity Research, 11*, 195–201.

Porcelli, P., Taylor, G. J., Bagby, R. M., & De Carne, M. (1999). Alexithymia and functional gastrointestinal disorders. A comparison with inflammatory bowel disease. *Psychotherapy & Psychosomatics, 68*, 263–269.

Porcelli, P., Bagby, R. M., Taylor, G. J., De Carne, M., Leandro, G., & Todarello, O. (2003). Alexithymia as a predictor of treatment outcome in patients with functional gastrointestinal disorders. *Psychosomatic Medicine, 65*, 911–918.

Porcelli, P., De Carne, M., & Todarello, O. (2004). Prediction of treatment outcome of patients with functional gastrointestinal disorders by the diagnostic criteria for psychosomatic research. *Psychotherapy & Psychosomatics, 73*, 166–173.

Posse, M., & Haellstroem, T. (1998). Alexithymia, personality, characteristics, and somatization tendency in different physical diseases. *European Journal of Psychiatry, 12*, 215–224.

Posse, M., Hällström, T., & Backenroth-Ohsako, G. (2004). Psychosocial predictors of alexithymia examined over a 12-month period in a non-patient female population. *European Journal of Psychiatry, 18*, 133–141.

Reich, J. W., Zautra, A. J., & Davis, M. (2003). Dimensions of affect relationships: models and their integrative implications. *Review of General Psychology, 7*, 66–83.

Roedema, T. M., & Simons, R. F. (1999). Emotion-processing deficit in alexithymia. *Psychophysiology, 36*, 379–387.

Rosenblum, A., Cleland, C., Magura, S., Mahmood, D., Kosanke, N., & Foote, J. (2005). Moderators of effects of motivational enhancements to cognitive behavioral therapy. *American Journal of Drug and Alcohol Abuse, 31*, 35–58.

Rufer, M., Hand, I., Braatz, A., Alsleben, H., Fricke, S., & Peter, H. (2004). A prospective study of alexithymia in obsessive-compulsive patients treated with multimodal cognitive-behavioral therapy. *Psychotherapy & Psychosomatics, 73*, 101–106.

Saarijarvi, S., Salminen, J. K., & Toikka, T. (2006). Temporal stability of alexithymia over a five-year period in outpatients with major depression. *Psychotherapy & Psychosomatics, 75*, 107–112.

Salminen, J. K., Saarijarvi, S., Aarela, E., Toikka, T., & Kauhanen, J. (1999). Prevalence of alexithymia and its association with sociodemographic variables in the general population of Finland. *Journal of Psychosomatic Research, 46*, 75–82.

Sayar, K., Ebrinc, S., & Ak, I. (2001). Alexithymia in patients with antisocial personality disorder in a military hospital setting. *Israel Journal of Psychiatry & Related Sciences, 38*, 81–87.

Sifneos, P. E. (1967). Clinical observations on some patients suffering from a variety of psychosomatic diseases. *Acta Medicina Psychosomatica, 7*, 1–10.

Solano, L., Donati, V., Pecci, F., Persichetti, S., & Colaci, A. (2003). Postoperative course after papilloma resection: effects of written disclosure of the experience in subjects with different alexithymia levels. *Psychosomatic Medicine, 65*, 477–484.

Spalletta, G., Pasini, A., Costa, A., De Angelis, D., Ramundo, N., Paolucci, S., et al. (2001). Alexithymic features in stroke: Effects of laterality and gender. *Psychosomatic Medicine, 63*, 944–950.

Stone, L. A., & Nielson, K. A. (2001). Intact physiological response to arousal with impaired emotional recognition in alexithymia. *Psychotherapy & Psychosomatics, 70*, 92–102.

Taylor, G. J., Ryan, D., & Bagby, R. M. (1985). Toward the development of a new self-report alexithymia scale. *Psychotherapy & Psychosomatics, 44*, 191–199.

Taylor, G. J., Bagby, R. M., & Parker, J. D. A. (1997). *Disorders of affect regulation: alexithymia in medical and psychiatric illness*. Cambridge: Cambridge University Press.

Todarello, O., Casamassima, A., Marinaccio, M., La Pesa, M. W., Caradonna, L., Valentino, L., et al. (1994). Alexithymia, immunity and cervical intraepithelial neoplasia: A pilot study. *Psychotherapy & Psychosomatics, 61*, 199–204.

Todarello, O., Taylor, G. J., Parker, J. D., & Fanelli, M. (1995). Alexithymia in essential hypertensive and psychiatric outpatients: A comparative study. *Journal of Psychosomatic Research, 39*, 987–994.

Todarello, O., Casamassima, A., Daniele, S., Marinaccio, M., Fanciullo, F., Valentino, L., et al. (1997). Alexithymia, immunity and cervical intraepithelial neoplasia: replication. *Psychotherapy & Psychosomatics, 66*, 208–213.

Tojek, T. M., Lumley, M. A., Barkley, G., Mahr, G., & Thomas, A. (2000). Stress and other psychosocial characteristics of patients with psychogenic nonepileptic seizures. *Psychosomatics, 41*, 221–226.

Torosian, T., Lumley, M. A., Pickard, S. D., & Ketterer, M. W. (1997). Silent versus symptomatic myocardial ischemia: the role of psychological and medical factors. *Health Psychology, 16*, 123–130.

Valkamo, M., Hintikka, J., Honkalampi, K., Niskanen, L., Koivumaa-Honkanen, H., & Viinamaki, H. (2001). Alexithymia in patients with coronary heart disease. *Journal of Psychosomatic Research, 50*, 125–130.

Van Dijk, M., Grootenhuis, M. A., de Boer, M., Bermond, B., & Last, B. F. (2002). Alexithymia in long-term survivors of childhood cancer. *Pediatric Rehabilitation, 5*, 203–207.

Vermeulen, N., Luminet, O., & Corneille, O. (2006). Alexithymia and the automatic processing of affective information: evidence from the affective priming paradigm. *Cognition & Emotion, 20*, 64–91.

Waldstein, S. R., Kauhanen, J., Neumann, S. A., & Katzel, L. I. (2002). Alexithymia and cardiovascular risk in older adults: psychosocial, psychophysiological, and biomedical correlates. *Psychology & Health, 17*, 597–610.
Watson, D., & Pennebaker, J. W. (1989). Health complaints, stress, and distress: exploring the central role of negative affectivity. *Psychological Review, 96*, 234–254.
Wearden, A. J., Lamberton, N., Crook, N., & Walsh, V. (2005). Adult attachment, alexithymia, and symptom reporting. An extension to the four category model of attachment. *Journal of Psychosomatic Research, 58*, 279–288.
Wehmer, F., Brejnak, C., Lumley, M. A., & Stettner, L. (1995). Alexithymia and physiological reactivity to emotion-provoking visual scenes. *Journal of Nervous & Mental Disease, 183*, 351–357.
Williams, K. R., Galas, J., Light, D., Pepper, C., Ryan, C., Kleinmann, A. E., et al. (2001). Head injury and alexithymia: implications for family practice care. *Brain Injury, 15*, 349–356.
Wise, T. N., & Mann, L. S. (1994). The relationship between somatosensory amplification, alexithymia, and neuroticism. *Journal of Psychosomatic Research, 38*, 515–521.
Zeitlin, S. B., McNally, R. J., & Cassiday, K. L. (1993). Alexithymia in victims of sexual assault: an effect of repeated traumatization? *American Journal of Psychiatry, 150*, 661–663.
Zlotnick, C., Mattia, J. I., & Zimmerman, M. (2001). The relationship between posttraumatic stress disorder, childhood trauma and alexithymia in an outpatient sample. *Journal of Traumatic Stress, 14*, 177–188.
Zonnevylle-Bender, M. J. S., Van Goozen, S. H. M., Cohen-Kettenis, P. T., Van Elburg, A., & Van Engeland, H. (2002). Do adolescent anorexia nervosa patients have deficits in emotional functioning? *European Child & Adolescent Psychiatry, 11*, 38–42.
Zonnevylle-Bender, M. J. S., Van Goozen, S. H. M., Cohen-Kettenis, P. T., Van Elburg, A., De Wildt, M., Stevelmans, E., et al. (2004). Emotional functioning in anorexia nervosa patients: adolescents compared to adults. *Depression and Anxiety, 19*, 35–42.
Zonnevylle-Bender, M. J. S., Van Goozen, S. H. M., Cohen-Kettenis, P. T., Jansen, L. M. C., Van Elburg, A., & Van Engeland, H. (2005). Adolescent anorexia nervosa patients have a discrepancy between neurophysiological responses and self-reported emotional arousal to psychosocial stress. *Psychiatry Research, 135*, 45–52.

Chapter 5
Current Issues in Repressive Coping and Health

Lynn B. Myers, John W. Burns, Naz Derakshan, Erin Elfant, Michael W. Eysenck, and Sean Phipps

Introduction

The year 2004 marked 25 years since Weinberger, Schwartz and Davidson (1979) published their seminal paper identifying individuals who possess a repressive coping style (*repressors*). Repressors are identified by their low scores on self-report measures of trait anxiety (measured by various trait anxiety scales, e.g., the Bendig version of the Manifest Anxiety Scale; Bendig, 1956) and high scores on defensiveness (usually measured with the Marlowe-Crowne Social Desirability Scale; Crowne & Marlowe, 1964). Apart from the repressor group, three control groups are usually identified using the same typology: a further low trait anxiety group that is low on defensiveness *(low-anxious)* and two high trait anxiety groups, one that is low on defensiveness *(high-anxious)* and one that is high on defensiveness (*defensive high-anxious*) (Table 5.1).

One of the defining characteristics of repressors is that when they are put in potentially stressful situations, they report low levels of distress but are physiologically very reactive (e.g., increased heart rate, raised blood pressure) as well as behaviorally very reactive. This "repressive dissociation" was noted in the original Weinberger et al. (1979) study and is a widely replicated finding in both male and female participants; in students samples, the general population and patients, and using different measures of anxiety and defensiveness (e.g., Asendorpf & Scherer, 1983; Benjamins, Schuurs, & Hoogstraten, 1994; Derakshan & Eysenck, 1997; 2001a; 2001b; Newton & Contrada, 1992). None of the nonrepressor groups exhibit this repressive style. A recent ISI Web of Knowledge search indicated that nearly 600 published papers have cited the original Weinberger et al. paper, and there are probably many more papers not included in that database. Thus, the Weinberger et al. methodology was very influential in starting a whole new area of repression research.

One of the defining features of repressors is that they tend to avoid negative affect. There is considerable evidence from various studies that repressors use an avoidant style of processing negative information and have a capacity to avoid socially threatening information. For example, in one study, undergraduate students watched either an unpleasant film about the aftereffects of atomic bomb testing on a Pacific island or a neutral film about Yellowstone National Park. Afterward,

A. Vingerhoets et al., (eds.), *Emotion Regulation.*

Table 5.1 A fourfold classification of coping styles

	Defensiveness score	
Anxiety score	Low	High
Low	Low anxious	Repressors
High	High anxious	Defensive high-anxious

Source: Weinberger, D. A., Schwartz, G. E., & Davidson, R. J., (1979). Low-anxious, high anxious and repressive coping styles: psychometric patterns and behavioral responses to stress. *Journal of Abnormal Psychology*, *88*, 369–380.

participants were asked to recall a happy memory. Repressors were faster at recalling happy memories after watching the unpleasant film than after the neutral film. Nonrepressors exhibited the opposite effect (Boden & Baumeister, 1997). So it seems as if repressors use happiness effectively as a way of distracting themselves from distressing information. Avoiding processing negative emotional material may result in poor recall of unpleasant memories, and a number of studies have demonstrated links between repressive coping and the accessibility of negative memories (e.g., Davis, 1987; Myers & Derakshan, 2004a; Myers & Brewin, 1994). Other memory studies have found that (a) repressors' own memories are emotionally impoverished, with repressors reporting experiencing less unpleasant affect during daily reporting of moods compared with nonrepressors (Cutler, Larsen, & Bunce, 1996) and (b) repressors have a distinctive style of processing negative material that affects more than their own personal histories. Repressors were significantly worse than nonrepressors in recalling negative material in both intentional and incidental recall tasks (Myers, 2004; Myers & Brewin, 1995; Myers, Brewin, & Power, 1998; Myers & Derakshan, 2004b). Consequently, repressors are conceptualized as a group who avoid negative affect.

Although repressors appear to be psychologically healthy, this is not the same for physical health, and there is considerable evidence indicating that the repressive coping style as defined by Weinberger et al. (1979) may be associated with adverse physical health. This is potentially serious as repressors account for between 10% and 20% of the nonclinical population (e.g., Myers & Reynolds, 2000; Myers & Vetere, 1997; Phipps & Srivastava, 1997).

In what follows, the evidence linking repressive coping to coronary heart disease, cancer, asthma, diabetes, and pain is summarized and discussed, followed by the description of a set of recent experiments designed to try and understand the mechanism underlying the "repressive dissociation" and repressors' processing of negative information.

Repressive Coping and Coronary Heart Disease

There is good evidence linking repressive coping with cardiovascular disease. For example, Shaw et al. (1986) examined the relationship between repressive coping, cardiac information, and medical complications in patients undergoing treatment for narrowed coronary arteries. Six months after treatment, repressors with high knowledge levels about cardiac disease and no history of myocardial infarction had a significantly higher risk of medical complications (e.g., hospitalization for chest pain, myocardial infarction). In an earlier study Shaw, Cohen, Doyle, and Palasky, (1985) studied the impact of repressive coping and cardiac knowledge on hospitalized patients who were recovering from myocardial infarction. They found that repressors gained less information about cardiac risk factors. Six months later, it was found that repressors, with high risk information, reported more complications (e.g., arrhythmias, fluid retention) and poorer functioning (sleep disturbance, depression, tension).

One of the criticisms of research into the link of repressive coping and physical health is that the majority of studies are cross-sectional, implying that no causal link can be made. However, two longitudinal studies on repressive coping and coronary heart disease (CHD) have indicated that repressive coping is a risk factor for mortality in CHD. The Montreal Heart Attack Readjustment Trial was a randomized control trial of monthly telephone monitoring of psychological distress and home nursing visits in 1,376 patients. At 5 years follow-up, repressors and two control groups, low-anxious and high-anxious, were identified. The program was associated with significantly worse survival in both male and female repressors. Other results suggested that the program caused distress in repressors, as they were more likely to be prescribed benzodiazepines and to have visited emergency rooms without being readmitted than those in the control group (Frasure-Smith, Lesperance, Gravel, Masson, Juneau, & Bourassa, 2002). Similarly, Denollet (1999) followed up 409 patients with CHD at 6 to 10 years after the original study. Significantly more repressors died than controls. After controlling for low exercise tolerance and three-vessel disease, repressive coping was retained as an independent predictor associated with long-term mortality in patients with CHD.

These studies strongly suggest that having a repressive coping style is associated with poor prognosis in CHD patients (Frasure-Smith et al., 2002; Denollet, 1999). In addition, standard interventions may be detrimental to repressors' health (Frasure-Smith et al., 2002; Shaw et al. 1985; 1986). Further studies are needed to ascertain what type of interventions would be beneficial to repressors.

Recently, a preliminary study investigated whether endogenous opioids have a role to play in the relationship between repressive coping and hypertension (Younger, Lawler-Roe, Moe, Kratz, & Keenan, 2006). Eighteen participants were given either an opioid antagonist (naltrexone) or a placebo in a randomized, double-blind trial that took place in the laboratory. Repressors were assessed during a laboratory stressor task. Interestingly, it appeared that opioid antagonism reduced repression. These results suggest a physiologic mechanism that may help to explain the relationship between CHD and repressive coping. However, this study needs replication.

Repressive Coping and Cancer

There are a number of studies that suggest a link between repressive coping and cancer. Jensen (1987) conducted a prospective study of women with a history of breast carcinoma who were followed up for 2 years. Patients exhibiting a repressive coping style were at greater risk of death from cancer: of 11 patients who died during follow-up, 8 were repressors, and repressors also displayed more rapid progression of the disease than nonrepressors (1,755 days remission for nonrepressors vs. 1,204 days for repressors). Other studies have found an increased incidence of repressors among cancer sufferers in children (Phipps & Srivastava, 1997) adolescents (Canning, Canning, & Boyce, 1992), and women with breast cancer (Kreitler, Chaitchik, & Kreitler, 1993). Findings from a later longitudinal study on women with metastatic breast cancer suggest poorer survival of repressive copers (Giese-Davis, DiMiceli, Sephton, & Spiegel, 2006; Giese-Davis, Sephton, Abercrombie, Duran, & Spiegel, 2004).

Phipps and co-workers have run a systematic set of studies on repressive coping in children. Some of these are described below.

Repressive Coping in Children with Cancer

Children undergoing treatment for cancer face a multitude of stressors that occur in the context of a significant threat to their own survival. In such a stressful life situation, one might expect to see high levels of depression and other symptoms of affective distress in these children. However, studies utilizing child self-report have consistently indicated surprisingly low levels of distress in this population. In studies of depressive symptoms that utilize self-report, a few have found no differences in levels of depressive symptoms in children with cancer relative to controls or test norms (Noll, Gartstein, Vannatta, Correll, Bukowski, & Davies, 1999), but the majority have shown significantly *lower* levels of depression in the children with cancer (Canning et al., 1992; Phipps & Srivastava, 1997; Worchel, Nolan, Wilson, Purser, Copeland, & Pfefferbaum, 1988). These findings are not limited to measures of depression but have been found with measures of anxiety, self-esteem, behavioral problems, general psychopathology, and even somatic distress (Elkin, Phipps, Mulhern, & Fairclough, 1997; Phipps, Brenner, Heslop, Krance, Jayawardene, & Mulhern, 1995). Indeed, it appears that children with cancer tend to report relatively low levels of disturbance on any self-report measures of experienced distress.

These findings raise questions regarding the validity of self-report measures in pediatric oncology populations. Of course, it is possible that the positive self-reports of children with cancer may be a valid reflection of their exceptionally high level of functioning. An alternative explanation is that the self-reports of children with cancer are biased toward minimization of distress. According to this hypothesis, the absence of affective disturbance in children with cancer may be reflective only of "illusory mental health" resulting from psychological defenses (Shedler, Maymen, & Manis, 1993). Support for this comes from studies that show children with cancer not only obtain lower scores on depression inventories than their healthy peers, but also that they rate themselves as less depressed than do their parents, nurses, or physicians (Phipps & Srivastava, 1997; Worchel et al., 1988). The first researchers to comment on this suggested that these findings are indicative of high levels of denial in the children with cancer, which is mobilized in response to questioning regarding their emotional state (Worchel et al., 1988). This is consistent with typical descriptions of childhood cancer patients that have been put forth over the past two decades. A more comprehensive explanation involves application of the repressive coping paradigm of Weinberger et al. (1979). In several studies, Phipps and co-workers have documented high levels of repressors and relatively low levels of high-anxious children in the pediatric cancer population. Using the repressive coping paradigm, the low levels of distress reported by children with cancer would reflect a distinct personality profile, characterized by avoidance of awareness of threat and a motivation to maintain a self-image as someone who is well adjusted and nondistressed.

Canning, Canning, and Boyce (1992) were the first to utilize this approach. They found significantly lower levels of self-reported depressive symptoms in a group of adolescent cancer patients compared with healthy controls. They also found a significantly higher proportion of repressors in the cancer population. Further, repressor status was associated with lower depression scores and accounted for significant variance in depression beyond that explained by group (cancer vs. control) status. This finding was replicated by Phipps & Srivastava (1997) in a much larger sample of pediatric cancer patients and across a wider age range from 7 to 16 years. The study utilized a cross-sectional design, including patients who were recently diagnosed and others who were several years from diagnosis and off therapy. The percentage of repressors in the cancer group was double that of the controls (36% vs. 18%). Children with cancer obtained significantly lower scores than controls on the Children's Depression Inventory (CDI), and differences in adaptive style accounted in part for this finding. Repressors obtained the lowest CDI scores in both groups, and there was not a single child identified as a repressor in either group who obtained a CDI score large enough to be considered clinically depressed. These findings have been replicated several times subsequently in new cohorts (Phipps & Steele, 2002; Phipps, Steele, Hall, & Leigh, 2001).

Repressive coping style is assessed in children in a manner similar to that developed by Weinberger et al. (1979) for assessment of adults. Anxiety measures appropriate for children are readily available, but measurement of defensiveness presents more of a challenge. Phipps and co-workers have used an adaptation of the Children's Social Desirability scale (CSD; Crandall, Crandall, & Katkovsky, 1965), which is similar conceptually and in item-content to the Marlowe-Crowne scale (Crowne & Marlowe, 1964), but more appropriate for children. However, clear developmental differences are seen on the CSD, with younger children obtaining higher scores than older children. Correlations with age are typically between –.30 and –.40. Thus, age must be corrected for before making cutoffs to categorize coping style.

Repressive Coping and Asthma

Asthma is a common chronic condition characterized by inflammation of the airways and reversible airflow obstruction resulting in four main symptoms: cough, chest tightness, wheezing, and shortness of breath. Asthma is a leading health problem in both developed and developing countries. According to World Health Organization (2006a) estimates, 300 million people worldwide suffer from asthma and 255,000 people died of asthma in 2005. In addition, asthma is the most common chronic disease among children (WHO, 2006a). The goals of treatment are freedom from symptoms day and night, restoration and maintenance of normal or best-possible peak flow, a reduction in acute attacks, and minimization of absence from work or school.

Only a few studies have investigated repressive coping in the adult asthma patient population. For example, Steiner, Higgs, Fritz, Laszlo, and Harvey (1987) reported that repressive asthma patients tended to have reduced sensitivity to changes in the severity of their symptoms. Cooke, Myers, and Derakshan (2003) investigated objective lung function (FEV_1 levels) and adherence (self-report measure). Repressors had a significantly lower FEV_1 score than nonrepressors, indicating poorer asthma control. Repressors reported high levels of adherence to treatment, supporting previous findings that repressors tend to answer self-report measures in a positive fashion (see Myers [2000] for a review).

In a later study, Myers, Davies, Evans, and Stygall (2005) found that repressors compared with nonrepressors reported significantly fewer asthma symptoms and reported being more calm and content, less tense and worried, and more in control of their asthma. No repressor attributed any symptom to anxiety. However, asthma physicians rated repressors as more anxious then nonrepressors.

Both Cooke et al. (2003) and Myers et al. (2005) found a high number of repressors in the sample: 33% and 38% of repressors, respectively, compared with an expected 10% to 20% found in nonclinical populations (e.g., Myers & Reynolds, 2000; Myers & Vetere, 1997).

Repressive Coping and Diabetes

The World Health Organization (2006b) estimates that more than 180 million people worldwide have diabetes. This number is likely to more than double by 2030. In 2005, an estimated 1.1 million people died from diabetes and its complications. A full and healthy life is possible with diabetes, but it is of vital importance to keep blood glucose levels within the "normal" range. This requires good self-management of the condition. Patients with Type 1 diabetes and a subgroup of patients with Type 2 diabetes have to take insulin and balance this with diet and exercise. The majority of Type 2 diabetics may have to follow a weight-reducing diet and take medication to potentiate the action of the insulin they have in their bodies. All people with diabetes need to monitor their blood glucose levels (see, e.g., Mertig, 2007).

Myers et al. (2005) measured metabolic control in a study of 87 participants with either Type 1 or Type 2 diabetes. The measure of metabolic control (glycosylated hemoglobin) indicates the level of blood glucose control over the previous 4–6 weeks. In this study, 50.6% (44) of participants were classified as repressors. The high number of repressors in this patient sample is in concordance with previous studies of other patient groups discussed in this chapter (e.g., Canning et al., 1992; Cooke et al., 2003; Phipps & Steele, 2002). However, repressors exhibited significantly *better* metabolic control than nonrepressors. These results are obviously contrary to other findings presented in this chapter concerning repressors' health.

It is possible that repressors are good at behaviors that require high levels of self-control. This would seem to fit with the repressors' personality profile. These findings are preliminary and need replication. However, to the authors' knowledge, this is the first study to suggest that in a chronic illness that requires high levels of regular self-monitoring, repressors may be better at self-management than nonrepressors.

Repressive Coping and Pain

The role of emotional repression has long been debated in the literature on pain. Repression is defined as a process whereby anxiety aroused by a host of threatening memories, impulses, and other desires is avoided or ameliorated by driving the provocative material from consciousness. Starting with Freud's theory of "conversion hysteria" (Breuer & Freud, 1955), a number of theories developed around the core notion that pain—chronic pain, in particular—could be a manifestation of repressed emotional distress and conflict converted intrapsychically into physical symptoms (Engel, 1959; Szasz, 1957). Repression, however, has proved very difficult to observe and assess (Holmes, 1990).

The most well-developed and deliberate attempts to provide empirical support for the role of repression in chronic pain explored the incidence of "conversion-V" profiles on the Minnesota Multiphasic Personality Inventory (MMPI) (e.g., Armentrout, Moore, Parker, Hewett, & Feltz, 1982; Bradley, Prokop, Margolis, & Gentry, 1978; Bradley & Van der Heide, 1984). Such a profile is believed to reflect tendencies toward somatic preoccupation and the exaggeration of physical symptoms, coupled with the repression of emotional difficulties (Gough, 1946). A preponderance of conversion-V profiles was initially taken as evidence that pain patients do indeed transform repressed emotional pain into physical pain (Sternbach, Wolf, Murphy, & Akeson, 1973). This particular configuration, however, has shown suspect construct validity in medical populations, and so attempts to study repression with this instrument have borne little fruit (Burns, 2000a; Prokop, 1986). Still, research focusing on constructs somewhat related to repression, such as anger suppression (Burns, Johnson, Mahoney, Devine, & Pawl, 1996; Kerns, Rosenberg, & Jacob, 1994), alexithymia (Lumley, Asselin, & Norman, 1997; Sriram, Chaturvedi, Gopinath, & Shanmugam, 1987), and the release of concealed memories and suppressed negative affect through verbal or written expression (Kelley, Lumley, & Leisen, 1997), has met with some success in documenting effects of emotional inhibition on chronic pain.

Recently, the study of repression and pain has been revived (Burns, 2000b; Jamner & Schwartz, 1986) through the use of contemporary notions of repressive coping style (Weinberger et al., 1979). According to this model, the tendency to repress may be profitably viewed as a stable trait. Repressive copers see themselves as composed, even-tempered, disposed to rational behavior, and not prone to strong negative emotion. They use manifold strategies to avoid awareness of appraisals, emotions, and urges that are incongruent with this self-concept, despite revealing signs of arousal through physiologic and behavioral reactions.

The experience of pain is intertwined with suffering and emotional distress (Bonica, 1990). Given that repressive copers demonstrate effortful attempts to avoid experiencing negative emotions (Eysenck, 1997; Myers, 1998; Myers et al., 1996) and use distraction strategies to inhibit their awareness of negative emotions (Myers, 1998), it can be expected that they will report low pain and distress when undergoing painful stimuli. That is, based on the repressive coping construct, it may be predicted that repressors would be stoic in the face of pain and—at least in the short-term—may cope well. Indeed, Jamner and Schwartz (1986) found that among healthy participants, repressors judged the electrical stimulation they received as less uncomfortable and painful and showed higher tolerance to it than nonrepressors, with repressors requiring twice the voltage of nonrepressors to elicit comparable affective responses. These results, however, seem discordant with expectations of long-term emotional and physical health problems based on more psychodynamic notions of repression (Engel, 1959; Szasz, 1957) and with recent results suggesting that emotional inhibition carries deleterious effects (e.g., Kelley et al., 1997).

Among chronic pain patients, evidence does suggest that repressive coping is associated with poor adjustment in the long-term (Burns, Kubilus, Bruehl, & Harden, 2001; Burns, 2000b). Burns et al. (2001) expanded cluster analyses of Multidimensional Pain Inventory (MPI; Kerns, Turk, & Rudy, 1985) subscales by adding a measure of defensiveness (i.e., Balanced Inventory of Desirable Responding, or BIDR; Paulhus, 1984). A number of studies have shown a stable three-cluster solution of the nine MPI subscales among patients with chronic pain that includes a "dysfunctional" group described by a consistent profile of poor adjustment composed of high pain, low activity, and high distress. Burns et al. (2001) hypothesized that inclusion of the BIDR would allow the emergence of a repressor-like group in a sample of pain patients characterized not only by high defensiveness but also by a discrepant profile of high pain/low activity contrasted by low distress. Results supported this contention. Further, Burns (2000b), in a study of chronic pain patients participating in a 4-week treatment program, found that repressors showed negligible pre-to posttreatment gains in pain severity, depression, and lifting capacity, the changes being generally smaller than those shown by high-anxious patients. Although these data do not address whether repressive coping was instrumental in the development of chronic pain, findings indicate that repressor chronic pain patients adjust poorly in the long-term, even when aided by multidisciplinary pain treatment. Moreover, they appear to do worse in the domains of physical pain and disability than in terms of emotional distress; findings consistent with the notions of "conversion" asserted by psychodynamic theorists. Thus, on the one hand, repressors evince high tolerance to acute pain, but on the other hand, they report high chronic pain severity and activity limitations. It is our contention that these apparently contradictory findings between responses to acute and chronic pain may be reconciled by demonstrating that they are immediate and delayed effects of the same process: namely, thought suppression. Long-standing beliefs that emotional repression "produces" physical pain and other symptoms may, therefore, be conceptualized and empirically evaluated in terms of well-founded cognitive/affective models.

Wegner and colleagues (1990; 1992; 1994) argue that attempts to suppress unwanted thoughts have the ironic effect of making these thoughts more insistent and salient. Thought suppression involves an intentional, effortful "operating process" that works to avoid unwanted thoughts through conscious use of distracters. However, a second unconscious "monitoring process" searches for mental contents that signal a failure to avoid the unwanted material. The irony of the unconscious monitor is that by searching for failure to suppress, accessibility of the undesired thought actually increases (for a review, see Wenzlaff & Wegner [2000]). Similarly, suppression of pain-related thoughts (and emotions) may unintentionally render them more salient and accessible. Although suppression may subdue pain-related thoughts in the short-term, it may lead paradoxically to exaggerated sensitivity to pain in the long-term as the unconscious monitoring system works to find more and more unwanted pain-related intrusions.

Results of Cioffi and Holloway (1993) support these contentions. First, participants who were instructed to suppress pain-related thoughts did not differ on tolerance to a cold pressor from participants assigned to use other coping strategies, suggesting that no substantial immediate effects emerged. However, suppression participants revealed a vulnerability to "rebound effects," such that they not only evinced slower recovery from the cold pressor than others, but they also rated a subsequent nonpain stimulus as more unpleasant. Thus, suppression led to a host of delayed effects on pain perception.

Evidence suggests that repressors may use thought suppression as part of their repertoire of strategies to avoid awareness of threatening information. In a study of projection, Newman, Duff, and Baumeister, (1997) found that repressors rated others as more likely to have negative traits that they denied in themselves (i.e., they "projected"), a process exacerbated when explicitly instructed to suppress thoughts of such traits. Finally, nonrepressors increased their attribution of negative traits to others only when they were told to suppress thoughts of such traits. If repressors routinely suppress thoughts of threatening material, such as pain, they may experience short-term (immediate) tolerance, but they also may fall victim to long-term (delayed) sensitivity. The accessibility of pain-related thoughts may increase over time as the unconscious monitoring system scans for failures to suppress.

To test the notion that repression and physical pain are linked via the adverse effects of thought suppression, Elfant, Burns, and Zeichner (in press) assigned 222 nonpatient participants to suppression and nonsuppression conditions, administered a cold pressor, followed them through pain recovery, and then exposed them to an innocuous physical stimulus (massage device). During acute pain, repressors in both conditions had nearly identical (relatively high) tolerance, suggesting no immediate detrimental effects. It was also found that repressors not told to suppress during the cold pressor showed a pattern of slow recovery (i.e., prolonged elevations of self-reported pain and mean arterial pressure) immediately after the pain stimulus that was similar to that of high-anxious participants told to suppress, and which was markedly slower than that shown by high-anxious individuals not instructed to suppress. Moreover, repressors told to suppress during the cold pressor revealed the most protracted recovery of all groups, suggesting that the deliberate and exaggerated practice of suppression among a susceptible group exacerbated ironic effects. Finally, unpleasantness ratings of the innocuous massage device for the repressor and high-anxious groups followed this pattern of effects. Results draw a distinction between responses during acute pain and those exhibited after pain. Findings suggest that repressors may experience long-term pain sensitivity as a function of delayed rebound effects after attempts to suppress pain-related thoughts during acute episodes of pain.

Extrapolating from this laboratory model, it may be surmised that people prone to avoid awareness of threatening information—such as painful suffering—may do so, in part, via thought suppression. A vicious spiral may be set in motion whereby acute pain is suppressed, but pain-related material becomes ironically hyperaccessible after pain (due to the operation of the automatic monitor), producing conscious intrusions, which are then, in turn, suppressed. Devotion of increasingly greater cognitive resources to suppression and increased sensitivity to pain are the paradoxical effects. Direct evidence that repression actually causes chronic pain has not been reported. Nonetheless, using contemporary models of repressive coping style coupled with viable cognitive/affective mechanisms has already provided insights into this persistent question. In sum, repressors may be victims of a maladaptive strategy in handling acute episodes of pain. Efforts to defend against the unpleasantness of pain with thought suppression may lead paradoxically to a chronic preoccupation with and increasing sensitivity to painful episodes.

Can the Mechanism Behind Repressors' Avoidance of Negative Affect Be Understood?

There is much evidence indicating that repressors show discrepancies between their (low) reported anxiety and their (high) levels of physiologic and behavioral indicators of anxiety, especially under stressful situations (see beginning of chapter). Below, we discuss the few attempts to understand the underlying mechanisms responsible for the lack of concordance found in repressors. Understanding these mechanisms could shed light on the nature and time course of the processes involved in the experience and minimization of reported anxiety levels.

The investigation of the time course of emotional information processing becomes important in this context and will permit a more detailed and thorough examination of the cognitive, behavioral, and psychophysiologic processes involved in early (unconscious) stages and later (conscious) stages of information processing (Eysenck, 1997). When exactly do repressors experience anxiety? and when do they manage to minimize such an experience? Is it the case that repressors experience anxiety below the level of conscious awareness, hence the heightened levels of physiologic and behavioral anxiety, and only at later stages of consciousness manage to minimize the experience of anxiety?

The experience of anxiety at conscious levels of awareness has been assessed through performance on complex cognitive tasks. It has been reasoned that impaired performance on tasks demanding working memory capacity is related to the existence of conscious anxiety-related thoughts removing attention from task demands (see Eysenck [1997] for a review). Derakshan and Eysenck (1998; 1999; 2005) found that repressors' performance on complex cognitive tasks demanding attentional control is at least as good as low-anxious controls. More recent evidence suggests that repressors while performing on cognitive tasks show low levels of self-focused attention contributing to low levels of reported anxiety under such conditions (Derakshan & Eysenck, 2001a). Repressors are reasonably good at monitoring attentional processes on task-related material that enhance their performance on tasks involving complex problem-solving processes. In a related manner, repressors are particularly good at forgetting anxiety-related material that is self-relevant under private conditions (Myers & Derakshan, 2004b). They also have superior strategies in suppressing self-relevant negative information in a potentially nonthreatening manner under normal conditions (Derakshan, Myers, Hansen, & O'Leary, 2004).

Repressors are avoidant of socially threatening material (Fox, 1993; Mogg, Bradley, Dixon, Fisher, Twelftree, & McWilliams, 2000; Newman & McKinney, 2002). In tasks such as the emotional Stroop, where latency in naming the color of an emotional word is indexed as an attentional bias toward or away from the salient meaning of that word, repressors take longer in color naming the threat-related word. In the Visual Dot Probe task, where reaction times to probes that do or do not replace emotional cues are indexed as attentional bias toward or away from the emotional cue, repressors also take longer to detect the probe that replaces a threatening cue (e.g., a socially threatening word). In a more general sense, it has been argued that repressors are hypersensitive to emotional material (negative and positive) when such material threatens self-esteem (Mendolia, 2002).

The evidence on the conscious experience of anxiety discussed so far indicates that repressors are particularly good at making use of avoidant strategies in dealing with anxiety-related material. However, it does not show clearly *when* in processing such disengagement occurs. As a result, it has not been possible to provide a comprehensive picture of early and later processing of emotional material. Furthermore, such avoidant strategies have been indexed with cognitive indicators alone and have not been coupled with behavioral or psychophysiologic measures. In order to reach a detailed understanding of the time course of processing, it is essential to provide a moment-by-moment analysis of early and later stages of processing indexed by cognitive, physiologic, and behavioral measures simultaneously.

There is some evidence to show that the avoidance in repressors is preceded by vigilance toward threat at earlier stages of processing (e.g., Derakshan, Feldman, Campbell, & Lipp, 2003; Hock and Egloff, 1998; Kline, Schwartz, Allen, & Dikman, 1998). For example, Hock and Egloff (1998) asked participants to perform an affective priming task combined with a lexical-decision task. At the end of the task, participants performed an unexpected recognition-memory test. Repressors showed enhanced performance for primed threat-related words presented on the lexical decision task but showed poor memory for such words on the recognition-memory test. This finding shows that initial vigilance in repressors was followed by avoidance. Kline et al. (1998) varied the duration of masked presented words and asked participants to identify the word. They found that repressors were able to identify the "potentially threatening" words at shorter stimulus durations compared with longer exposure durations indicating vigilance.

There are also a few studies that have examined the time course of interpretive bias in repressors. Calvo and Eysenck (2000) assessed interpretive bias at various intervals of time after the presentation of an ambiguous sentence. Repressors showed vigilance in the form of interpretive bias at a short interval. However, this effect disappeared at longer intervals, presumably because repressors made use of inhibitory processes. Speculatively, the initial vigilance response of repressors may be associated with increased physiologic arousal, whereas the subsequent inhibitory processes serve to minimize consciously experienced anxiety. Caldwell and Newman (2005) obtained similar findings using a very different paradigm. They presented participants with short ambiguous passages that described negative and positive traits about people and then asked their participants to make favorable or unfavorable inferences about them. The key manipulation was to make these inferences under time pressure or longer periods of time. Under time pressure, repressors made more negative (unfavorable) inferences compared with other groups. They showed the opposite pattern, made more favorable inferences, when simply asked to respond quickly with no time pressure. Repressors were the only group showing a shift in interpretive bias in the direction of more positive inferences over time.

Recently, Derakshan, Feldman, Campbell, and Lipp (2003) have provided a more detailed and systematic investigation of the time course of emotional information processing. They used a modified version of a visual cueing paradigm called the Inhibition of Return Paradigm (IOR; Posner & Cohen, 1984) that enabled the examination of early versus late processing of emotional material. In this paradigm, it is possible to examine how quickly or slowly participants detect a target (e.g., a cross) that replaces a cue (e.g., an emotional cue such as an angry or happy face). Thus, reaction times to targets replacing the cue index engagement toward the cue. More importantly, this paradigm also measures the time needed to detect targets that do not replace such cues (i.e., how they are inhibited to return to where they have looked before). In this case, it measures how reaction times can be used as an index of disengagement from cue. Different patterns of engagement and disengagement depend on the cue-target-interval (CTI), that is, the time between onset of cue and onset of target (see Klein [2000] and Pratt, Hillis, & Gold [2001] for a review). In the seminal study of Posner and Cohen (1984), it was shown that if the CTI is less than 200 milliseconds (i.e., short interval), then patterns of engagement toward the cue are observed. However, if this interval exceeds 500 milliseconds, a pattern of inhibition of return (IOR) is found, that is, patterns of disengagement from cue are observed. In an elegant experiment, Danziger and Kingstone (1999) revealed that if a person is motivated to disengage from cue, IOR will happen earlier.

In a series of experiments with emotional faces as cues, Derakshan et al. (2002; 2003) examined patterns of engagement and disengagement in repressors. At short intervals, repressors were faster than anyone else to detect emotional faces but also were faster to disengage from them. This early engagement and disengagement occurred for angry and happy faces but not for neutral faces or other neutral cues. Derakshan and Bose (unpublished) argued that with appropriate manipulations of

CTI in the IOR paradigm, it is possible to detect patterns of engagement toward emotional material in repressors, a finding not reported before but consistent with a central hypothesis within the repressor research (Eysenck, 1997).

A key feature of the above experiments is the inclusion of moment-by-moment psychophysiologic analysis of the time course of processing. The authors not only obtained behavioral data as indexed by reaction times to target but also provided an online measurement of event-related potentials (ERPs) for cues and for targets throughout the tasks. ERPs, averaged electrical brain wave signals measured in microvolts, have been shown to be sensitive measures of the amount of processing resources allocated for the processing of emotional material (Carretie, Martin-Loeches, Hinojosa, & Mercado, 2001; Carretie, Mercado, Tapia, & Hinojosa, 2001; Smith, Cacioppo, Larsen, & Chartrand, 2003). The peak latency and peak amplitude of such waves are of particular interest in emotion research and indicate the speed and amount of processing, respectively (Duncan-Johnson & Donchin, 1982) (see also Kok [2001] for a review). ERP recordings in the experiments of Derakshan et al. found greater peak amplitudes for repressors when processing emotional faces (angry and happy) compared with everyone else. Repressors also had shorter peak latencies when disengaging from angry and happy faces indicating a faster disengagement pattern that matched the reaction time behavioral data that was discussed above. Current work is trying to replicate and extend these findings.

What can be concluded about the time course of emotional information processing in repressors? Can it be argued for a pattern of vigilance for emotional material at early stages of processing followed by avoidant mechanisms operating at later stages of processing? Such a pattern may indeed exist, but it appears that such biases operate much earlier in processing that was previously thought. Very early processing of emotional material below the level of conscious awareness is currently being investigated (Derakshan & Shoker, in preparation). There is the exciting prospect that further research on the time course of underlying mechanisms will allow us to develop a complete understanding of the various phenomena such as poor physical health associated with the repressive coping style.

Conclusion

This chapter has discussed current research in repressive coping and health. A valid criticism of earlier research was that studies were mainly cross-sectional, implying that it could not be established whether repressors had worse health outcomes because of their earlier repressive coping style (see Myers, 2000; Myers & Derakshan, 2004c). However, longitudinal studies in both coronary heart disease and breast cancer have now established that repressors tend to have worse health outcomes (Denollet, 1999; Frasure-Smith et al., 2002; Giese-Davis et al., 2004; Giese-Davis et al., 2006; Jensen, 1987). In addition, Phipps and colleagues are improving our understanding of emotional reactions in children with cancer and have established a link with repressive coping. There are a substantial number of repressors in asthma and diabetes samples, similar to cancer patients. The asthma study results suggest worse outcomes in the repressor group, whereas the diabetes study results suggest a better health outcome in the repressor group, which may be due to high levels of self-management required for good diabetic control.

Even though it has been known for many years that repressive coping is linked with impaired pain perception, the research of Burns and colleagues emphasizes the importance of identifying repressors in chronic pain sufferers, as they may not react well to intervention programs. Also, these investigators are working toward explaining the mechanisms of repressors' impaired pain perception. At a more basic level, it is important to understand the cognitive and neuropsychological processes by which repressors are able to avoid negative information. This exciting new step is being explored by Derakshan and colleagues in their ERP studies.

The first 25-plus years of research on repressive coping as defined by Weinberger et al. (1979) have produced a host of important findings. We expect the next 25 years will explain many more of the health-related-findings, and that researchers will be able to design successful health interventions to improve repressors' physical health.

References

Armentrout, D., Moore, J., Parker, J., Hewett, J., & Feltz, C. (1982). Pain-patients MMPI subgroups: the psychological dimensions of pain. *Journal of Behavioral Medicine, 5*, 201–211.

Asendorpf, J. A., & Scherer, K. R. (1983). The discrepant repressor: Differentiation between low anxiety, high anxiety, and repression of anxiety by autonomic-facial-verbal patterns of behaviour. *Journal of Personality and Social Psychology, 45,* 1334–1346.

Bendig, A. W. (1956). The development of a short form of the Manifest Anxiety Scale. *Journal of Consulting Psychology, 20*, 384.

Benjamins, C., Schuurs, A. H. B., & Hoogstraten, J. (1994). Skin conductance, Marlowe-Crowne defensiveness and dental anxiety. *Perceptual and Motor Skills, 79*, 611–622.

Boden, J. M., & Baumeister, R. M. (1997). Repressive coping: Distraction using pleasant thoughts and memories. *Journal of Personality and Social Psychology, 73*, 45–62.

Bonica, J. J. (1990). Definitions and taxonomy of pain. In J. J. Bonica (Ed.), *The management of pain* (pp 18–27). Philadelphia, PA: Lea & Febiger.

Bradley, L., Prokop, C., Margolis, R., & Gentry, W. (1978). Multivariate analyses of the MMPI profiles of low back pain patients. *Journal of Behavioral Medicine, 1*, 253–257.

Bradley, L. A., & Van der Heide, L. H. (1984). Pain-related correlates of MMPI profile subgroups among back pain patients. *Health Psychology, 3,* 157–174.

Breuer, J., & Freud, S. (1955; 1895). *Studies on hysteria.* Standard edition of the complete psychological works of Sigmund Freud (Vol. II). London: Hogarth Press.

Burns, J. W. (2000a). Repression in chronic pain: an idea worth recovering. *Applied and Preventive Psychology, 9,* 173–190.

Burns, J. W. (2000b). Repression predicts outcome following multidisciplinary treatment or chronic pain. *Health Psychology, 19*, 75–84.

Burns, J. W., Johnson, B. J., Mahoney, N., Devine, J., & Pawl, R. (1996). Anger management style, hostility and spouse responses: Gender differences in predictors of adjustment among chronic pain patients. *Pain, 64*, 445–453.

Burns, J. W., Kubilus, A., Bruehl, S., & Harden, R. N. (2001). A fourth empirically-derived cluster of chronic pain patients based on the Multidimensional Pain Inventory: evidence for repression within the dysfunctional group. *Journal of Consulting and Clinical Psychology, 69*, 663–673.

Caldwell, T. L., & Newman, L. S. (2005). The timeline of threat processing in repressors: More evidence for early vigilance and late avoidance. *Personality and Individual Differences, 38,* 1957–1967.

Calvo, M. G., & Eysenck, M. W. (2000). Early vigilance and late avoidance of threat processing: Repressive coping versus low/high anxiety. *Cognition and Emotion, 14*, 763–787.
Canning, E. M., Canning, R. D., & Boyce, T. (1992). Depressive symptoms and adaptive style in children with cancer. *Journal of American Child and Adolescent Psychiatry, 31,* 1120–1124.
Carretie, L., Martin-Loeches, M., Hinojosa, J. A., & Mercado, F. (2001). Emotion and attention interaction studied through event-related potentials. *Journal of Cognitive Neuroscience, 13,* 1109–1128.
Carretie, L., Mercado, F., Tapia, M., & Hinojosa, J. A. (2001). Emotion, attention, and the 'negativity bias,' studied through event-related potentials. *International Journal of Psychophysiology, 41,* 75–85.
Cioffi, D., & Holloway, J. (1993). Delayed costs of suppressed pain. *Journal of Personality and Social Psychology, 64,* 274–282.
Crandall, V. C., Crandall, V., & Katkovsky, W. (1965). A children's social desirability questionnaire. *Journal of Consulting & Clinical Psychology, 29*, 27–36.
Cooke, L., Myers, L. B., & Derakshan, N. (2003). Adherence, repressive coping and denial in asthma patients. *Psychology, Health & Medicine, 8,* 35–44.
Crowne, D. P., & Marlowe, D. A. (1964). *The approval motive: studies in evaluative dependence.* New York: Wiley.
Cutler, S. E., Larsen, R. J., & Bunce, S. C. (1996). Repressive coping style and the experience and recall of emotion: A naturalistic study of daily affect. *Journal of Personality, 64,* 381–405.
Danziger, S., & Kingstone, A. (1999). Unmasking the inhibition of return phenomenon. *Perception & Psychophysics, 61,* 1024–1037.
Davis, P. J. (1987). Repression and the inaccessibility of affective memories. *Journal of Personality and Social Psychology, 53*, 585–593.
Denollet, J. K. L. (1999). Repressive coping predicts mortality in patients with coronary heart disease (CHD). *Psychosomatic Medicine, 61,* 125.
Derakshan, N., & Eysenck, M. W. (1997). Interpretive biases for one's own behaviour and physiology in high trait-anxious individuals and repressors. *Journal of Personality and Social Psychology, 73,* 816–825.
Derakshan, N., & Eysenck, M. W. (1998). Working memory capacity in high trait-anxious and repressor groups. *Cognition and Emotion, 12,* 697–713.
Derakshan, N., & Eysenck, M. W. (1999). Are repressors self-deceivers or other-deceivers? *Cognition and Emotion, 13,* 1–17.
Derakshan, N., & Eysenck, M. W. (2001a). Manipulation of focus of attention and its effects on anxiety in high-anxious individuals and repressors. *Anxiety, Stress, and Coping, 14,* 173–191.
Derakshan, N., & Eysenck, M. W. (2001b). Effects of focus of attention on experienced anxiety in high-anxious, low-anxious, defensive high-anxious, and repressor individuals. *Anxiety, Stress, and Coping, 14,* 285–300.
Derakshan, N., & Eysenck, M. (2005). When the bogus pipeline interferes with self-deceptive strategies: Effects on state anxiety in repressors. *Cognition and Emotion, 19,* 83–100.
Derakshan, N., & Bose, S. (unpublished). Sensitivity to threat in represors: an investigation using the Inhibition of Return paradigm.
Derakshan, N. & Shoker, L. (in preparation). Attentional bias for threat in repressors: evidence from eye-movements.
Derakshan, N., Feldman, M., & Campbell, T. (2002). Don't look back to emotion: inhibited to return to emotion. *Psychophysiology, 39,* S31.
Derakshan, N., Feldman, M., Campbell, T., & Lipp, O. V. (2003). Can I have attention please: repressors and enhanced P3 to emotional stimuli. *Psychophysiology, 40,* S36.
Derakshan, N., Myers, L. B., Hansen J., & O'Leary, M. (2004). Defensiveness and attempted thought suppression of negative material. *European Journal of Personality, 18*, 521–535.
Elfant, E., Burns, J. W., & Zeichner, A. (in press). Repressive coping style and suppression of pain-related thoughts: Effects on responses to acute pain induction. *Cognition and Emotion.*
Elkin, T. D., Phipps, S., Mulhern, R. K., & Fairclough, D. (1997). Psychological functioning of adolescent and young adult survivors of pediatric malignancy. *Medical and Pediatric Oncology, 29*, 582–588.

Engel, G. (1959). "Psychogenic" pain and the pain prone patient. *American Journal of Medicine, 26*, 899–918.
Eysenck, M. W. (1997). *Anxiety and cognition: a unified theory*. Hove, England: Psychology Press.
Fox, E. (1993). Allocation of visual attention and anxiety. *Cognition and Emotion, 7*, 207–215.
Frasure-Smith, N, Lesperance, F, Gravel, G, Masson, Juneau, M, & Bourassa, M. (2002). Long term survival differences among low-anxious, high-anxious and repressive copers enrolled in the Montréal Heart Attack Readjustment Trial. *Psychosomatic Medicine, 64*, 571–579.
Giese-Davis, J., Sephton, S. E., Abercrombie, H., Duran, R. E. F., & Spiegel, D. (2004). Repression and high anxiety are associated with aberrant diurnal cortisol rhythms in women with metastatic breast cancer. *Health Psychology, 23*, 645–650.
Giese-Davis, J., DiMiceli, S., Sephton, S., & Spiegel, D. (2006). Emotional expression and diurnal cortisol slope in women with metastatic breast cancer in supportive-expressive group therapy *Biological Psychology, 73*, 190–198.
Gough, H. E. (1946). Diagnostic patterns on the Minnesota Multiphasic Personality Inventory. *Journal of Clinical Psychology, 2*, 23–37.
Hock, M., & Egloff, B. (1998). Interindividuelle Differenzen in Priming-und Gedächtniseffekten bedrohungsbezogener Stimuli: Der Einfluss kognitiv vermeidender und vigilanter Angstbewältigung. *Zeitschrift für Experimentelle Psychologie, 45*, 149–166.
Holmes, D. S. (1990). The evidence for repression: An examination of sixty years of research. In J. L. Singer (Ed.),*Repression and dissociation: implications for personality theory, psychopathology, and health* (pp. 85–102). Chicago, IL: The University of Chicago Press.
Jamner, L. D., & Schwartz, G. E. (1986). Selfdeception predicts selfreport and endurance to pain. *Psychosomatic Medicine, 48*, 211–223.
Jensen, M. R. (1987). Psychobiological factors predicting the course of breast cancer.*Journal of Personality, 55*, 317–342.
Kelley, J. E., Lumley, M. A., & Leisen, J. C. C. (1997). Health effects of emotional disclosure among rheumatoid arthritis patients. *Health Psychology, 16*, 331–340.
Kerns, R. D., Turk, D. C., & Rudy, T. E. (1985). The West Haven-Yale Multidimensional Pain Inventory (WHYMPI). *Pain, 23*, 345–356.
Kerns, R. D., Rosenberg, R., & Jacob, M. C. (1994). Anger expression and chronic pain. *Journal of Behavioral Medicine, 17*, 57–67.
Klein, R. M. (2000). Inhibition of Return. *Trends in Cognitive Sciences, 4*, 138–147.
Kline, J. P., Schwartz, G. E., Allen, J. J. B., & Dikman, Z. V. (1998). Perceptual and electroencephalographic registration of masked emotional words in defensiveness: an exploratory study. *Personality and Individual Differences, 24*, 499–512.
Kok, A. (2001). On the utility of the P3 amplitude as a measure of processing capacity. *Psychophysiology, 38*, 557.
Kreitler, S., Chaitchik, S., & Kreitler, H. (1993). Repressiveness: cause or result of cancer? *Psychooncology, 2*, 43–54.
Lumley, M. A., Asselin, L. A., & Norman, S. (1997). Alexithymia in chronic pain patients. *Comprehensive Psychiatry, 38*, 160–165.
Mendolia, M. (2002). An index of self-regulation of emotion and the study of repression in social contexts that threaten or do not threaten self-concept. *Emotion, 2*, 215–232.
Mertig, R. G. (2007). *Teaching diabetes self-management: what nurses need to know*. New York: Springer.
Mogg, K., Bradley, B. P., Dixon, C., Fisher, S., Twelftree, H., & McWilliams, A. (2000). Trait anxiety, defensiveness and selective processing of threat: an investigation using two measures of attentional bias. *Personality and Individual Differences, 28*, 1063–1077.
Myers, L. B. (1998). Repressive coping, trait anxiety and reported avoidance of negative thoughts. *Personality and Individual Differences, 24*, 299–303.
Myers, L. B. (2000). Identifying repressors: a methodological issue for health psychology. *Psychology and Health, 15*, 205–214.
Myers, L. B. (2004). Repressive coping and health. In N. Anderson (Ed.), *Encyclopedia of health & behavior* (Vol. 2). Thousand Oaks, CA: Sage.

Myers, L. B., & Brewin, C. R. (1994). Recall of early experience and the repressive coping style. *Journal of Abnormal Psychology, 103*, 288–292.

Myers, L. B., & Brewin, C. R. (1995). Repressive coping and the recall of emotional material. *Cognition and Emotion, 9*, 637–642.

Myers, L. B., & Brewin, C. R. (1996). Illusions of well-being and the repressive coping style. *British Journal of Social Psychology 33*, 443–457.

Myers, L. B., & Derakshan, N. (2004a). Do childhood memories colour social judgements of today? *European Journal of Personality, 18*, 321–330.

Myers, L. B., & Derakshan, N. (2004b). To forget or not to forget: what do repressors forget and when do they forget? *Cognition and Emotion 18*, 495–511.

Myers, L. B., & Derakshan, N. (2004c). Repressive coping and avoidance of negative affect. In I. Nyklicek, L. Temoshok, & A. J. J. M. Vingerhoets (Eds.), *Emotional expression and health. Advances in theory, assessment and clinical applications*. (pp. 169–184). Hove, UK: Brunner-Routledge.

Myers, L. B., & Reynolds, R (2000). How optimistic are repressors? The relationship between repressive coping, controllability, self-esteem and comparative optimism for health-related events. *Psychology and Health, 15*, 667–688.

Myers, L. B., & Vetere, A. L. (1997). Repressors' responses to health-related questionnaires. *British Journal of Health Psychology, 2*, 245–257.

Myers, L. B., Brewin, C. R., & Power, M. J. (1998). Repressive coping and the directed forgetting of emotional material. *Journal of Abnormal Psychology, 107*, 141–148.

Myers, L. B. Davies, A., Evans, E, & Stygall, J. (2005). How successful are repressors at self-care behaviour? *Psychology and Health, 20*, 188–189.

Newman, L. S., & McKinney, L. C. (2002). Repressive coping and threat-avoidance: an idiographic Stroop study. *Personality and Social Psychology Bulletin, 28*, 409–422.

Newman, L. S., Duff, K. J., & Baumeister, R. F. (1997). A new look at defensive projection: thought suppression, accessibility and biased person perception. *Journal of Personality and Social Psychology, 72*, 980–1001.

Newton, T. L., & Contrada, R. J. (1992). Repressive coping and verbal-autonomic response dissociation: the influence of social context. *Journal of Personality and Social Psychology, 62*, 159–167.

Noll, R. B., Gartstein, M. A., Vannatta, K., Correll, J., Bukowski, W. M., & Davies, W. H. (1999). Social, emotional, and behavioral functioning of children with cancer. *Pediatrics, 103*, 71–78.

Paulhus, D. L. (1984). Two-component models of socially desirable responding. *Journal of Personality and Social Psychology, 46*, 598–609.

Phipps, S., & Srivastava, D. K. (1997). Repressive adaptation in children with cancer. *Health Psychology, 16*, 521–528.

Phipps, S., & Steele, R. G. (2002). Repressive adaptation in children with chronic illness. *Psychosomatic Medicine, 64*, 1–9.

Phipps, S., Brenner, M., Heslop, H., Krance, R., Jayawardene, D., & Mulhern, R. (1995). Psychological effects of bone marrow transplantation on children and adolescents: preliminary report of a longitudinal study. *Bone Marrow Transplantation, 15*, 829–835.

Phipps, S., Steele, R. G., Hall, K., & Leigh, L. (2001). Repressive adaptation in children with cancer: a replication and extension. *Health Psychology, 20*, 445–451.

Posner, M. I., & Cohen, Y. P. C. (1984). Components of visual orienting. In H. Bouma & D. Bouwhuis (Eds.), *Attention and performance X: control of language processes* (pp. 531–556). Hillsdale, NJ: Erlbaum.

Pratt, J., Hillis, J., & Gold, J. M. (2001). The effect of physical characteristics of cues and targets on facilitation and inhibition. *Psychonomic Bulletin and Review, 8*, 489–495.

Prokop, C. K. (1986). Hysteria scale elevations in low back pain patients: a risk factor for misdiagnosis? *Journal of Consulting and Clinical Psychology, 54*, 558–562.

Shaw, R. E., Cohen, F., Doyle, B., & Palasky, J. (1985). The impact of denial and repressive style on information gain and rehabilitation outcomes in myocardial infarction patients. *Psychosomatic Medicine, 47*, 262–273.

Shaw, R. E., Cohen, F., Fishman-Rosen, J., Murphy, M. C., Stertzer, S., Clark, D. A., & Myler, R. K. (1986). Psychologic predictors of psychosocial and medical outcomes in patients undergoing coronary angioplasty. *Psychosomatic Medicine, 48*, 582–597.

Shedler, J., Maymen, M., & Manis, M. (1993). The *illusion* of mental health. *American Psychologist, 48*, 1117–1131.

Smith, N. K., Cacioppo, J. T., Larsen, J. T. & Chartrand, T. L. (2003). May I have your attention, please: electrocortical responses to positive and negative stimuli. *Neuropsychologia, 41*, 171–183.

Steiner, H., Higgs, C. M. B., Fritz, G. K., Laszlo, G., & Harvey, J. E. (1987). Defense style and the perception of asthma. *Psychosomatic Medicine, 49*, 35.

Sriram, T. G., Chaturvedi, S. K., Gopinath, P. S., & Shanmugam, V. (1987). Controlled study of alexithymic characteristics in patients with psychogenic pain disorder. *Psychotherapy and Psychosomatics*, *47*, 11–17.

Sternbach, R. A., Wolf, S. R., Murphy, R. W., & Akeson, W. H. (1973). Aspects of chronic low back pain. *Psychosomatics*, *14*, 52–56.

Szasz, T.S. (1957). *Pain and pleasure: a study of bodily feelings*. London: Tavistock.

Wegner, D. M., & Erber, R. (1992). The hyperaccessibility of suppressed thoughts. *Journal of Personality and Social Psychology, 63*, 903–912.

Wegner, D. M., & Zanakos, S. (1994). Chronic thought suppression. *Journal of Personality, 62*, 615–640.

Wegner, D. M., Shortt, J. W., Blake, A. W., & Page, M. S. (1990). The suppression of exciting thoughts. *Journal of Personality and Social Psychology, 58*, 409–418.

Weinberger, D. A., Schwartz, G. E., & Davidson, R. J. (1979). Low-anxious, high anxious and repressive coping styles: psychometric patterns and behavioral responses to stress. *Journal of Abnormal Psychology*, *88*, 369–380.

Wenzlaff, R. M., & Wegner, D. M. (2000). Thought suppression. *Annual Review of Psychology, 51*, 59–91.

Worchel, F. F., Nolan, B. F., Wilson, V. L., Purser, J., Copeland, D. R., & Pfefferbaum, B. (1988). Assessment of depression in children with cancer. *Journal of Pediatric Psychology 13*, 101–112.

World Health Organization. (2006a). Asthma. Fact sheet number 307. Available at http://www.who.int/mediacentre/factsheets/fs307/en/index.html.

World Health Organization. (2006b). Diabetes. Fact sheet number 312. Available at http://www.who.int/mediacentre/factsheets/fs312/en/index.html.

Younger, J., Lawler-Roe, K., Moe, A., Kratz, A., & Keenan, A. (2006). Effects of naltrexone on repressive coping and disclosure of emotional material: a test on the opioid-peptide hypothesis of repression and hypertension. *Psychosomatic Medicine, 68*, 734–741.

Chapter 6
Why Crying Improves Our Well-being: An Attachment-Theory Perspective on the Functions of Adult Crying

Michelle C.P. Hendriks, Judith K. Nelson, Randolph R. Cornelius, and Ad J.J.M. Vingerhoets

Introduction

Crying is a common and apparently universal form of human emotional expression. Whereas no other species has the ability to shed emotional tears, people of all ages and from all cultures cry on certain occasions to express their emotions. Despite the widespread occurrence of crying, no truly comprehensive theory of the origins and functions of adult crying has been established. In this chapter, an attachment-theory perspective on crying is presented in which crying is hypothesized to serve a variety of interpersonal functions, foremost among these being to communicate distress to others and to facilitate social bonding. It is argued that by way of these interpersonal benefits, crying improves the physiologic and psychological well-being of the crying person. Empirical studies of adult crying are reviewed with an eye toward what they reveal about the role of crying as an attachment behavior.

A Model of Adult Crying

Vingerhoets, Cornelius, Van Heck, & Becht (2000) were the first to present a comprehensive, albeit preliminary, model of adult crying. This model mainly focused on the antecedents of crying and considered crying to be the result of the interaction between several psychobiological, cognitive, and social processes. Crying was further seen as having an impact both on psychobiological processes in the crying individual himself or herself (*intra*personal effects) and on the crying person's social environment (*inter*personal effects). In other words, the act of crying may lead to tension relief and may facilitate the physiologic and psychological recovery after distress via psychobiological mechanisms. At the same time, crying may communicate the need for help and may stimulate others to offer this help and support, which may indirectly have an effect on the well-being of the crying individual.

Crying and Health

The belief that crying brings tension relief and helps to regain emotional and physical balance is an old one. Cornelius (1986) reviewed how popular American and British magazines described crying from 1848 until 1985. It appears that people have always been convinced that crying is good for one's health. In current literature and popular psychology, it is still often stated that crying is healthy or at least that it makes people feel better.

Empirical studies on the effects of crying on mood and physiologic functioning have yielded mixed results, apparently depending on the design of the study. Quasi-experimental laboratory studies exposing subjects to sad films have mostly found a negative effect of the shedding of emotional tears; people who cried while watching a sad film felt sadder and more depressed afterward than people who did not cry (Cornelius, 1997). Physical functions such as heart rate and blood pressure also did not recover more rapidly after a crying spell (for a review, see Cornelius [2001]; Vingerhoets & Scheirs [2001]). Only Rottenberg, Wilhelm, Gross, & Gotlib (2003) and Hendriks, Rottenberg, and Vingerhoets (2007) found that crying might be associated with a parasympathetic rebound mechanism that facilitates the recovery of homeostasis. However, the source of parasympathetic activation was ambiguous, and although heart rate decreased rapidly after the onset of crying, it did not decrease to below baseline levels (Hendriks et al., 2007). Nevertheless, if you ask people how they generally feel after a crying episode, they most often report feeling better (Cornelius, 1997).

Research has also been done on the relationship between general crying frequency and subjective well-being, thereby focusing on the long-term effects of crying. These studies again yielded little evidence in support of the hypothesis that crying is healthy. Rather, the few studies that have been conducted suggest that crying is negatively related to one's physical well-being (for a review, see Vingerhoets & Scheirs [2001]).

In short, crying does not seem to have immediately observable or direct beneficial effects on the crying person. Perhaps, as suggested by Cornelius (2001) and by Hendriks (2005), crying may only have a positive effect on well-being when the shedding of tears leads to a positive change in the situation. Nelson (2005) also noted that the benefits may come not so much from actually shedding tears but rather because tears bring us physical contact and solace from others. It is well-known that social support has positive benefits on psychological and physical well-being (Uchino, 2004). This implies that crying does not automatically (e.g., via biopsychological pathways) lead to tension and/or emotional relief. Rather, the social context in which crying occurs, in particular the reactions of others, may predominately determine its intrapersonal effects. For example, a crying individual might only feel better afterward if his or her tears result in emotional support and understanding rather than when he or she meets disapproval and negative reactions. The first question that should be answered then is how people from the social environment react to tears. This chapter aims to provide an answer to this question based on attachment theory.

Attachment-Theory Perspective on Adult Crying

Attachment behaviors are designed to elicit caregiving responses from significant others (Bowlby, 1969). Repeated experience of the interlocking attachment and caregiving systems serve to establish and maintain the parent-child bond (Ainsworth, Blehar, Waters, & Wall, 1978) and romantic adult bonds as well (Hazan & Zeifman, 1999). Attachment theory and research have shown that crying is an inborn behavior that functions to call for and ensure the protective and nurturing presence of caregivers (Bell & Ainsworth, 1972; Bowlby, 1969; Cassidy, 1999; Zeifman, 2001). As suggested by Bowlby (1969), crying continues to be an attachment behavior throughout life.

Social-psychological theories have likewise asserted that crying is an expressive display whose primary function is to communicate to others in an unambiguous way that one is vulnerable, suffering, and/or in need of aid (Cornelius & Labott, 2001; Fridlund, 1992; Frijda, 1997; Yik & Russell, 1999). Crying is a powerful elicitor of sympathy and empathy that is difficult for others to ignore, especially for those who share a close relationship with the crying person. The main function of crying may be to beckon others to help remove a given source of discomfort, to elicit attention, empathy, and support, and to facilitate social bonding (Frijda, 1997; Kottler & Montgomery, 2001; Vingerhoets et al., 2000).

When observing the behaviors of infants separated from their caregivers, Bowlby (1960) noted that babies first responded with protest that included loud crying and active thrashing about. If there was no reunion, protest eventually gave way to the more prolonged distress of grief characterized by despair and quiet crying. If there was still no reunion with a caregiver, then the infants entered a silent state referred to as detachment. When Bowlby (1961) later studied bereaved adults, he noted that in reaction to the loss of a close loved one, adults went through similar stages of protest and despair. The symptomatic absence of crying in adults when it would be an appropriate and expected reaction to loss might be considered a form of detachment (Nelson, 2005). Bereaved adults, unlike infants, are optimally able to work through their grief to a stage Bowlby called reorganization. Each type of (non)crying (i.e., protest crying, crying of despair, and detached inhibited crying) is hypothesized to represent a different internal grief response on the part of the crier and, subsequently, to trigger different caregiving responses from others.

Protest Crying

The purpose of protest crying, whether for the baby left alone in the crib or the adult first hearing of the unexpected loss of a loved one, is to undo the loss and bring about a reunion (Bowlby, 1960). As Bowlby pointed out, the vast majority of separations from loved ones are temporary: protest crying after separation is typically followed by reunion. Protest crying in infancy is loud and active, and in suddenly bereaved adults, it is often accompanied by vocalized crying, as opposed to silent weeping

(Nelson, 2000). If words are spoken, they are often plaintive denials of the news such as “No! No!” or in the case of a bereaved man quoted in the newspaper, “I want my mother back!” (Newsham, 2000). There is a lot of energy behind these cries, and it is directed at reestablishing the threatened connection and at fighting any sign that the loss is permanent.

Protest crying, according to Nelson (2005), causes the most interpersonal difficulties. In the presence of protesting infants or traumatically bereaved loved ones, caregivers usually feel sympathy and a parallel wish to undo the loss. However, protest crying over everyday losses often has a hostile, negative, accusatory edge that can result in alienating potential caregivers, particularly when the protest is aimed at the caregiver. Protest crying in adults can leave potential caregivers feeling manipulated, guilty, or apathetic instead of sympathetic and caring and may evoke negative reactions from others such as anger, frustration, and irritation (Frijda, 1986, 1997; Hill & Martin, 1997; Vingerhoets et al., 2000). Moreover, even if sympathy is felt or offered, Nelson (2005) has observed clinically that protest criers often reject sympathy outright because accepting comfort of any kind implies acceptance of the loss. Protest criers want action rather than comfort; they want caregivers to do something to undo their loss. Unless their demands are satisfactorily met, protest criers typically do not feel better after their crying spell.

Sad Crying of Despair

Crying in despair has more of a sad, quiet energy in both children and adults. The hope for a reunion, reconciliation, or restoration is abandoned, which leads to a deep, heavy sadness (Nelson, 2005). Bowlby (1960) noted that infants’ cries at this stage were a quiet, low wail. Sad crying in adulthood signifies surrender to or acceptance of the loss (Nelson, 2005): the boyfriend loves another woman or the tumor is indeed a malignancy. Nelson (2005) has postulated that it is this type of crying that promotes healing and the working through of grief as the bereaved person acknowledges the painful permanence of the loss and reestablishes a symbolic connection with the lost attachment figure, object, or quality (for instance, by establishing an award in honor of the deceased or by forming a support group for others going through a similar loss). Through this process, the grieving person is eventually able to connect with new attachment figures, reconfigure relationships with surviving ones, and reorganize life anew.

Unlike crying in protest, sad crying in despair evokes positive caregiving feelings and a desire to comfort in even the most distant observer (Nelson, 2005). It exerts a sympathetic pull toward the sufferer that transcends words and crosses cultures. Touching, hugs, words of sympathy, and offers of help are among the caregiving behaviors of adults. However, feelings of needing or giving care can also evoke feelings of awkwardness in some people. Then, caregiving may take the form of false reassurance, distraction, or even deciding the crier prefers to be “left alone.” People who are uncomfortable with intimacy may pull away when comfort is needed or, in extreme cases, react to sad crying with hostility.

Detached Inhibited Crying

In infancy, the final stage of response to separation from the caregiver is silence. For babies, this may be life-threatening, because helpless children will die if they fail to connect with a caregiver. Bowlby called this stage detachment and noted the eerie absence of crying. Detached inhibited crying, as Nelson (2005) describes it in adults, is typically associated with withdrawal, blocked or denied grief, and depression. There is no hope of resolution or healing after a significant loss. Detachment in adults may also be life-threatening if it involves excessive consumption of alcohol or drugs, refusal of food, or suicidal behavior. Interpersonally, detached inhibited crying is problematic because it defies connection and deflects support and caring while isolating the griever. Potential caregivers become frustrated and may even feel rejected. However, not all inhibited adult crying represents detachment. Some inhibited criers are able to show their sadness in alternative ways (e.g., by verbalizing their feelings) and to receive caregiving when they experience a loss even though they do not cry.

Review of Empirical Studies Concerning Adult Crying as an Attachment Behavior

Antecedents of Crying

Evidence for the perspective that crying is an attachment behavior can be found by examining the situations that most likely induce crying in adults. According to Nelson (2005), most adult crying is triggered by situations analogous to the separations and vulnerabilities of infancy, and the common denominator of crying throughout life is grief over separation or loss. For example, funerals or memorials for family members or other intimates, situations involving the dissolution of romantic relationships or conflicts within such relationships, and sad films or television programs that have loss as a main theme are the situations in which people most often report crying (Nelson, 1998; 2000; Vingerhoets et al., 2000; Vingerhoets, Van Geleuken, Van Tilburg, & Van Heck, 1997). Among positive situations, weddings, music, and reunions occupy the top positions. These so-called tears of joy (Avery, 1983; Feldman, 1956; Weiss, 1952) that are associated with accomplishments, victories, and happy endings also touch intimately on themes of loss and grief. Victory instead of loss at an athletic competition, reunion instead of permanent separation after a child is kidnapped, and the end of childhood or the separation between child and parent at a wedding all represent happy outcomes combined with losses that have been averted, outlived, or overcome.

Although adult crying may be an expression of different emotions such as sadness, anger, joy, or fear, these emotions are typically accompanied by feelings of powerlessness (Vingerhoets, Boelhouwer, Van Tilburg, & Van Heck, 2001; Vingerhoets et al., 2000). Evidence further suggests that we are most likely to cry in the presence of someone with whom we share a close relationship of some sort (Cornelius, 1981). Vingerhoets and colleagues (Vingerhoets et al., 2000; Vingerhoets et al., 1997) have found that adult crying typically occurs at home where intimates may be expected to be present. In short, the kinds of situations in which adults cry most frequently are those that would be predicted by an attachment approach to crying.

Social Reactions to Crying

Most important to the understanding of how crying enhances well-being through its interpersonal benefits is to review how people respond to the tears of others. In a study by Cornelius (1982), most individuals reported that they stop their ongoing activities to pay attention to the crying person. People reported that they try to physically or verbally comfort the crying individual or start to cry themselves. Wagner, Hexel, Bauer, & Kropiunigg (1997) demonstrated that, in response to a crying patient, doctors, nurses, and medical students mostly try to soothe the patient with words, hold the hand of the patient, and/or become personally affected. When Wagner et al. (1997) asked the hospital staff how other colleagues responded to their tears at work, it appeared that health professionals were mostly either comforted or left to themselves. However, a fifth of the medical students reported that they were ridiculed, screamed at, or looked at with contempt.

In addition to these real-life observations, some quasi-experimental studies have been carried out. In the study by Hill & Martin (1997), confederates (in this study, only women) acted as if they were crying or not crying in reaction to a film. The results showed that crying confederates elicited more sympathy and more crying from the participants (also only women) than did noncrying confederates. Hendriks, Croon, and Vingerhoets (2007) had participants respond to vignettes describing several situations in which the main character cried or did not cry. It appeared that participants tended to give more emotional support to and express less negative affect toward a crying than a noncrying person.

Cornelius and Lubliner (2003) and Hendriks & Vingerhoets (2006) both examined the so-called signal value of crying faces; that is, the social messages they convey to others. Cornelius and Lubliner (2003) found that most participants (60.0%) felt that crying people communicated the message that they want help, comfort, or to be taken care of. A smaller, albeit substantial, percentage (50.0%) of those who viewed the same faces with the tears digitally removed ("nontearful faces") gave the same answer. Cornelius and Lubliner (2003) additionally asked participants to indicate how they would respond to the person on the photo. The majority of participants who viewed a tearful face (59.0%) indicated that they would comfort the person, whereas the majority of respondents who viewed a nontearful face (52.1%) indicated that they would ask the person what was wrong. A larger percentage of those who saw a nontearful face (26.0%) reported they would leave the person alone compared with those who saw a crying face (19.6%). In the study of Hendriks &

Vingerhoets (2006), the reactions to crying faces were compared with the reactions to neutral, angry, and fearful faces. Respondents tended to give more emotional support to a crying person and to avoid a crying person less than people expressing the other emotions.

Concerning sex differences in reactions to crying, Jesser (1989) demonstrated that most female respondents reported crying along with a crying person, whereas male respondents were more likely to report ignoring a crying person. Respondents were more inclined to comfort and help a crying woman than a crying man (Cretser, Lombardo, Lombardo, & Mathis, 1982; Jesser, 1989). A crying man was more likely to be helped by female than by male respondents and was more looked down on by male than by female respondents (Cretser et al., 1982). In contrast, in the studies of Cornelius and colleagues (Cornelius and Lubliner, 2003; Cornelius, Nussbaum, Warner, & Moeller, 2000) and of Hendriks and colleagues (Hendriks & Vingerhoets, 2006; Hendriks, Croon, et al., in press), the sex of the respondent and of the crying person did not substantially influence the social reactions to crying. In the study by Cornelius and Lubliner (2003), there was some indication that men more likely than women leave a crying person alone, particularly if that person is another man. However, this interaction effect was quite small.

In short, most findings of the studies on social reactions to crying are in accordance with what the attachment perspective on adult crying would predict. As expected, crying mainly elicited sympathy and support, and crying people were perceived as communicating the message that they are in need of help. In addition, however, evidence was found for negative reactions from the social environment in reaction to tears. These negative findings do not necessarily contradict the attachment-theory perspective. Protest crying can evoke feelings of guilt and irritation in others, who subsequently may express their anger or frustration. Also, people who cry out of sadness may evoke feelings of awkwardness in potential caregivers, which may result in their pulling away. The sex of the potential caregiver might partially determine the amount of awkwardness that is experienced in the presence of a crying person. Because women are more comfortable with intimacy and a nurturing role, they may experience fewer feelings of awkwardness in the presence of a crying person than men. This might explain why women reacted with sympathy and support while men tended to feel irritated and confused in the presence of a crying person (Cretser et al., 1982; Jesser, 1989).

Hendriks et al. (in press) demonstrated that reactions from the social environment to crying were partially determined by the situation (i.e., the context) in which the person cried. Whether or not others perceive the crying as appropriate might be especially relevant in this regard. Anecdotal evidence has suggested that tears that are considered as inappropriate or manipulative may evoke strong negative reactions and even may be considered as blackmail (Frijda, 1997; Kottler, 1996). As an example, crying on the job is often considered as inappropriate (Hoover-Dempsey, Plas, & Wallston, 1986), which might explain the findings of Wagner et al. (1997) that crying medical students were sometimes ridiculed, looked at with contempt, or screamed at by their colleagues.

Conclusion

This chapter focused on the question whether adult crying acts as an attachment behavior; that is, whether crying elicits support and facilitates social bonding. It is posited that these caregiving responses may subsequently improve the well-being of the crying person. The research findings here presented support the view that crying is a very compelling communicative signal with a high potential to elicit caregiving responses and to strengthen social bonds. Crying appears to be an important attachment behavior throughout life that is primarily designed to communicate the need for help and to stimulate others to offer this comfort and help.

However, the commonly made assumption that crying is a clear and unambiguous phenomenon generally yielding the same interpersonal functions does not seem to hold. In certain conditions, people also responded negatively to the tears of others. These discrepant reactions confirm the validity of distinguishing between different types of crying (i.e., protest crying and sad crying of despair). Protest crying might lead to interpersonal difficulties, whereas sad crying might primarily elicit positive reactions in others. Unfortunately, until now, researchers have made no distinction between these kinds of crying. Future research should therefore explicitly examine the social reactions to different kinds of crying, for instance, by manipulating the auditory aspects of the crying spell; protest crying could be presented by a loud cry and sad crying could be presented by a quiet wail. Another possibility is to manipulate or analyze the social context of crying.

Future research should also combine the study of the intrapersonal and interpersonal consequences of crying. In this way, it could be determined whether the alleged beneficial health effects of crying depend upon the reactions from people in the social environment. The effects of crying on physiologic and psychological functioning should be investigated both in situations in which crying has positive interpersonal effects and in situations in which crying has no or negative interpersonal effects. Given the social reactions to the different types of crying, it can be expected that protest crying will be less beneficial for one's well-being than sad crying of despair.

References

Ainsworth, M. D. S., Blehar, M., Waters, E., & Wall, S. (1978). *Patterns of attachment: a psychological study of the strange situation*. Hillsdale, NJ: Lawrence Erlbaum Associates.

Avery, N. (1983). Tears of joy. *Journal of the American Academy of Psychoanalysis, 11*, 251–263.

Bell, S. M., & Ainsworth, M. D. S. (1972). Infant crying and maternal responsiveness. *Child Development, 43*, 1171–1190.

Bowlby, J. (1960). Grief and mourning in infancy and early childhood. *Psychoanalytic Study of the Child, 15*, 9–52.

Bowlby, J. (1961). Processes of mourning. *The International Journal of Psycho-analysis, 42*, 317–339.

Bowlby, J. (1969). *Attachment*. New York: Basic Books.

Cassidy, J. (1999). The nature of the child's ties. In J. Cassidy & P. R. Shaver (Eds.), *Handbook of attachment. Theory, research and clinical applications* (pp. 3–20). New York: The Guilford Press.

Cornelius, R. R. (1981). *Weeping as social interaction: the interpersonal logic of the moist eye*. Amherst, MA: Unpublished doctoral dissertation, University of Massachusetts.

Cornelius, R. R. (1982). *Weeping as social interaction.* Paper presented at the fifty-third annual meeting of the Eastern Psychological Association, Baltimore, Maryland.

Cornelius, R. R. (1986). *Presience in the pre-scientific study of weeping: a history of weeping in the popular press from the mid-1800's to the present.* Paper presented at the 75th Annual Meeting of the Eastern Psychological Association, New York.

Cornelius, R. R. (1997). Toward a new understanding of weeping and catharsis? In A. J. J. M. Vingerhoets, F. J. Van Bussel, & A. J. W. Boelhouwer (Eds.), *The (non)expression of emotions in health and disease* (pp. 303–321). Tilburg, The Netherlands: Tilburg University Press.

Cornelius, R. R. (2001). Crying and catharsis. In A. J. J. M. Vingerhoets & R. R. Cornelius (Eds.), *Adult crying: a biopsychosocial approach* (pp. 199–211). Hove, United Kingdom: Brunner-Routledge.

Cornelius, R. R., & Labott, S. M. (2001). The social psychological aspects of crying. In A. J. J. M. Vingerhoets & R. R. Cornelius (Eds.), *Adult crying: a biopsychosocial approach* (pp. 159–176). Hove, United Kingdom: Brunner-Routledge.

Cornelius, R. R., & Lubliner, E. (2003). *The what and why of others' responses to our tears: Adult crying as an attachment behavior.* Paper presented at the Third international conference on The (Non)Expression of Emotions in Health and Disease, Tilburg, The Netherlands.

Cornelius, R. R., Nussbaum, R., Warner, L., & Moeller, C. (2000). *'An action full of meaning and of real service': the social and emotional messages of crying.* Paper presented at the XIth Conference of the International Society for Research on Emotions, Quebec City, Canada.

Cretser, G. A., Lombardo, W. K., Lombardo, B., & Mathis, S. (1982). Reactions to men and women who cry: a study of sex differences in perceived societal attitudes versus personal attitudes. *Perceptual and Motor Skills, 55*, 479–486.

Feldman, S. (1956). Crying at the happy ending. *Journal of the American Psychoanalytic Association, 4*, 477–485.

Fridlund, A. J. (1992). The behavioral ecology and sociality of human faces. In M. S. Clark (Ed.), *Emotion* (pp. 90–121). Newbury Park: Sage Publications.

Frijda, N. H. (1986). *The emotions*. Cambridge: Cambridge University Press.

Frijda, N. H. (1997). On the functions of emotional expression. In A. J. J. M. Vingerhoets, F. J. Van Bussel & A. J. W. Boelhouwer (Eds.), *The (non)expression of emotions in health and disease* (pp. 1–14). Tilburg, The Netherlands: Tilburg University Press.

Hazan, C., & Zeifman, D. M. (1999). Pair bonds as attachments. Evaluating the evidence. In J. Cassidy & P. R. Shaver (Eds.), *Handbook of attachment. Theory, research, and clinical implications* (pp. 336–354). New York: The Guilford Press.

Hendriks, M. C. P., & Vingerhoets, A. J. J. M. (2006). The social messages of crying faces: their influence on anticipated person perception, emotions and behavioural responses. *Cognition and Emotion, 20*, 878–886.

Hendriks, M. C. P., Croon, M. A., & Vingerhoets, A. J. J. M. (in press). Social reactions to adult crying: the help-soliciting function of tears. *Journal of Social Psychology.*

Hendriks, M. C. P., Rottenberg, J., & Vingerhoets, A. J. J. M. (2007). Can the distress-signal and arousal-reduction views of crying be reconciled? Evidence from the cardiovascular system. *Emotion, 7*, 458–463.

Hill, P., & Martin, R. B. (1997). Empathic weeping, social communication, and cognitive dissonance. *Journal of Social and Clinical Psychology, 16*, 299–322.

Hoover-Dempsey, K. V., Plas, J. M., & Wallston, B. S. (1986). Tears and weeping among professional women: In search of new understanding. *Psychology of Women Quarterly, 10*, 19–34.

Jesser, C. J. (1989). Men and crying. *Changing Men,* Winter/spring, 12, 15.

Kottler, J. A. (1996). *The language of tears*. San Francisco: Jossey-Bass Publishers.

Kottler, J. A., & Montgomery, M. J. (2001). Theories of crying. In A. J. J. M. Vingerhoets & R. R. Cornelius (Eds.), *Adult crying: a biopsychosocial approach* (pp. 1–17). Hove, United Kingdom: Brunner-Routledge.

Nelson, J. K. (1998). The meaning of crying based on attachment theory. *Clinical Social Work Journal, 26*, 9–22.

Nelson, J. K. (2000). Clinical assessment of crying and crying inhibition based on attachment theory. *Bulletin of the Menninger Clinic, 64*, 509–529.
Nelson, J. K. (2005). *Seeing through tears. Crying and attachment*. New York: Brunner-Routledge.
Newsham, B. (2000, May 22). Somebody's mother. *San Francisco Chronicle*, D8.
Rottenberg, J., Wilhelm, F. H., Gross, J. J., & Gotlib, I. H. (2003). Vagal rebound during resolution of tearful crying among depressed and nondepressed individuals. *Psychophysiology, 40*, 1–6.
Uchino, B. N. (2004). *Social support and physical health: understanding the health consequences of relationships*. New Haven, CT: Yale University Press.
Vingerhoets, A. J. J. M., & Scheirs, J. G. M. (2001). Crying and health. In A. J. J. M. Vingerhoets & R. R. Cornelius (Eds.), *Adult crying: a biopsychosocial approach* (pp. 227–246). Hove, United Kingdom: Brunner-Routledge.
Vingerhoets, A. J. J. M., Van Geleuken, A. J. M. L., Van Tilburg, M. A. L., & Van Heck, G. L. (1997). The psychological context of adult crying: towards a model of adult crying. In A. J. J. M. Vingerhoets, F. J. Van Bussel, & A. J. W. Boelhouwer (Eds.), *The (non)expression of emotions in health and disease* (pp. 323–336). Tilburg, The Netherlands: Tilburg University Press.
Vingerhoets, A. J. J. M., Cornelius, R. R., Van Heck, G. L., & Becht, M. C. (2000). Adult crying: a model and review of the literature. *Review of General Psychology, 4*, 354–377.
Vingerhoets, A. J. J. M., Boelhouwer, A. J. W., Van Tilburg, M. A. L., & Van Heck, G. L. (2001). The situational and emotional context of adult crying. In A. J. J. M. Vingerhoets & R. R. Cornelius (Eds.), *Adult crying: a biopsychosocial approach* (pp. 71–89). Hove, United Kingdom: Brunner-Routledge.
Wagner, R. E., Hexel, M., Bauer, W. W., & Kropiunigg, U. (1997). Crying in hospitals: a survey of doctors', nurses' and medical students' experience and attitudes. *Medical Journal of Australia, 166*, 13–16.
Weiss, J. (1952). Crying at the happy ending. *Psychoanalytic Review, 39*, 338.
Yik, M. S. M., & Russell, J. A. (1999). Interpretation of faces: a cross-cultural study of a prediction from Fridlund's theory. *Cognition and Emotion, 13*, 93–104.
Zeifman, D. M. (2001). Developmental aspects of crying: infancy, and beyond childhood. In A. J. J. M. Vingerhoets & R. R. Cornelius (Eds.), *Adult crying: a biopsychosocial approach* (pp. 37–53). Hove, United Kingdom: Brunner-Routledge.

Chapter 7
Emotional Intelligence: Relationships to Stress, Health, and Well-being

Guus L. van Heck and Brenda L. den Oudsten

Introduction

Recently, the concept of *emotional intelligence* (EI), involving the perception, assimilation, comprehension, and management of emotions, has been introduced as an explanatory concept of behavior. EI is, according to its proponents, substantially distinct from general cognitive ability and personality.

This chapter addresses first the following question: What is EI and how is it different from other established constructs? After mentioning the debate about the adaptive versus maladaptive qualities of emotion and a brief sketch of some precursors of EI, the general scope and origin of EI will be described as well as the major theories of EI, focusing on the work of Mayer and Salovey (1993, 1997), Bar-On (1997, 2000), and Goleman (1995). Thereafter, a scheme will be presented containing the components of EI as distinguished in the various EI models. Then, in a critical evaluation of EI, the relationships of EI with other intelligences (traditional IQ, social intelligence, and practical intelligence) and personality will be the focus of analysis, addressing questions regarding the discriminant and incremental validity of EI against other cognitive abilities and personality variables as well as EI-related constructs like alexithymia and psychological mindedness. An intriguing question is whether it is possible to express EI in terms of a standard trait model.

The assessment of EI will then be described. This section will contain descriptions of the major EI instruments as well as a critical evaluation of their psychometric qualities. The chapter continues with an analysis of the contribution of EI to understanding the relationship between stress and health variables. For this purpose, EI will first be scrutinized with respect to the cognitive-motivational-emotive model that has been developed by Lazarus and others (e.g., Lazarus & Folkman, 1984). Special attention will be given to EI as a moderator in the stress process. Here, the major questions concern the role of EI regarding appraisal and coping strategies. The chapter will provide a thorough overview of health correlates of EI with emphasis on mental health, depression, propensity to burnout, psychological adaptation to chronic diseases, and health habits. In addition, the current status of research outcomes regarding the associations between EI and health-related quality of life, life satisfaction, and emotional well-being will be discussed. The chapter will end with a sketch of future prospects.

A. Vingerhoets et al., (eds.), *Emotion Regulation.*

The Emotion Systems

Emotions have a tremendous impact on our beliefs, inform our decision making, and guide how we adapt our behavior to the world around us. Hence, they play a powerful role in people's lives (Gratch & Marsella, 2004).

Emotions can impair or facilitate psychological adaptation (Lazarus, 2006). They sometimes interfere with a reasoned examination of adaptation tasks. For instance, threat-based anxiety can hinder accurate judgment and task performance. Feelings of depression can elicit rumination and attempts to use reasoning to escape from unpleasant private experiences, which in turn can make the depression stronger. Anger can obstruct rational actions leading to retaliation. Envy and jealousy can undermine friendships and intimate relationships. Sadness, annoyance, and remorse can block redefinition of situations and redirection of personal goals. On the other hand, emotions can reveal what is personally important (Nussbaum, 2001). They can serve as a barometer of how well or poorly people are doing in advancing their values, goals, and beliefs (Lazarus, 2006). Therefore, it is not surprising that Schultz, Izard, and Abe (2005) have proposed that the starting point for considering the development of the construct *emotional intelligence* (EI) is the emotion system. According to Schultz et al., emotion responses, positive as well as negative affects, are helpful in responding intelligently and adaptively to the many challenges of daily life. When describing the adaptive function of emotions, they point at processes like focusing attention on important environmental stimuli, providing internal cues about the status of interactions with the environment, priming bodily parts to respond, and motivating facial and bodily expressions that communicate important information to others. Schultz et al. are rather critical concerning the construct of EI. In their view, many components of EI overlap with facets of temperament and intelligence. Moreover, they express doubts regarding the coherence of EI and suggest that EI components actually reflect the functioning of the emotion systems. Be it as it is, most models of EI are more heavily influenced by intelligence than by emotions (Schulze & Roberts, 2005). The overlap of EI with prominent structural models of intelligence will be discussed in the next section.

Intelligence Defined

Historically, intelligence has been defined in various ways. Traditionally, the focus of the majority of intelligence researchers has been on cognitive aspects, such as memory and problem solving. Others, however, have tried to include nonintellective, that is affective and conative abilities, into total intelligence. For instance, Wechsler (1950, 1958) has emphasized the capacities to act purposefully, to think rationally, and to deal effectively with the environment, while in Sternberg's (1985) view, intelligence is purposive adaptation to, shaping of, and selection of real-world environments relevant to one' s life.

Thus, there is a wide range of conceptions of intelligence. A prominent approach in the study of intelligence, supported by psychologists like Galton, Spearman, and Jensen, uses the intercorrelations of tests of mental ability in order to isolate a global general factor, known as *g*, from other aspects of cognitive ability (see, e.g., Carroll [1993] for a review). Proponents of the opposing approach, like Thurstone, Gardner, and Sternberg, think that there are three, seven, or even more different intelligences that are rather independent of each other. Sternberg's (1985) theory makes a distinction between (i) analytical intelligence, which is similar to the standard psychometric definition of intelligence, (ii) creative intelligence, which consists of the ability that allows people to adjust creatively and effectively to new situations, and (iii) practical intelligence, reflecting the ability to grasp, understand, and deal with everyday tasks. Gardner's (1983) theory of multiple intelligences distinguishes seven different forms of intelligence: linguistic, musical, spatial, bodily, interpersonal, intrapersonal, and logico-mathematical.

What is the predictive value of *g*? The answer is rather easy: general cognitive ability tends to be a good predictor of academic performance. For instance, Neisser et al. (1996) found that traditional tests of intelligence typically account for around 25% of the variance of academic performance, depending on the test used.

Intelligence as measured by IQ tests, however, is not just a narrow academic skill that is only related to academic performance. It is also linked to various health behaviors and outcomes. An impressive series of epidemiologic studies has taken advantage of the fact that in 1932 in Scotland, IQ testing was conducted on nearly a complete year-of-birth cohort. This research reveals that psychometric intelligence is an important factor in public health (Gottfredson & Deary, 2004). Hart et al. (2003a; 2003b) found that lower childhood IQ predicted significantly higher likelihood of dying from cardiovascular disease in general, coronary heart disease, and lung cancer. Whalley and Deary (2001) suggest several possible mechanisms that could be responsible for associations between IQ and longevity. IQ might be a record of perinatal or childhood insults, a record of the integrity of the body, a predictor of health behaviors, or a predictor of entry into healthy environments. Gottfredson and Deary (2004) focus on the third possibility by pointing at the links between psychometric intelligence and learning, reasoning, and problem-solving skills, which they conceive of as useful in preventing chronic disease and accidental injury and in adhering to complex treatment regimens.

Recently, it has been stated that the emotional, personal, social, and survival dimensions of intelligence are often more important for daily functioning than the more traditional cognitive aspects of intelligence (Bar-On, 1997). For instance, Goleman (1995) has argued that to get along in the world requires more than just cognitive abilities.

The idea that people differ in their ability to understand and make use of their emotions and the emotions of others in order to interact with the environment is a fairly recent development (e.g., Mayer, 2001). More than 80 years ago, Thorndike (1920) proposed that intelligence could be categorized in three broad dimensions: mechanical, abstract, and social. A person's level of mechanical intelligence reflected the ability to manage things and mechanisms. Abstract intelligence referred to the ability to manage and understand ideas and symbols, whereas social intelligence referred to the ability to understand and manage people, for instance, the ability to handle interpersonal situations. Social intelligence is related to a narrower construct: emotional intelligence (EI). Although emotional intelligence is usually regarded as a construct within the broad framework of human cognitive abilities (Goleman, 1995; Mayer, Caruso, & Salovey, 1999; Mayer & Geher, 1996; Mayer & Salovey, 1993; Mayer, Salovey, & Caruso, 2000; Salovey & Mayer, 1994), it is currently unclear whether EI should be regarded as an "intelligence." For instance, Mayer et al. (1999) assert that the construct indeed meets the criteria of a new intelligence (see also Mayer & Geher, 1996; Mayer, Salovey, Caruso, & Sitarenios, 2002). In their view, EI is operationalized as a set of abilities; it is objective in that answers on the test are either right or wrong as determined by consensus or expert scoring; its scores increase with age and correlate with existing intelligences while also showing unique variance (Derksen, Kramer, & Katzko, 2002; Mayer & Geher, 1996; Mayer et al., 1999; Mayer et al., 2002). Others (e.g., Locke, 2005), however, partly focusing on different conceptualizations of EI, argue that EI is not another form or type of intelligence but simply intelligence applied to a particular life domain: emotions. In this view, being intelligent *about* emotions is just a skill, not a new intelligence.

Conceptualization of Emotional Intelligence

Over the past decade, the concept of EI has become increasingly popular. Although the literature is growing, researchers are still involved in a hot debate how to conceptualize EI. Petrides and Furnham (2001; 2003; see also Neubauer & Freudenthaler, 2005) have suggested that existing conceptualizations of EI can be classified into two predominant models: *ability* models and *mixed (trait)* models. Whereas ability models focus on the interplay of emotion and intelligence as traditionally defined, mixed models describe a broader conception of intelligence that combines mental abilities with a wide range of personality characteristics (Mayer et al., 2000). However, all EI models do have overlapping core features, for example, mood regulation (Austin & Saklofske, 2005).

Abilities-Based Model

The definitions of EI as proposed by Salovey and Mayer's (1990; see also Mayer & Salovey, 1997) fit the ability model. They labeled EI as a form of social intelligence (SI), separable from the traditional intelligence construct, which lies in the intersection between emotion and cognitions (Mayer et al., 2000). The original conceptualization of EI (1990) comprised three related mental processes, namely (i) the appraisal and expression of emotion; (ii) the regulation and control of emotion; and (iii) the use of emotion in psychological adaptation. Appraisal and expression as well as the regulation and control are subdivided according to the self and other perspective. For instance, the appraisal of one's own emotions reflects a specific form of self-knowledge, while the appraisal of the emotions of others mainly reflects empathy.

In the revised model of EI (Mayer & Salovey, 1997), the same distinction can be recognized. It distinguishes four branches (Fig. 7.1). The first branch, "perception, appraisal, and expression of emotion," comprises the most emotion-related skills that are required in order to process emotional information and eventually to solve problems. This branch involves the ability to identify one's own emotions as well as emotions in other people. It also deals with the ability to express emotions and related needs accurately as well as the ability to discriminate between emotions. The second branch, "emotional facilitation of thinking," involves emotions that focus on important information that may facilitate reasoning. This branch describes the use of emotions in prioritizing thinking by directing attention to important information, and facilitating reasoning, judgment, and the consideration of multiple points of view. The third branch, "understanding, analyzing, and employing emotional knowledge," describes four abilities involving abstract understanding and reasoning about emotions. This branch involves the abilities to label emotions, to recognize relations among the words and the emotions themselves, to interpret the meanings that emotions convey regarding relationships, to understand complex combinations of feelings, and to recognize likely transitions among emotions. Finally, the fourth branch, "reflective regulation of emotions," comprises the most advanced skills and stands for the ability to manage emotions in oneself, and in others, in order to promote emotional and intellectual growth.

This modified model gives more emphasis on cognitive processes by defining EI in terms of the ". . . ability to recognize the meanings of emotions and their relationships, and to reason and problem-solve on the basis of them. Emotional

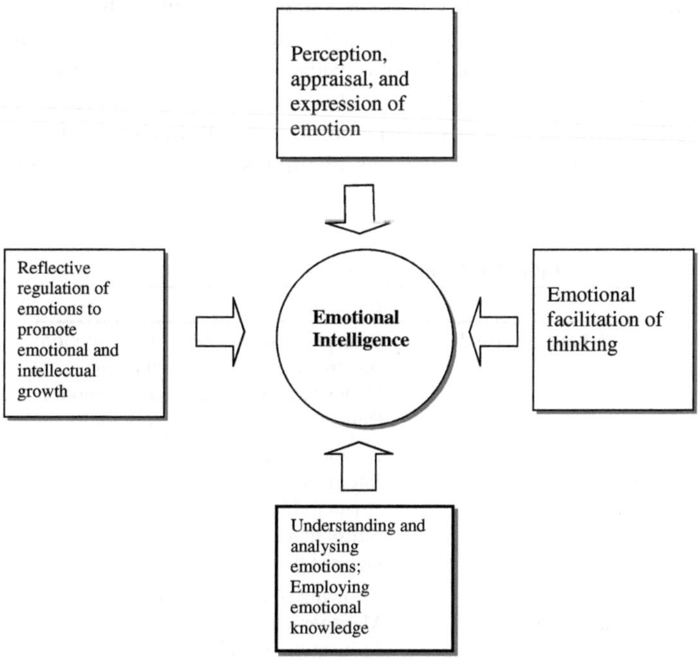

Fig. 7.1 Schematic presentation of Mayer and Salovey's 1997 model of emotional intelligence.

intelligence is involved in the capacity to perceive emotions, assimilate emotion-related findings, understand the information of those emotions, and manage them." (Mayer & Salovey, 1997, p. 267). Mayer and Salovey (1997) have suggested that EI qualifies as an intelligence because some people are better than others in problem solving and monitoring emotions in themselves and others.

Mixed Models

In contrast with the ability model, as formulated by Mayer and Salovey (1997), the mixed model is represented by, for instance, Bar-On (1997) and Goleman (1995). The mixed model of EI refers to a group of personality characteristics that tries to predict success in several domains, for example, academic achievements. EI is used as an umbrella term to designate a wide array of competencies. For instance, Bar-On (1997) defined EI as "an array of non-cognitive capabilities, competencies, and skills that influence one's ability to succeed in coping with environmental demands and pressures" (p. 14). Three years later, Bar-On (2000) revised the conceptualization of his EI model. The original model comprised 15 facets along five broad dimensions: intrapersonal skills, interpersonal skills, adaptability, stress management, and general mood. The revised model, labeled "a model of emotional and social intelligence," consists of 10 constituent components also found in the original concept: self-regard, emotional self-awareness, assertiveness, empathy, interpersonal relationship, stress tolerance, impulse control, reality testing, flexibility, and problem solving. The other five components of the original model (i.e., self-actualization, independence, social responsibility, optimism, and happiness) are considered as facilitators instead of constituent components. Goleman (1995, p. xii) goes one step further in his definition and includes also the components "self-control, zeal, and persistence, and the ability to motivate oneself." Table 7.1 presents the elements of EI as distinguished in the most prominent EI models.

Table 7.1 Elements of emotional intelligence

	Elements of EI
Mayer & Salovey (1997)	Perception and expression of emotion Assimilating emotion in thought Understanding and analyzing emotion Reflective regulation of emotion
Bar-On (1997)	Intrapersonal skills Interpersonal skills Adaptability skills Stress-management skills General mood
Goleman (1995)	Knowing one's emotions Management of emotions Motivating oneself Recognizing emotions in others Handling relationships

Related Constructs

In some ways, EI is not new. In fact, it is based on a long history of theory building and research in personality and social psychology. For instance, skilful recognition of others' emotional reactions has been studied for decades in empathy research. Other relevant aspects, clearly related to EI, are stress tolerance and impulse control. The most closely related concepts, however, are undoubtedly social and practical intelligence (Kang, Day, & Meara, 2005), alexithymia, and psychological mindedness (Denollet & Nyklíček, 2004).

Social and Practical Intelligence

The purposive and essentially adaptive nature of human actions is a fundamental assumption of the social intelligence model (Zirkel, 2000). Social intelligence (SI) reflects the acquired declarative and procedural knowledge about social events. SI is not just general intelligence applied to social situations; it is distinct from academic intelligence (Kang et al., 2005). SI refers to the capacity to understand, interact, and deal with people (see, e.g., Cantor & Kihlstrom, 1987). It refers to social sensitivity, social insight, prosocial attitudes, a genuine understanding of people, as well as the ability to deal well with people in warm and caring ways. SI incorporates work from both personality psychology and social psychology.

Practical intelligence (PI) refers to the ability to deal with real-life problems and relates to the procedural tacit knowledge, not formally acquired, that serves to establish and maintain a good person-environment fit (e.g., Sternberg, Wagner, & Okagaki, 1993). PI serves "to find a more optimal fit between the individual and the demands of the individual's environment, by adapting to the environment, changing (or shaping) the environment, or selecting a different environment" (Hedlund & Sternberg, 2000, p. 150).

SI and PI are not conceptualized as being specifically emotional. In contrast with EI, they also do not explicitly cover internal regulatory processes (Austin & Saklofske, 2005).

Alexithymia

A conceptual similar construct, but somewhat narrower in scope than EI, is alexithymia. Alexithymia, originating from clinical observations of characteristic features of patients with psychosomatic disorders, involves the absence rather than the presence of emotional abilities. When alexithymia is translated literally, it stands for "lacking words for feelings" (Sifneos, 1973). This construct includes difficulties in identifying and describing one's own feelings to others, and differentiating one's feeling from physiologic sensations. Alexithymia is associated with a cognitive style characterized by operative thinking that includes constricted imaginal processes, limited dreaming, and an externally oriented style of thinking (Taylor, Bagby, & Parker, 1997). In addition, several other characteristics have been observed in alexithymic individuals, such as a limited capacity for empathy. Several neurobiological grounds for alexithymia have been suggested, reflecting, for instance, deficits in the connections between the limbic system and the neocortex or deficits in interhemispheric integration (see Taylor [2004] for an overview).

Parker, Taylor, and Bagby (2001) studied the empirical association between EI and alexithymia, using Bar-On's (1997) model of EI. Results revealed that the two constructs are independent, but overlap considerably: $r = -.72$. This outcome is consistent with the finding of Schutte et al. (1998) that EI and alexithymia are strongly ($r = -.65$) correlated (inversely) constructs.

Psychological Mindedness

Psychological mindedness can be defined in terms of the intrinsic motivation to be in touch with one's inner feelings and thoughts by monitoring and analyzing them in an adaptive way (Denollet & Nyklíček, 2004). The concept refers to the ability to have access to one's feelings, a willingness to talk about one's feelings and interpersonal problems, an active interest in other persons, and a capacity for behavioral change. From this description, it becomes clear that there is a considerable overlap between psychological mindedness and EI (Parker, 2005).

EI and Personality

Among the theories of personality, one of the most prominent is the Five Factor Model (FFM; e.g., Costa & McCrae, 1992; John & Srivastava, 1999). The Five Factor Model or Big Five structure contains the following dimensions: (i) Extraversion, (ii) Agreeableness, (iii) Conscientiousness, (iv) Emotional Stability versus Neuroticism, and (v) Openness to New Experiences. This structure of five dimensions of interpersonal and intrapersonal conduct "... captures, at a broad level of abstraction, the commonalities among most of the existing systems of personality description, and provides an integrative descriptive model for personality research" (John, 1990, p. 96). Austin, Saklofske, and Egan (2005) found that EI is more strongly associated with social network size when compared with the Big Five personality traits. The latter, however, appeared to be more strongly related with social network quality, life satisfaction, alcohol consumption, number of doctor consultations, and health status. These findings indicate that EI and personality have different well-being and health correlates. They also suggest that it is worthwhile to investigate the construct validity of EI by examining its relations to academic intelligence and personality, as others (e.g., Schulte, Ree, & Carretta, 2004) have questioned the uniqueness of EI.

Interestingly, the evidence for a relationship between EI and personality variables is much stronger than the evidence for a relationship with academic intelligence

(Van der Zee, Thijs, & Schakel, 2002) (see, however, Schulte et al. [2004] for a moderate relationship between EI and *g*). Based on a conceptual analysis of possible links between the Big Five factors of personality and the EI facets that are most prominent in mixed models of EI (Bar-On, 1997; Goleman, 1995), McCrae (2000) expected high correlations with extraversion and neuroticism, and lower, but still significant positive correlations with agreeableness and conscientiousness. Several studies have supported these expectations (Dawda & Hart, 2000; Petrides & Furnham, 2001; Saklofske, Austin, & Minski, 2003; Schutte, Malouff, Hall et al., 1998). For instance, in a recent study, high-EI individuals tended to be considerably more extraverted and conscientious than low-scorers on EI (Day, Therrien, & Carroll, 2005). Dawda and Hart (2000) reported correlations between EI, measured by the Bar-On (1997) Emotional Quotient Inventory, and neuroticism, extraversion, agreeableness, and conscientiousness of −.62, .52, .43, and .51, respectively. Also, Warwick and Nettelbeck (2004) sought to identify psychological variables underlying EI. Using two EI measures (the Trait Meta-Mood Scale [TMMS]; Salovey, Mayer, Goldman et al., 1995) and the Mayer Salovey Caruso Emotional Intelligence Test (MSCEIT), they found that the total TMMS score correlated moderately with extraversion and agreeableness and weakly with conscientiousness, emotional stability, and openness, whereas the MSCEIT score was only associated with agreeableness. Lopes, Salovey, and Straus (2003) reported a general pattern of low correlations between EI (MSCEIT), on the one hand and personality traits and verbal intelligence on the other, providing some evidence of discriminant validity. In contrast, Schulte et al. (2004) reported a corrected multiple *R* exceeding .80, showing that EI can be largely predicted from sex and personality. Such relationships with personality do raise the question of the distinctness of trait EI from the personality domain. Therefore, De Raad (2005) explored to what extent EI can be expressed in terms of a standard trait model. He classified a huge set of more than 400 items from several EI instruments into the categories of a Big Five circumplex model (AB5C; De Raad, Hendriks, & Hofstee, 1992). It turned out that the majority of the EI items were classifiable, especially in categories delineated by the factors Agreeableness and Emotional Stability. Furthermore, a joint factor analysis of a large pool of EI items and Big Five items yielded a four-factor structure that was strongly related to four of the Big Five factors. Only Conscientiousness did not play a prominent role. De Raad concluded that "rational and organized information processing is not captured by understandings of emotional intelligence" (p. 673) and that "emotional intelligence represents a stripped Big Five" (p. 685).

The Assessment of Emotional Intelligence

Assuming that EI is important in predicting success in life domains, it becomes important to discuss the assessment of EI. As we have seen before, there is a division in the field of EI regarding the conceptualization of the construct. Similarly, the attempts to measure EI are also twofold (Petrides & Furnham, 2001; 2003). Trait EI is measured exclusively by self-report measures comprising items that assess one's typical levels of EI. In contrast, ability EI is measured by questionnaires that assess one's maximal levels of EI. The instruments based on ability models (Salovey & Mayer, 1990; Mayer & Salovey, 1997) have been developed to assess relevant aspects of individuals' perception of their emotional competencies (e.g., the Trait Meta-Mood Scale [TMMS]; Salovey et al., 1995). On the other hand, tests reflecting trait models focus predominately on "noncognitive" factors such as social skills, self-esteem, and personality dimensions (Emotional Quotient Inventory [EQ-I]; Bar-On, 1997; Trait Emotional Intelligence Questionnaire [TEIQue]; Petrides, Frederickson, & Furnham, 2004).

Trait-Meta Mood Scale

The Trait Meta-Mood Scale (TMMS; Salovey et al., 1995) is a 30-item self-report measure[1] that was designed to assess general beliefs about attention to mood, the clarity of one's own experiences of mood, and one's efforts to repair mood states. It is composed of three subscales: Attention to Feelings, Clarity in Discrimination of Feelings, and Mood Repair. Attention to Feelings indexes the amount of attention individuals feel they allot to experienced emotions and the importance of attending to mood. It consists of items like "I pay a lot of attention to how I feel" and "I never give in to my emotions" (reversed scoring). Clarity in Discrimination of Feelings measures how clearly and distinctly individuals feel and experience their emotions, for example, "I am rarely confused about how I feel." The final subscale, Mood Repair, reflects an individual's efforts to repair negative mood in a way that maintains a generally positive outlook. A characteristic item of this subscale is "When I become upset I remind myself of all the pleasures in life." Internal consistencies for the three subscales are all exceeding .80: $\alpha = .86$, .88, and .82 for Attention to Feelings, Clarity of Discrimination of Feelings, and Mood Repair, respectively (Salovey et al., 1995). Confirmatory factor analysis has demonstrated the robustness of the theoretical three-factor structure (Goldman, Kraemer, & Salovey, 1996). Findings revealing that the factors are sufficiently differentiated from related constructs such as neuroticism and repression provide evidence for the conceptual distinctiveness of the three factors (Salovey et al., 1995). Recently, Pérez, Petrides, and Furnham (2005) have indicated that there is convincing empirical support for predictive validity of the TMMS with respect to depression, mood recovery, and goal orientation. The TMMS was not designed to cover the entire trait EI sampling domain. Accordingly, it overlooks many core facets of EI (Pérez et al., 2005).

---

[1] Salovey et al. (1995) started with a 48-item scale. They next tried to evaluate whether a shorter version could be derived by dropping items with low loadings. The resulting, more efficient 30-item version is now recommended (Salovey et al., 1995).

Mayer-Salovey-Caruso Emotional Intelligence Test, Version 2.0

The Mayer-Salovey-Caruso Emotional Intelligence Test, Version 2.0 (MSCEIT V2.0; Mayer, Salovey, & Caruso, 2002) is a 141-item scale designed to measure EI. Scores represent (i) a general level of EI; (ii) two area scores, Experiencing EI reflecting the ability to identify emotions and to assimilate emotions in thought, and Strategic EI reflecting the ability to understand and manage emotions; and (iii) four branch scores, each measured by two subscales, that assess the four branches of EI, that is, perceiving emotions, using emotions to facilitate thought, understanding emotions, and managing emotions (Fig. 7.1). The MSCEIT V2.0 measures perception of emotions with the Faces and Picture subscales in which persons are asked to rate how much of a particular emotion is being expressed in photographed faces expressing a basic emotion, photographed landscapes, or abstract designs. Emotional facilitation of thought is assessed by the Sensations and Facilitations subscales asking persons to imagine certain emotions and to indicate the extent to which they match different sensations and would assist cognitive tasks or behaviors. Understanding emotions is measured by the Blends and Changes subscales, which ask people how emotions combine to form more complex feelings and how emotional reactions result from the intensification of certain feelings. Finally, the MSCEIT V2.0 measures emotion management by the Emotional Management and Emotional Relationships subscales that ask to indicate how effective certain actions might be in regulating one's own moods and emotions and those of others. The reliability of the MSCEIT V2.0 at the total scale, area, and branch levels was found to be good; for example, split-half reliability coefficients at the branch level ranged from .76 to .91, at the area level from .86 to .90, and at the full-scale level from .91 to .93 (Mayer, Salovey, Caruso, & Sitarenios, 2003). Recently, Palmer, Gignac, Manocha, and Stough (2005) examined the psychometric properties of the MSCEIT V2.0. They reported that the reliability was good at the level of the total scale, as well as at area and branch levels, but rather low at the level of the separate subscales. Moreover, in contrast with earlier findings (Mayer et al., 2003), they could only obtain partial support for the original four-factor model of EI (Fig. 7.1). Palmer et al. (2005) found convincing support for a distinct four-factor model with a general EI-factor and three branch factors (i.e., Perceiving Emotions, Understanding Emotions, and Managing Emotions). There was no support for the Experiential Area level factor and the Facilitating Branch level factor.

Bar-On Emotional Quotient Inventory

A popular trait test is the Bar-On Emotional Quotient inventory (EQ-I; Bar-On, 1997). The theoretical background is "somewhat vague" (Pérez et al., 2005, p. 187), due to the fact that the EQ-I has been converted from a well-being scale to an EI assessment instrument. The EQ-I consists of 133 items arranged on a 5-point Likert-type scale. The instrument has 15 subscales: Emotional Self-Awareness,

Assertiveness, Self-Regard, Self-Actualization, Independence, Empathy, Interpersonal Relationships, Social Responsibility, Problem Solving, Reality Testing, Flexibility, Stress Tolerance, Impulse Control, Happiness, and Optimism. The response scale ranges from "not true of me" (1) to "true of me" (5). Persons are asked to indicate the degree to which each statement is true of the way they feel, think, and act in most situations. According to Bar-On (1997), the instrument assesses five aspects of EI: (i) Interpersonal (i.e., the ability to be aware of and understand others' emotions); (ii) Intrapersonal (i.e., the ability to be aware of and understand one's own emotions); (iii) Adaptability (i.e., the capacity to be flexible and to change one's own emotions); (iv) Stress Management (i.e., the ability to cope with stressors and to control one's own emotions); and (v) General Mood (i.e., the capacity to be optimistic and to express positive emotions). Petrides and Furnham (2001) have questioned this higher-order structure, presenting evidence that the questionnaire is essentially unifactorial. The reliability and validity of the measures have been examined extensively (see the EQ-I technical manual; Bar-On, 1997). The internal consistency is generally good: across many studies, the Cronbach alpha (α) is about .85. Predictive validity is reflected in substantial associations with mental health, preferences for particular coping strategies, and work and marital satisfaction (Pérez et al., 2005).

Emotional Competencies Inventory

The Emotional Competencies Inventory (ECI; Boyatsis, Goleman, & Hay/McBer Group, 1999; Boyatzis, Goleman, & Rhee, 2000; Sala, 2002) is especially popular in the field of human resources management. The ECI contains 110 items (Version 1, 7-point Likert scale) or 73 items (version 2, 6-point Likert scale). There are forms for self-report and ratings by others (peers, supervisors). The ECI assesses 20 emotional competencies that are organized into four domains: (i) Self-Awareness, (ii) Social Awareness, (iii) Self-Management, and (iv) Social Skills. The internal consistency coefficients of the self-assessment ECI scales range from .61 to .85. For the peer and supervisor rating scales, the range is .80 to .95. There is little information about its validity properties in scientific journals (Pérez et al., 2005).

Self-Report Emotional Intelligence Test

The Self-Report Emotional Intelligence Test (SREIT; Schutte et al., 1998) contains a set of 33 self-report items reflecting Salovey and Mayer's (1990) early model of EI. Schutte et al. conceive of this inventory as a one-dimensional scale. However, Petrides and Furnham (2000) have presented data that point into the direction of four scales: Optimism and Mood Regulation, Appraisal of Emotions, Social Skills, and Utilization of Emotions.

Trait Emotional Intelligence Questionnaire

The Trait Emotional Intelligence Questionnaire (TEIQue; Petrides et al., 2004) focuses primarily in trait EI. The inventory contains 153 items, providing scores on 15 subscales, four factors (Well-being, Self-control Skills, Emotional Skills, and Social Skills), and global trait EI. The 15 subscales reflect the EI model of Petrides and Furnham (2001). This model features Adaptability, Assertiveness, Emotion Appraisal (self and others), Emotion Expression, Emotion Management (others), Emotion Regulation, Impulsiveness (low), Relationships Skills, Self-esteem, Self-motivation, Social Competence, Stress Management, Trait Empathy, Trait Happiness, and Trait Optimism. According to Pérez et al. (2005), the internal consistency (about .85) and the test-retest reliability (.78 for global EI across 12-month interval) are generally good. Evidence for predictive validity is available with respect to depression, personality disorders, dysfunctional attitudes, adaptive coping styles, job stress, job performance, organizational commitment, deviant behavior at school, and sensitivity to mood induction.

Swinburne University Emotional Intelligence Test

The 64-item Swinburne University Emotional Intelligence Test (SUEIT; Palmer & Stough, 2001) contains five scales, which correspond with the ability model: Emotional Recognition and Expression, Understanding of Emotions, Emotions Direct Cognition, Emotional Management, and Emotional Control. Test-retest correlations (interval = 1 month) ranged between .81 and .94, internal consistency coefficients for the subscales ranged from .80 to .89, and the Cronbach's α for the total scale was .92 (Palmer & Stough, 2001).

Convergent, Discriminant, and Incremental Validity of EI Measures

The different ways of defining the EI construct have resulted in different types of assessment procedures and instruments. Ability-based measures are more distinct from basic personality measures than self-report EI measures reflecting so-called mixed models. In addition, ability-based instruments generally have higher correlations with general mental ability compared with the trait-based questionnaires covering mixed models. Taking these associations into account, one would expect, first of all, that the various measures lack comparability, and, furthermore, that especially a self-report personality-based approach would be successful in predicting health-related outcomes. The latter expectation is grounded in empirical findings demonstrating substantial links between temperament, personality, and health (Van Heck, 1997).

Brackett and Mayer (2003; see also Brackett, Mayer, & Warner, 2004) investigated the convergent, discriminant, and incremental validity of the ability-based MSCEIT (Mayer et al., 2002) and two self-report tests: the EQ-I (Bar-On, 1997) and the SREIT (Schutte et al., 1998). The MSCEIT showed weak associations with the other two instruments, whereas the latter two were moderately interrelated. The MSCEIT appeared to be relatively independent of basic personality dimensions. For instance, correlations with Neuroticism and Extraversion were – .08 and .11, respectively. The corresponding correlations were – .57 and .37 in case of the EQ-I and –.19 and .32 for the SREIT. Given these associations, it does not come as a big surprise that EQ-I and SREIT are more strongly related to psychological well-being featuring self-acceptance, environmental mastery, purpose in life, positive relations with others, personal growth, and autonomy, than MSCEIT: .54 and .69 versus .28. More similar semantic content between the EQ-I, the SREIT, and measures of personality and well-being, compared with the MSCEIT, seems to be the most plausible explanation of this pattern of associations.

Emotional Intelligence and Health

In health psychology, psychologists study the relationship between mind and body, as well as the ways in which these two elements respond to environmental challenges to produce either illness or health (Larsen & Buss, 2002). Some researchers in this field focus on personality and individual differences in susceptibility to disease and in recovery from diseases or surgical interventions. More recently, the construct of EI is also studied in order to explain individual differences between persons in the field of health/illness. In this section, these two important constructs, personality and EI, and their influence on health are discussed.

Personality

Personality is one of the constructs associated with individual differences found in the processes of getting ill, staying healthy, or recovery from a disease. How can personality be related with such health-related outcomes? There are several ideas about the way personality can influence a person's health, namely (i) personality can affect the way persons cope in stressful situations, (ii) personality can influence how the person appraises or interprets events, (iii) personality can influence the exposure to stressful events themselves, (iv) personality can affect health indirectly, through health-promoting or health-degrading behaviors, and, finally, (v) personality can influence the degree to which a person perceives and pays attention to bodily sensations and the degree to which the person interprets and labels those sensations in terms of illness (Larsen & Buss, 2002). Thus, personality is associated with factors that cause disease, may lead to behaviors that protect or diminish health, or may relate to the successful implementation of health-related coping efforts and adherence to treatment regimens (Caspi, Roberts, & Shiner, 2005; Contrada, Cather, & O'Leary, 1999; Ozer & Benet-Martínez, 2006; Van Heck, 1997).

The Moderating Role of Emotional Intelligence

Does EI also moderate the relationship between stress and health? Some preliminary findings demonstrated that certain aspects of EI, for instance, skills on emotion management (Ciarrochi, Chan, & Caputi, 2000), protect people from stress and may lead to better adaptation (Ciarrochi, Deane, & Anderson, 2002). Other research, by Ciarrochi, Chan, and Bajgar (2001), suggests that persons who are good at perceiving and managing others' emotions tend to have more social support and tend to be more satisfied with that support. So, it seems reasonable to assume that high EI would be associated with better stress management and lower levels of psychological distress (Austin et al., 2005). On the other hand, persons who are poor at perceiving and regulating their emotions may actually tend to be less sensitive to the effects of stress (e.g., Ciarrochi et al., 2002). Recently, Gohm, Corser, and Dalsky (2005) studied the psychological states and processes involved in having a sense of control. They could show convincingly that individual differences in one's perceived ability to manage stressful person-environment relationships played a major moderating role with respect to the association between (i) EI, reflecting emotional task performance and emotional problem solving ability, not perceived EI (cf. Mayer, Salovey, & Caruso, 2002), and (ii) stress, assessed by feelings of inability to control life events. Gohm et al. found that EI predicts stress for individuals whose emotions are intense and well understood and persons characterized by rather mild emotions, which are only poorly understood. In contrast, EI did not predict stress in the case of persons who are typically overwhelmed by unclear intense emotions or cerebral types whose emotions are rather mild but very well understood. These outcomes suggest that personality plays a decisive role in determining whether EI under stress is useful, unnecessary, or irrelevant.

Models of Stress-Illness Relationships

In the literature, several models have been suggested for the role of individual differences variables in stress-illness relationships (e.g., Van Heck, 1997; Wiebe & Smith, 1997). The health behavior model and the transactional model seem to be the most relevant models for indicating moderating roles of EI.

Figure 7.2 describes the adapted health behavior model, expanded with paths indicating the role of EI. The model suggests that personality influences the degree to which a person engages in various health-promoting or health-degrading behaviors. For example, extraversion is associated with the tendency to smoke (Eysenck, 2000). Relationships between EI and health behaviors, like smoking and tobacco use, have also been found (Trinidad & Johnson, 2002). This suggests that there are substantial links between EI and personality and temperament. A growing body of studies (see, e.g., Tsaousis & Nikolaou, 2005) has demonstrated the effect

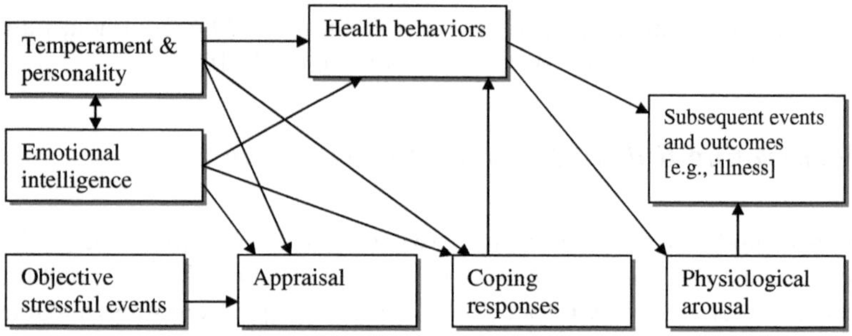

Fig. 7.2 Expanded Health Behavior model. (Adapted from Wiebe, D. J., & Smith, T. [1997]. Personality and health: progress and problems in psychosomatics. In R. Hogan, J. Johnson, & S. Briggs (Eds.), *Handbook of personality psychology* (pp. 892–918). San Diego, CA: Academic Press. See also Van Heck [1997]; Larsen & Buss [2002].)

of negative mood or unpleasant emotional experiences on a number of habits or health behaviors, like smoking (Brandon, 1994; Trinidad & Johnson, 2002), drinking (Cooper, Frone, Russell, & Mudar, 1995; Trinidad & Johnson, 2002), and other health behaviors. For instance, Goldman et al. (1996) found, in a natural stress situation, that individuals scoring low on a measure of Emotional Repair were more likely to visit a health center when stress was high, while in periods of low stress, scores on Emotional Repair did not predict health center visit.

In addition to the health behavior model, another model seems to be relevant. Different individuals do not experience the same level of stress. There are also huge differences in ways of dealing with environmental demands. Furthermore, people differ with respect to selection, creation, and manipulation of situations. The transactional stress-illness model takes these individual differences into account. An expanded transactional model, including EI, is presented in Figure 7.3.

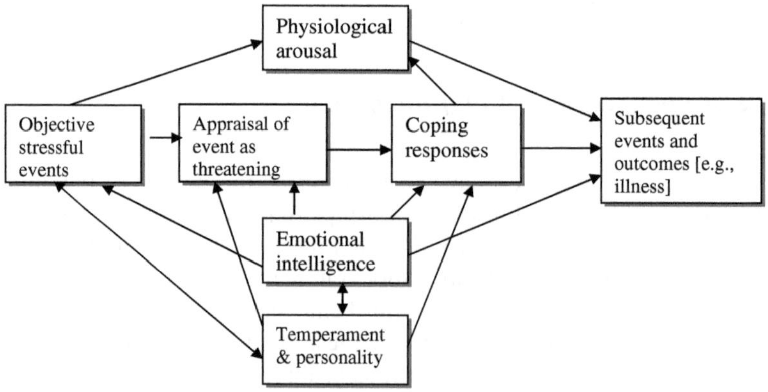

Fig. 7.3 Expanded transactional stress-illness model featuring temperament, personality, EI, and the appraisal-coping process. (Adapted from Wiebe, D. J., & Smith, T., [1997]. Personality and health: progress and problems in psychosomatics. In R. Hogan, J. Johnson, & S. Briggs (Eds.), *Handbook of personality psychology* (pp. 892–918). San Diego, CA: Academic Press. See also Van Heck [1997]; Larsen & Buss [2002].)

EI and Physical Health

Salovey, Bedell, Detweiler, and Mayer (1999) have claimed that EI can influence physical health by the failure of emotional self-management. Having low scores on EI could lead to, for example, excessive cardiovascular reactivity (Salovey, 2001), and high scores have been associated negatively with physical symptoms reporting (Salovey, Stroud, Woolery, & Epel, 2002). Furthermore, Extremera and Fernàndez-Berrocal (2002) found that middle-aged women with high scores on Clarity showed better self-reported physical functioning. They also had less role limitations due to physical health problems. High scores on Emotional Repair were associated with, among others, lower bodily pain.

Salovey et al. (2002) found that people who reported that they frequently attend to their moods showed attenuated cortisol, systolic blood pressure, and diastolic blood pressure reactivity to stress. In another study (Salovey et al., 1995), it was found that high-scorers on Clarity tend to experience more adaptive cardiovascular responses when they write about emotional life events. In a recent overview of these studies, Woolery and Salovey (2004) concluded that perceived EI may be linked to physical health problems through psychophysiologic stress reactivity.

Brown and Schutte (2006) reported that higher EI was associated with less disabling fatigue. Recently, Schutte, Malouff, Thorsteinsson, Bhullar, and Rooke (2007) published a meta-analytic investigation that convincingly demonstrated that higher EI is connected with better health.

EI and Psychological Health

A number of studies have shown that a positive relationship exists between EI and psychological health (Dawda & Hart, 2000; Extremera & Fernàndez-Berrocal, 2002; Salovey et al., 2002; Slaski & Cartwright, 2002). It is hypothesized that people with a high score on EI are skilled with respect to coping with the stressors and demands of everyday life (Bar-On, 1997; Taylor, 2001). Salovey et al. (1995) examined the relationship between the TMMS subscales and important life criteria. They found that individuals with high scores on Clarity showed greater rebound from induced negative mood and greater decline in ruminative thoughts after an experimental stressor.

Hunt and Evans (2004) found that high-scorers on EI reported fewer posttraumatic stress disorder (PTSD) symptoms, reflecting intrusion, avoidance, and hyperarousal related to their traumatic experiences, than low-scorers.

In recent years, EI has begun to attract the attention of researchers studying the relationships between DSM-IV personality disorder (PD) symptomatology and several aspects of EI. Leible and Snell (2004) found that individuals with borderline PD reported less emotional clarity and poorer emotional regulation, revealing "problems with their emotional adaptation, due to deficits in their emotional intelligence"

(p. 400). In addition to the finding that people with borderline PD symptomatology report less understanding of the nature of their emotions and a limited capacity to overcome negative emotional experiences, Leible and Snell (2004) reported other significant results encompassing PDs. For example, schizoid PD was linked to less emotional clarity, less emotional repair, less emotional attention, and less private emotional self-awareness, and high-scorers on a measure of narcissistic PD showed a lack of emotional control and poor emotional repair.

Both theory and research findings suggest a link between EI and emotional well-being. Theoretically, various authors have suggested that persons who are able to understand and regulate their emotions will have greater feelings of emotional well-being (Bar-On, 1997; Goleman, 1995; Salovey & Mayer, 1990). Empirically, several studies using self-report measures (e.g., EQ-I) and performance-based measures (e.g., MEIS) provide evidence that higher EI is associated with less depression (Martinez-Pons, 1997; Schutte et al., 1998), greater optimism (Schutte et al., 1998), and greater life satisfaction (Austin et al., 2005; Bar-On, 1997; Ciarrochi et al., 2000; Martinez-Pons, 1997; Mayer et al., 2002). Importantly, Carriochi et al. (2002) found that EI correlated with life satisfaction ($r = .22$, $p < .05$), even after controlling for IQ and personality variables, suggesting that EI accounts for unique variance. Bastian, Burns, and Nettelbeck (2005), however, found that controlling for personality and cognitive abilities substantially reduced the contribution of EI in the prediction of life satisfaction, regardless of the measure used (TMMS, SREIT, or MSCEIT). Furthermore, Spence, Oades, and Caputi (2004) reported that global trait EI, in spite of a substantial link between high levels of trait EI (SREIT) and more congruent, self-integrated personal goal systems, was nevertheless a rather poor predictor of global emotional well-being.

Previous research has reported that some dimensions of personality, specifically neuroticism, extraversion, and positive and negative affect, are strong predictors if not the major determinants of life satisfaction (Diener & Larsen, 1993; McCrae & Costa, 1991; Myers & Diener, 1995). A couple of years ago, Palmer, Donaldson, and Stough (2002) examined the associations between EI, positive and negative affect, and life satisfaction. They were able to show that a particular component of the EI construct, Clarity, added a statistically significant increase of approximately 5.5% in the prediction of life satisfaction over and above the percentage accounted for by personality. However, Gannon and Ranzijn (2005) demonstrated that EI predicted only a very small amount of unique variance in life satisfaction beyond personality and demographic variables. Due to substantial conceptual overlap between EI and personality, EI scores accounted only for a further 1.3%. This is quite remarkable, considering that the used EI measure, the SUEIT, is based on the ability model of EI rather than the mixed model.

Future Prospects

In a critical review, Matthews, Roberts, & Zeidner (2004) have listed seven myths about EI (Table 7.2).

Table 7.2 Seven myths about EI

Definitions of EI are conceptually coherent
Measures of EI meet standard psychometric criteria
Self-report EI is distinct from existing personality constructs
Ability tests or EI meet criteria for a cognitive intelligence
EI relates to emotion as IQ relates to cognition
EI predicts adaptive coping
EI is critical for real-world success

Source: Matthews, G., Roberts, R. D., & Zeidner, M. (2004). Seven myths about emotional intelligence. *Psychological Inquiry*, *15*, 179–196.

It speaks for itself that the aim of Matthews et al. (2004) was not to dismiss work on EI out of hand. The goal of their analysis of the state-of-the-art in EI was to "examine where the first wave of research of the construct is meeting barriers to progress and whether those barriers can be overcome" (p. 179).

One year later, in the final chapter of a new (international) handbook of EI (Schulze & Roberts, 2005), Roberts, Schulze, Zeidner, and Matthews (2005) provide a new synthesis of the current state of theory, research, and applications of EI. Pointing at the many conflicting views and perspectives on the nature of EI, they propose that future research should be guided by clearer conceptual and psychometric discrimination of the multiple constructs related to EI, a stronger focus on mediating mechanisms and situational moderators of EI constructs, and a greater emphasis on developing causal models using data from experimental and longitudinal studies.

We agree with these guidelines. With respect to the need for greater conceptual coherence, we would like to emphasize that such coherence can only be attained when EI will be "liberated" from elements that do not represent forms of intelligence and facets that are already encapsulated by existing personality and temperament models. Ability-based EI measures appear to be most promising. However, many unresolved issues remain even regarding these instruments (Conte, 2005). Therefore, the use of EI measures in clinical psychology, health psychology, clinical health psychology, and related fields should be accompanied by great caution. We feel that this may not be in line with the many populist accounts of EI, but it certainly reflects the opinion of some of the most prominent EI proponents (see, e.g., Mayer et al., 2003). To use the words of Zeidner, Roberts, and Matthews (2004): "As EI grows up from its flashy adolescence, it may need to trade in the bandwagon for some more modest but better engineered form of transportation" (p. 247).

References

Austin, E. J., & Saklofske, D. H. (2005). Far too many intelligences? On the communalities and differences between social, practical, and emotional intelligences. In R. Schulze & R. D. Roberts (Eds.), *Emotional intelligence. An international handbook* (pp. 107–128). Göttingen, Germany: Hogrefe & Huber Publishers.

Austin, E. J., Saklofske, D. H., & Egan, V. (2005). Personality, well-being and health correlates of trait emotional intelligence. *Personality and Individual Differences*, *38*, 547–558.

Bar-On, R. (1997). *Emotional Quotient Inventory: technical manual.* Toronto, ON: Multi-Health Systems.
Bar-On, R. (2000). Emotional and social intelligence: insights from the Emotional Quotient inventory. In R. Bar-On & J. D. A. Parker (Eds.), *The handbook of emotional intelligence: theory, development, assessment, and application at home, school, and in the workplace* (pp. 363–388). San Francisco, CA: Jossey-Bass.
Bastian, V. A., Burns, N. R., & Nettelbeck, T. (2005). Emotional intelligence predicts life skills, but not as well as personality and cognitive abilities. *Personality and Individual Differences, 39*, 1135–1145.
Boyatsis, R. E., Goleman, D., & Hay/McBer Group (1999). *Emotional Competence Inventory.* Boston, MA: Hay/McBer Group.
Boyatzis, R. E., Goleman, D., & Rhee, K. S. (2000). Clustering competence in emotional intelligence: Insights from the Emotional Competence Inventory. In R. Bar-On & J. D. A. Parker (Eds.), *The handbook of emotional intelligence: theory, development, assessment, and application at home, school, and in the workplace* (pp. 343–362). San Francisco, CA: Jossey-Bass.
Brackett, M. A., & Mayer, J. D. (2003). Convergent, discriminant, and incremental validity of competing measures of emotional intelligence. *Personality and Social Psychology Bulletin, 29*, 1147–1158.
Brackett, M. A., Mayer, J. D., & Warner, R. M. (2004). Emotional intelligence and its relation to everyday behavior. *Personality and Individual Differences, 36*, 1387–1402.
Brandon, T. H. (1994). Negative affect as a motivation to smoke. *Current Directions in Psychological Science, 3*, 33–37.
Brown, R. F., & Schutte, N. S. (2006). Direct and indirect relationships between emotional intelligence and subjective fatigue in university students. *Journal of Psychosomatic Research, 60*, 585–593.
Cantor, N., & Kihlstrom, J. (1987). *Personality and social intelligence.* Englewood Cliffs, NJ: Erlbaum.
Carroll, J .B. (1993). *Human cognitive abilities: a survey of factor-analytic studies.* New York: Cambridge University Press.
Caspi, A., Roberts, B. W., & Shiner, R. L. (2005). Personality development: stability and change. *Annual Review of Psychology, 56*, 453–484.
Ciarrochi, J., Chan, A., & Caputi, P. (2000). A critical evaluation of the emotional intelligence construct. *Personality and Individual Differences, 28*, 539–561.
Ciarrochi, J., Chan, A., & Bajgar, J. (2001). Measuring emotional intelligence in adolescents. *Personality and Individual Differences, 31*, 1105–1119.
Ciarrochi, J., Deane, F. P., & Anderson, S. (2002). Emotional intelligence moderates the relationship between stress and mental health. *Personality and Individual Differences, 32*, 197–209.
Conte, J. M. (2005). A review and critique of emotional intelligence measures. *Journal of Organizational Behavior, 26*, 433–440.
Contrada, R. J., Cather, C., & O'Leary, A. (1999). Personality and health: dispositions and processes in disease susceptibility and adaptation to illness. In L. A. Pervin & O. P. John (Eds.), *Handbook of personality. Theory and research* (pp. 576–604). New York: The Guilford Press.
Cooper, M. L., Frone, M. R., Russell, M., & Mudar, P. (1995). Drinking to regulate positive and negative emotions: a motivational model of alcohol use. *Journal of Personality and Social Psychology, 69*, 990–1005.
Costa, P. T., Jr., & McCrae, R. R. (1992). *NEO-PI-R: Professional manual.* Odessa, FL: Psychological Assessment Resources.
Dawda, D., & Hart, S. D. (2000). Assessing emotional intelligence: reliability and validity of the Bar-On Emotional Quotient inventory (EQ-i) in university students. *Personality and Individual Differences, 28*, 797–812.

Day, A. L., Therrien, D. L., & Carroll, S. A. (2005). Predicting psychological health: assessing the incremental validity of emotional intelligence beyond personality, type A behavior, and daily hassles. *European Journal of Personality, 19*, 519–536.

Denollet, J., & Nyklíček, I. (2004). Psychological mindedness. A new index to assess a major emotion-focused coping style. In I. Nyklíček, L. Temoshok, & A. Vingerhoets (Eds.), *Emotional expression and health. Advances in theory, assessment and clinical applications* (pp. 185–203). Hove and New York: Brunner-Routledge.

De Raad, B. (2005). The trait-coverage of emotional intelligence. *Personality and Individual Differences, 38*, 673–687.

De Raad, B., Hendriks, A. A. J., & Hofstee, W. K. B. (1992). Towards a refined structure of personality traits. *European Journal of Personality, 6*, 301–319.

Derksen, J., Kramer, I., & Katzko, M. (2002). Does a self-report measure for emotional intelligence assess something different than general intelligence? *Personality and Individual Differences, 32*, 37–48.

Diener, E., & Larsen, R. J. (1993). The experience of emotional well-being. In M. Lewis & J. M. Haviland (Eds.), *Handbook of emotions* (pp. 404–415). New York The Guilford Press.

Eysenck, H. J. (2000). *Smoking, health, and personality*. New York: Transaction.

Extremera, N., & Fernàndez-Berrocal, P. (2002). Relation of perceived emotional intelligence and health-related quality of life of middle-aged women. *Psychological Reports, 91*, 47–59.

Gannon, N., & Ranzijn, R. (2005). Does emotional intelligence predict unique variance in life satisfaction beyond IQ and personality? *Personality and Individual Differences, 38*, 1353–1464.

Gardner, H. (1983). *Frames of mind*. New York: Basic Books.

Gohm, C. L., Corser, G. C., & Dalsky, D. J. (2005). Emotional intelligence under stress: useful, unnecessary, or irrelevant? *Personality and Individual Differences, 29*, 1017–1028.

Goldman, S. L., Kraemer, D. T., & Salovey, P. (1996). Beliefs about mood moderate the relationship of stress to illness and symptom reporting. *Journal of Psychosomatic Research, 41*, 115–128.

Goleman, D. (1995). *Emotional intelligence*. New York, NY: Bantam Books.

Gottfredson, L. S., & Deary, I. J. (2004). Intelligence predicts health and longevity, but why? *Current Directions in Psychological Science, 13*, 1–4.

Gratch, J., & Marsella, S. (2004). A domain-independent framework for modeling emotion. *Cognitive Systems Research, 5*, 269–306.

Hart, C. L., Deary, I. J., Taylor, M. D., MacKinnon, P. L., Davey Smith, G., Whaley, L. J., Wilson, V., Hole, D. J., & Star, J. M. (2003a). The Scottish Mental Survey 1932 linked to the Midspan studies: a prospective investigation of childhood intelligence and future health. *Public Health, 117*, 187–195.

Hart, C. L., Taylor, M. D., Davey Smith, G., Whalley, L. J., Starr, J. M., Hole, D. J., Wilson, V., & Deary. I. J. (2003b). Childhood IQ, social class, deprivation and their relationships with mortality and morbidity risk in later life. *Psychosomatic Medicine, 65*, 877–883.

Hedlund, J., & Sternberg, R. J. (2000). Too many intelligences? Integrating social, emotional, and practical intelligence. In R. Bar-On & J. D. A. Parker (Eds.), *The handbook of emotional intelligence: theory, development, assessment, and application at home, school, and in the workplace* (pp. 136–167). San Francisco, CA: Jossey-Bass.

Hunt, N., & Evans, D. (2004). Predicting traumatic stress using emotional intelligence. *Behavior Research and Therapy, 42*, 791–798.

John, O. P. (1990). The "Big Five" factor taxonomy: dimensions of personality in the natural language and in questionnaires. In L. A. Pervin (Ed.), *Handbook of personality. Theory and research* (pp. 66–100). New York: The Guilford Press.

John, O. P., & Srivastava, S. (1999). The Big Five trait taxonomy: history, measurement, and theoretical perspectives. In L. A. Pervin & O. P. John (Eds.), *Handbook of personality. Theory and research* (pp. 102–138). New York: The Guilford Press.

Kang, S.-M., Day, J. D., & Meara, N. M. (2005). Social and emotional intelligence: Starting a conversation about their similarities and differences. In R. Schulze & R. D. Roberts (Eds.),

Emotional intelligence: an international handbook (pp. 91–105). Göttingen, Germany: Hogrefe & Huber Publishers.

Larsen, R. J., & Buss, D. M. (2002). *Personality psychology: domains of knowledge about human nature*. New York: McGraw-Hill.

Lazarus, R. S. (2006). Emotions and interpersonal relationships: toward a person-centered conceptualization of emotions and coping. *Journal of Personality, 74*, 9–46.

Lazarus, R. S., & Folkman, S. (1984). *Stress, appraisal, and coping*. New York: Springer.

Leible, T. L., & Snell, W. E., Jr. (2004). Borderline personality disorder and multiple aspects of emotional intelligence. *Personality and Individual Differences, 37*, 393–404.

Locke, E. A. (2005). Why emotional intelligence is an invalid concept. *Journal of Organizational Behavior, 26*, 425–431.

Lopes, P. N., Salovey, P., & Straus, R. (2003). Emotional intelligence, personality, and perceived quality of social relationships. *Personality and Individual Differences, 35*, 641–658.

Matthews, G., Roberts, R. D., & Zeidner, M. (2004). Seven myths about emotional intelligence. *Psychological Inquiry, 15*, 179–196.

Martinez-Pons, M. (1997). The relationship of emotional intelligence with selected areas of personal functioning. *Imagination, Cognition and Personality, 17*, 3–13.

Mayer, J. D. (2001). A field guide to emotional intelligence. In J. Ciarrochi, J. P. Forgas, & J. D. Mayer (Eds.), *Emotional intelligence in everyday life* (pp. 3–24). New York: Psychological Press.

Mayer, J. D., & Geher, G. (1996). Emotional intelligence and identification of emotion. *Intelligence, 22*, 89–113.

Mayer, J. D., & Salovey, P. (1993). The intelligence of emotional intelligence. *Intelligence, 17*, 443–450.

Mayer, J. D., & Salovey, P. (1997). What is emotional intelligence? In P. Salovey & D. J. Sluyter (Eds.), *Emotional development and emotional intelligence: educational implications* (pp. 3–31). New York: Basic Books.

Mayer, J. D., Caruso, D. R., & Salovey, P. (1999). Emotional intelligence meets traditional standards for an intelligence. *Intelligence, 27*, 267–298.

Mayer, J. D., Salovey, P., & Caruso, D. R. (2000). Models of emotional intelligence. In R. Sternberg (Ed.), *Handbook of intelligence* (pp. 396–420). Cambridge, UK: Cambridge University Press .

Mayer, J. D., Salovey, P., & Caruso, D. R. (2002). *Mayer-Salovey-Caruso Emotional Intelligence Test (MSCEIT) user's manual*. Toronto, ON: Multi-Health Systems.

Mayer, J. D., Salovey, P., Caruso, D. R., & Sitarenios, G. (2002). Emotional intelligence meets traditional standards for an intelligence. *Intelligence, 27*, 267–298.

Mayer, J. D., Salovey, P., Caruso, D. R., & Sitarenios, G. (2003). Measuring emotional intelligence with the MSCEIT V2.0. *Emotion, 3*, 97–105.

McCrae, R. R. (2000). Emotional intelligence from the perspective of the five-factor model of personality. In R. Bar-On & J. D. A. Parker (Eds.), *The handbook of emotional intelligence: theory, development, assessment, and application in home, school, and in the workplace* (pp. 263–276). San Francisco, CA: Jossey-Bass.

McCrae, R. R., & Costa, P. T., Jr. (1991). Adding Liebe und Arbeit: the full five-factor model and well-being. *Personality and Social Psychology Bulletin, 17*, 227–232.

Myers, D. G., & Diener, E. (1995). Who is happy? *Psychological Science, 6*, 10–19.

Neisser, U., Boodoo, G., Bouchard, T. J., Boykin, A. W., Brody, N., Ceci, S. J., Halpern, D. F., Loehlin, J. C., Perloff, R., Sternberg, R. J., & Urbina, S. (1996). Intelligence: knowns and unknowns. *American Psychologist, 51*, 77–101.

Neubauer, A. C., & Freudenthaler, H. H. (2005). Models of emotional intelligence. In R. Schulze & R. D. Roberts (Eds.), *Emotional intelligence: an international handbook* (pp. 31–50). Göttingen, Germany: Hogrefe & Huber Publishers.

Nussbaum, M. (2001). *Upheavals of thought: the intelligence of emotions*. Cambridge, UK: Cambridge University Press.

Ozer, D. J., & Benet-Martínez, V. (2006). Personality and the prediction of consequential outcomes. *Annual Review of Psychology, 57*, 401–421.

Palmer, B. R., & Stough, C. (2001). *Swinburne University Emotional Intelligence Test: interim technical manual.* Melbourne, Australia: Organisational psychology Research Unit, Swinburne University of Technology.

Palmer, B. R., Donaldson, C., & Stough, C. (2002). Emotional intelligence and life satisfaction. *Personality and Individual Differences*, *33*, 1091–1100.

Palmer, B. R., Gignac, G., Manocha, R., & Stough, C. (2005). A psychometric evaluation of the Mayer-Salovey-Caruso Emotional Intelligence Test Version 2.0. *Intelligence*, *33*, 285–305.

Parker, J. D. A. (2005). The relevance of emotional intelligence for clinical psychology. In R. Schulze & R. D. Roberts (Eds.), *Emotional intelligence. An international handbook* (pp. 271–287). Göttingen, Germany: Hogrefe & Huber Publishers.

Parker, J. D. A., Taylor, G. J., & Bagby, R. M. (2001). The relationship between emotional intelligence and alexithymia. *Personality and Individual Differences*, *30*, 107–115.

Pérez, J. C., Petrides, K. V., & Furnham, A. (2005). Measuring trait emotional intelligence. In R. Schulze & R. D. Roberts (Eds.), *Emotional intelligence. An international handbook* (pp. 181–201). Göttingen, Germany: Hogrefe & Huber Publishers.

Petrides, K. V., & Furnham, A. (2000). On the dimensional structure of emotional intelligence. *Personality and Individual Differences*, *29*, 313–320.

Petrides, K. V., & Furnham, A. (2001). Trait emotional intelligence: psychometric investigation with reference to established trait taxonomies. *European Journal of Personality*, *15*, 425–448.

Petrides, K. V., & Furnham, A. (2003). Trait emotional intelligence: behavioral validation in two studies of emotion recognition and reactivity to mood induction. *European Journal of Personality*, *17*, 39–57.

Petrides, K. V., Frederickson, N., & Furnham, A. (2004). The role of trait emotional intelligence in academic performance and deviant behavior at school. *Personality and Individual Differences*, *36*, 277–293.

Roberts, R. D., Schulze, R., Zeidner, M., & Matthews, G. (2005). Understanding, measuring, and applying emotional intelligence: What have we learned? What have we missed? In R. Schulze & R. D. Roberts (Eds.), *Emotional intelligence. An international handbook* (pp. 311–341). Göttingen, Germany: Hogrefe & Huber Publishers.

Saklofske, D. H., Austin, E. J., & Minski, P. S. (2003). Factor structure and validity of a trait emotional intelligence measure. *Personality and Individual Differences*, *34*, 1091–1100.

Sala, F. (2002). *Emotional Competence Inventory: technical manual*. Boston, MA: Hay/McBer Group.

Salovey, P. (2001). Applied emotional intelligence: regulating emotions to become healthy, wealthy, and wise. In J. Ciarrochi, J. P. Forgas, & J. D. Mayer (Eds.), *Emotional intelligence in everyday life: a scientific inquiry* (pp. 168–184). Philadelphia, PA: Psychology Press.

Salovey, P., & Mayer, J. D. (1990). Emotional intelligence. *Imagination, Cognition and Personality*, *9*, 185–211.

Salovey, P., & Mayer, J. D. (1994). Some final thoughts about personality and intelligence. In R. J. Sternberg (Ed.),*Personality and intelligence* (pp. 303–318). New York: Cambridge University Press.

Salovey, P., Mayer, J. D., Goldman, S. L., Turvey, C., & Palfai, T. P. (1995). Emotional attention, clarity, and repair: exploring emotional intelligence using the Trait Meta-Mood Scale. In J. W. Pennebaker (Ed.), *Emotion, disclosure, and health* (pp. 125–154). Washington, DC: APA.

Salovey, P., Bedell, B. T., Detweiler, J. B., & Mayer, J. D. (1999). Coping intelligently: emotional intelligence and the coping process. In C. R. Snyder (Ed.), *Coping: the psychology of what works* (pp. 141–164). New York: Oxford Psychology Press.

Salovey, P., Stroud, L. R., Woolery, A., & Epel, E. S. (2002). Perceived emotional intelligence, stress reactivity, and symptom reports: further explorations using the Trait Meta-Mood Scale. *Psychology and Health*, *17*, 611–627.

Schulte, M. J., Ree, M. J., & Carretta, T. R. (2004). Emotional intelligence: not much more than *g* and personality. *Personality and Individual Differences*, *37*, 1059–1068.

Schultz, D., Izard, C. E., & Abe, J. A. A. (2005). The emotion systems and the development of emotional intelligence. In R. Schulze & R. D. Roberts (Eds.), *Emotional intelligence: an international handbook* (pp. 51–67). Göttingen, Germany: Hogrefe & Huber Publishers.
Schulze, R., & Roberts, R. D. (2005). *Emotional intelligence. An international handbook.* Göttingen, Germany: Hogrefe & Huber Publishers.
Schutte, N. S., Malouff, J. M., Hall, L. E., Haggerty, D. J., Cooper, J. T., Golden, C. J., & Dornheim, L. (1998). Development and validation of a measure of emotional intelligence. *Personality and Individual Differences, 25*, 167–177.
Schutte, N. S., Malouff, J. M., Thorsteinsson, E. B., Bhullar, N., & Rooke, S. E. (2007). A meta-analytic investigation of the relationship between emotional intelligence and health. *Personality and Individual Differences, 42,* 921–933.
Sifneos, P. E. (1973). The prevalence of "alexithymic" characteristics in psychosomatic patients. *Psychotherapy and Psychosomatics, 22*, 255–262.
Slaski, M., & Cartwright, S. (2002). Health, performance and emotional intelligence: an exploratory study of retail managers. *Stress and Health, 18*, 63–68.
Spence, G., Oades, L. G., & Caputi, P. (2004). Trait emotional intelligence and goal self-integration: important predictors of emotional well-being? *Personality and Individual Differences, 37,* 449–461.
Sternberg, R. J. (1985). *Beyond IQ: a triarchic theory of human abilities*. New York: Cambridge University Press.
Sternberg, R. J., Wagner, R. K., & Okagaki, L. (1993). Practical intelligence: the nature and role of tacit knowledge in work and at school. In J. M. Puckett & H. W. Reese (Eds.), *Mechanisms of everyday cognition* (pp. 205–27). Hillsdale, NJ: Erlbaum.
Taylor, G. J. (2001). Low emotional intelligence and mental health. In J. Ciarrochi, J. P. Forgas, & J. D. Mayer (Eds.), *Emotional intelligence in everyday life: a scientific inquiry* (pp. 67–81). Philadelphia, PA: Psychology Press.
Taylor, G. J. (2004). Alexithymia: 25 years of theory and research. In I. Nyklíček, L. Temoshok, & A. Vingerhoets (Eds.), *Emotional expression and health. Advances in theory, assessment and clinical applications* (pp. 137–153). Hove and New York: Brunner-Routledge.
Taylor, G. J., Bagby, R. M., & Parker, J. D. A. (1997). *Disorders of affect regulation: alexithymia in medical and psychiatric illness*. Cambridge: Cambridge University Press.
Thorndike, E. L. (1920). Intelligence and its uses. *Harper's Magazine*, *140*, 227–235.
Trinidad, D. R., & Johnson, C. A. (2002). The association between emotional intelligence and early adolescent tobacco and alcohol use. *Personality and Individual Differences, 32*, 95–105.
Tsaousis, I., & Nikolaou, I. (2005). Exploring the relationship of emotional intelligence with physical and psychological health functioning. *Stress and Health, 21*, 77–86.
Van Heck, G. L. (1997). Personality and physical health: toward an ecological approach to health-related personality research. *European Journal of Personality, 11*, 415–443.
Van der Zee, K., Thijs, M., & Schakel, L. (2002). The relationship of emotional intelligence with academic intelligence and the Big Five. *European Journal of Personality, 16,* 103–125.
Warwick, J., & Nettelbeck, T. (2004). Emotional intelligence is ...? *Personality and Individual Differences*, *37*, 1091–1100.
Wechsler, D. (1950). Cognitive, conative, and non-intellective intelligence. *American Psychologist, 5*, 78–83.
Wechsler, D. (1958). *The measurement and appraisal of adult intelligence* (4th ed.). Baltimore, MD: The Williams & Wilkins Company.
Whalley, L. J., & Deary, I. J. (2001). Longitudinal cohort study of childhood IQ and survival up to age 76. *British Medical Journal*, *322*, 1–5.
Wiebe, D. J., & Smith, T. (1997). Personality and health: progress and problems in psychosomatics. In R. Hogan, J. Johnson, & S. Briggs (Eds.), *Handbook of personality psychology* (pp. 892–918). San Diego, CA: Academic Press.
Woolery, A., & Salovey, P. (2004). Emotional intelligence and physical health. In I. Nyklíček, L. Temoshok, & A. Vingerhoets (Eds.), *Emotional expression and health. Advances in theory, assessment and clinical applications* (pp. 154–168). Hove and New York: Brunner-Routledge.

Zeidner, M., Roberts, R. D., & Matthews, G. (2004). The emotional intelligence bandwagon: too fast to live, too young to die? *Psychological Inquiry, 15*, 239–248.

Zirkel, S. (2000). Social intelligence. The development and maintenance of purposive behavior. In R. Bar-On & J. D. A. Parker (Eds.), *The handbook of emotional intelligence. Theory, development, assessment, and application at home, school, and in the workplace* (pp. 3–27). San Francisco, CA: Jossey-Bass.

Part II
Clinical Perspectives and Interventions

Chapter 8
Emotion Expression in Depression: Emerging Evidence for Emotion Context-Insensitivity

Jonathan Rottenberg and Christine Vaughan

Introduction

From cradle to grave, emotion expression powerfully shapes our adaptation to the environment (Keltner, Kring, & Bonanno, 1999). Often, emotion-expressive behavior promotes healthy outcomes, as when a hungry baby is fed after crying. At other times, emotion expressions are counterproductive, such as in the assaultive displays of anger seen in "road rage" (Connell & Joint, 1996). Over the past two decades, the "basic" emotion research of psychologists working in diverse subfields has illuminated the central role of emotion expression in adaptation (e.g., Ekman, 1993; Fridlund, 1992). Recently, psychopathology researchers have drawn upon this basic research, using it to connect abnormalities in emotion expression to the impaired social functioning that is observed across many clinical disorders (Keltner & Kring, 1998; Rottenberg & Johnson, 2007).

Depression, an often painful psychological disorder that is the leading cause of psychiatric hospitalization, and which affects nearly 20% of the population over the lifetime (Kessler, 2002), is an important place to apply the insights of basic emotion research. Depression is also a natural context to examine *interconnections* between emotion expression and social functioning, as it typically involves impairments in both of these domains (Rottenberg & Gotlib, 2004). Therefore, this chapter is directed toward describing depressed persons' emotion-expressive behavior and addressing the implications of abnormalities in expressive behavior for social functioning.

Our chapter has four parts. First, we will briefly consider what basic research on emotion teaches us about the major functions of expressive behavior. Second, we will review empirical findings (both naturalistic and experimental) concerning depressed individuals' emotion-expressive behavior. Third, to integrate these empirical findings, we will highlight the theme of emotion context-insensitivity: This theme states that depressed persons express emotions inflexibly and in ways that are inappropriate to dynamically changing environmental contexts. Finally, we will offer suggestions for future research designed to increase understanding of emotion context-insensitivity and its impact on social functioning.

A. Vingerhoets et al., (eds.), *Emotion Regulation.*

Defining Emotion Expression

Emotions are commonly understood as relatively brief-lived reactions that help us to respond to problems and challenges in our environment, organizing our thoughts and actions, and shaping our behavior (e.g., Frijda, 1986). Emotional reactions are triggered when an organism encounters a meaningful stimulus (which can be inside or outside the person). Most scientists view emotions as involving changes in multiple response components (Lang, 1978), such as emotion experience, central and peripheral physiology, as well as the component that is our focus here: behavior. Although these emotion response components are often coordinated, they can also diverge from one another (e.g., we can smile when we feel unhappy). Emotion expression, then, refers to the behavioral component of emotional reactions, indexed via several indicators, typically including facial expressive behavior, vocal characteristics (such as tone), posture, and gesture (reviewed in Russell, Bachorowski, & Fernandez-Dols, 2003).

What Are the Functions of Emotion Expression?

It has often been noted that the majority of emotion expressions occur during social interaction (e.g., Ekman, 1992; 1993). Following Darwin's seminal (1872) work on emotional expression, a surge of modern research has elucidated the critical role of emotional behavior in signaling conspecifics. Two primary types of signaling function have been emphasized. One function is *informative*. That is, many facial and vocal displays of emotion communicate information in a fairly reliable fashion to receivers about the senders' emotions and their social intentions (e.g., Ekman, 1993, Fridlund, 1992). For example, senders' displays of embarrassment communicate appeasement and a future intent to submit to the receivers' desires (Keltner & Anderson, 2000). A second function of emotional behaviors in social interactions is *evocative*. That is, emotional behaviors elicit responses from others that are relevant to the emotional situation or event. For example, smiling evokes affiliative tendencies (Keltner & Bonanno, 1997); displays of anger motivate fear responses in others (Dimberg & Öhman, 1996); and displays of sadness or distress typically elicit sympathy, helping, and increased proximity to the individual (see Rottenberg, Gross, Wilhelm, Najmi, & Gotlib, 2002). In this way, emotion expressions can in themselves be a potent emotional stimulus that alters feeling states (Bachorowski & Owren, 2001), behavior (Wexler, Levenson, Warrenburg, & Price, 1993), and/or physiology (Dimberg & Öhman, 1996).

It is important to acknowledge complexities in the instantiation of these informative and evocative functions. With respect to the informative function, emotion expressions often contain ambiguous information regarding a sender's internal state. This ambiguity may be due to a deceptive intent or simply because the relationship between emotion expressions and feelings is only probabilistic. For example, laughter can be emitted not only when a person experiences positive feelings, but also when negative feelings such as anger, anxiety, or sadness are felt (e.g., Keltner &

Bonanno, 1997). This ambiguity explains why observers so often rely upon contextual information to decode expressive behaviors like laughter. The *evocative* effects of emotion, similarly, are probabilistic and depend upon the surrounding context: Whereas laughing at a party is likely to evoke laughter from others, laughing at a funeral ceremony is likely to evoke anger.

In sum, as basic research elucidates the normal functions of expressive behavior (as well as complexities surrounding these functions), we are placed in a stronger position to understand the impact of clinical disorders on emotion-expressive behavior. Indeed, psychopathologists have conducted groundbreaking empirical studies of expressive behavior in several psychiatric conditions, including schizophrenia (Kring, 1999) and psychopathy (Patrick, Cuthbert, & Lang, 1994). The study of expressive behavior in depression has lagged relative to these other disorders; nevertheless, depression researchers have generated several noteworthy findings, which we review.

Empirical Studies of Emotion Expression in Depression

Major Depressive Disorder is formally classified among the mood disorders and includes several affective symptoms, such as persistent sad mood, a loss of interest or pleasure in daily activities, and guilt. Although expressive behavioral signs are not required for the diagnosis of depression, clinicians may use such signs as symptom indicators (e.g., sad facial and vocal cues; American Psychiatric Association, 2000). Depression is thus a disorder with strong affective features that warrant a systematic investigation of emotion expression.

Because only a small corpus of studies of emotion expression in depression focuses upon specific emotion expressions (e.g., fear or anger; Ekman, 1992), we structure our review using a broader distinction between positive and negative emotion expressions. This distinction is one that is embedded in many investigations, drawing from theories of motivation that delineate two systems of emotional activation (e.g., Gray 1982): an appetitive system associated with positive feeling states and prototypically expressed by behavioral approach, and a defensive system associated with negative feeling states and prototypically expressed by behavioral escape or avoidance.

Naturalistic Studies

Naturalistic, uncontrolled observations are one important source of information about emotion expression in depression. Naturalistic studies' signal virtue is ecological validity. Thus, naturalistic studies may be especially useful for connecting expressive behavior to real-life social impairments, especially when observations are made from important relationships, such as marriage (Segrin & Abramson, 1994).

Positive Emotions

Given the deficits in pleasure (anhedonia) reported by many depressed persons (American Psychiatric Association, 2000), investigators' focus on positive emotion expressive behavior makes good sense. Indeed, some commentators regard anhedonic deficits to be an "affective signature" of depression (e.g., Davidson, 1998). Several behavioral indices of positive emotion have been traditionally used: smiling, raised eyebrows, gaze at one's interaction partner, head movements, and amount of gesture.

Several types of naturalistic studies have demonstrated depression-related reductions in positive expressive behavior. One group of studies has assessed expressive behavior during clinical interviews. In one such investigation, the frequency and duration of smiling, eyebrow movements, head movements, and gaze (a measure of interest) were examined among recently admitted depressed or schizophrenic inpatients and healthy nonpsychiatric controls (Jones & Pansa, 1979). Depressed and schizophrenic inpatients smiled less frequently and for a shorter period of time during the interview than the control group. Depressed inpatients also demonstrated abnormalities in gaze, exhibiting shorter gaze duration than the other two groups and less frequent gaze than healthy controls. These results were largely replicated by Ellgring (1989), who found that depressed inpatients displayed less smiling behavior, eyebrow raising, and gazing at the interviewer than did nonpsychiatric controls. Finally, depressed outpatients also exhibit reduced levels of gaze and smiling during clinical interviews (Troisi & Moles, 1999), suggesting that these deficits also characterize less severe depression.

Depressed patients have also been observed as they freely behave in hospital settings (e.g., hallways and recreation rooms). Depressed patients on a hospital ward displayed fewer facial expressions conveying interest, nodded their head and gestured less frequently, and exhibited less gaze behavior than nondepressed psychiatric inpatients (Fossi, Faravelli, & Paoli, 1984). In short, depressed persons routinely exhibit reduced positive emotion-expressive behavior in clinical settings.

Observations recorded during unstructured social interactions, such as those that occur with strangers, may be more representative than clinically based observations of depressed persons' typical social interaction. For example, one study paired depressed and nondepressed undergraduate females (i.e., targets) with a nondepressed female undergraduate stranger: depressed targets smiled less frequently, demonstrated fewer hand gestures, and evinced fewer facial expressions connoting pleasantness and arousal than the nondepressed targets (Gotlib & Robinson, 1982). Another investigation of stranger interaction contrasted depressed subjects' nonverbal behavior during dyad and group interactions to that of nondepressed psychiatric subjects and nonpsychiatric controls (Youngren & Lewinsohn, 1980). Although no behavioral differences were observed for dyadic interactions, during group interactions (with members of the other participant groups), depressed participants displayed reduced eye contact and less pleasant and aroused facial expressions than the nonpsychiatric controls.

Mother-infant interactions afford a particularly valuable assessment context for the behavioral expression of positive emotion, as the verbal limitations of infants lead mothers to rely heavily on emotion-expressive behavior in their transactions with infants. Consistent with findings elsewhere of attenuated expression of positive emotion in depression, depressed mothers spend less time than nondepressed mothers expressing positive emotion while playing with their infants (e.g., Cohn, Campbell, Matias, & Hopkins, 1990; Field, Healy, Goldstein, & Guthertz, 1990). Moreover, depressed mothers are also less likely to appropriately modulate their expression of positive emotion as the play situation changes. Field (1984) compared the positive facial expressions of depressed and nondepressed mothers who interacted with their infants in three situations: "spontaneous," in which mothers were instructed to play normally with their infants; "depressed," in which the mother was instructed to look depressed; and "reunion," in which the mother was asked to return to her normal pattern of interaction with her infant. Interestingly, whereas nondepressed mothers modulated positive emotion appropriately to mirror situational changes (increased in the "spontaneous" and "reunion" conditions relative to the "depressed" condition), depressed mothers displayed similarly few positive facial expressions across situations. As we will see, depressed persons' lack of appropriate modulation of their expressive behavior is a recurrent theme of this chapter.

Depressed individuals also evidence attenuated positive emotional expression in spousal relations. For example, depressed persons' marital interactions have been found to be low in facilitative behavior (e.g., humor, approval, affirmation; Biglan, Hops, Sherman, Friedman, Arthur, & Osteen., 1985; Nelson & Beach, 1990). Because facilitative behavior is a composite of *both* nonverbal and verbal positive behaviors, it is unclear how nonverbal expressive behavior contributes to these findings. Mitigating this concern, however, Bradbury, Beach, Fincham, and Nelson (1996) found low levels of facilitative behavior in depressed spouses using a "pure" nonverbal measure of behavior. Ruscher & Gotlib (1988) used the same coding system as Bradbury et al. (1996) but found only non-significantly lower levels of positive nonverbal behavior in depressed spouses. Taken as a whole, however, naturalistic investigations provide good evidence of diminished expression of positive emotion in depression.

Negative Emotions

Although negative emotion is featured prominently in many theories of depression, cognitive theories (e.g., Beck, 1967) make perhaps the strongest predictions that depression will magnify expressive behaviors reflecting negative emotion. Naturalistic studies have addressed this prediction using several indices of negative emotion-expressive behavior: facial expressions of sadness, anger, fear, or disgust; crying; gaze down or away from one's interaction partner; slouched or slumped body posture; shaking or thrusting of the head; and self-grooming or self-touching behavior (a sign of anxiety).

Negative emotion-expressive behaviors in depressed patients have often been investigated in clinical settings. Results here have been mixed. Comparisons between recently admitted depressed and schizophrenic inpatients and nonpsychiatric controls in self-touching behavior and eyebrow furrowing (i.e., as in a frown) during a clinical interview revealed no group differences in eyebrow furrowing, but depressed inpatients engaged in more self-touching behaviors than the other groups (Jones & Pansa, 1979). In another study of interview behaviors, depressed participants exhibited *less* self-touching behavior than their nondepressed counterparts but greater frequency of eyebrow furrowing, shaking and thrusting of the head, and shoulder shrugging (Troisi & Moles, 1999). Finally, observations of free behavior of depressed and nondepressed psychiatric inpatients on a hospital ward revealed no group differences in body posture, but greater frequency of arm crossing and display of sad facial expressions in depressed patients (Fossi et al., 1984). In general, depressed individuals thus appear to express negative emotion more frequently than nondepressed individuals in clinical settings. The discrepancies in results for particular behaviors (e.g., eyebrow furrowing and self-touching) are likely due to several factors such as the inconsistent categorization of target behaviors, varying data-gathering procedures, and variations in the specific behavioral context that is assessed (Mash & Foster, 2001) Although these methodological issues fall outside the scope of this chapter, they are all important for future work to address.

Increased expression of negative emotion in depression has also been manifested in the less verbally centered context of mother-infant interactions. Depressed mothers evidence more expressions of negative emotion during play interactions with their infants relative to nondepressed mother-infant interactions (Cohn et al., 1990; Field et al., 1990). In addition, depressed mothers lack normal modulation of their negative emotional expression, displaying negative expressions in a flat, unchanging fashion. This was the pattern of results obtained in Field's (1984) aforementioned study in which depressed and nondepressed mothers interacted with their infants under "spontaneous," "depressed," and "reunion" conditions: in contrast with nondepressed mothers who displayed appropriate modulation of negative expressions (e.g., higher levels in the "depressed" condition than in the other two conditions), depressed mothers evinced similarly high levels of negative expression across all conditions.

Given the high prevalence of marital distress among depressed individuals (Beach, Whisman, & O'Leary, 1994), marital relationships are another important context to hypothesize elevated negative emotion expression in depressed individuals. Consistent with this expectation, it has been repeatedly found that depressed wives display greater levels of depressive behavior (a composite of verbal and nonverbal behavior) during discussion of a marital problem than their husbands or the wives of healthy comparison couples (Biglan et al., 1985; Nelson & Beach, 1990). Moreover, under the same conditions, depressed spouses demonstrate more overall negative nonverbal behaviors when compared with spouses in a healthy control group (Bradbury et al., 1996; Ruscher & Gotlib, 1988) and also display more negative affective expressions and more frequent crying than nondepressed spouses or nondepressed comparison couples (Hautzinger, Linden, & Hoffman, 1982).

In sum, robust support has been garnered for the proposition that depressed individuals evince more frequent displays of negative emotion in naturalistic settings. As was seen with positive expression, these findings generalize across a variety of social contexts and interaction partners, including health care providers, infants, and spouses.

Limitations of Naturalistic Studies

Although naturalistic studies provide a wealth of data demonstrating that emotion expression is altered in depression, they are poor at isolating the source of depression-related differences in emotion expression. In a clinical interview setting, for instance, depressed persons' greater negative emotion expression might simply reflect the fact that depressed persons have many more negative conversation topics at the ready (i.e., negative life events). Likewise, increased negative emotional responding during naturalistic interactions may be attributable to the unusual toxicity of the environments that often surround depressed persons (e.g., frequent attacks by a critical spouse). From this perspective, it is unclear whether differences in naturalistic studies expose the influence of situational factors or changes in the emotion system per se.

Experimental Studies

Stronger statements concerning group differences in emotional behavior are possible in experimental studies, which assess emotion under carefully controlled laboratory conditions. Typically, participants' expressive behavioral responses are measured during presentation of standardized emotional stimuli (e.g., films, photographs, etc.). Moreover, laboratory studies also have the advantage (over naturalistic studies) that emotion expression can readily be assessed in the same person under several different conditions in a within-subjects design, allowing for the sensitive measurement of behavioral change or reactivity.

Positive Emotions

Corroborating naturalistic studies, experimental findings largely indicate that depressed individuals express fewer positive emotions than their nondepressed counterparts. A study of depression and schizophrenia revealed that depressed participants and blunted schizophrenics produced fewer positive facial expressions in response to consuming drinks and viewing film clips intended to elicit positive emotion than did nondepressed participants and nonblunted schizophrenics (Berenbaum & Oltmanns, 1992). Depressed participants also evidenced fewer and less intense positive facial expressions than nondepressed participants when viewing positively valenced slide stimuli (Sloan, Strauss, & Wisner, 2001).

Other experimental investigations have objectively recorded facial behavior with facial electromyography (EMG); this technique can detect subtle changes in facial tonus that cannot be seen by observers (Fridlund & Cacioppo, 1986). Two regions that generate EMG activity have been emphasized: the zygomatic region, which falls between the mouth and the cheekbones and is activated in smiling, and the corrugator region, which lies above the bridge of the nose and is activated in expressions of negative emotions, including sadness, grief, pain, anger, and fear.

EMG studies of zygomatic activity are most pertinent to positive emotion expression. Greden and colleagues compared zygomatic activity of depressed inpatients with healthy controls who were instructed to generate happy and sad memories and reexperience the feelings associated with each memory; a neutral comparison condition asked participants to think of their activities during a typical day. As expected, normal controls' zygomatic activity fluctuated appropriately as a function of imagery condition (e.g., higher in happy than baseline imagery), but depressed inpatients generally did not differentiate these conditions (Greden, Genero, Price, Feinberg, & Levine, 1986). A lack of appropriate modulation of positive emotional expression has also been obtained when examining depressed persons' zygomatic responses to photographs of actors posing happy, sad, or neutral facial expressions: Normal control participants, but not depressed participants, exhibited appropriate stimuli-dependent changes in positive emotional expression (i.e., zygomatic activity higher while viewing happy faces than while viewing sad faces; Wexler et al., 1993). Finally, depressed individuals exhibit reduced overall levels of zygomatic activity when generating emotional imagery in response to standardized, hypothetical scenarios (Gehricke & Shapiro, 2000). Taken together, these EMG findings constitute robust evidence that depressed participants demonstrate a lack of modulation of positive expression in response to varying types of stimulation and (in some cases) lower overall levels of positive emotion expression.

Negative Emotions

Contrary to naturalistic studies and to the predictions of cognitive theories, there is little experimental evidence that depressed individuals respond to negative stimuli with more frequent or more intense expressions of negative emotion. The few experimental findings consistent with the potentiation of negative emotion are from methodologically weak studies, such as those that use highly contrived conditions to elicit emotion (e.g., the voluntary posing of negative facial expressions; Jaeger, Borod, & Peselow, 1986) or those that lack a neutral reference condition needed for a true assessment of emotional reactivity (e.g., Sloan, Strauss, Quirk, Sajatovic, 1997)

The experimental literature contains also several null findings for negative emotion expression (again consistent with a lack of evidence for potentiation). For example, depressed, schizophrenic, and healthy individuals who sampled negative-tasting (i.e., disgusting) drinks and viewed negative film clips exhibited no-depression related differences in negative facial expressions during any of these tasks (Berenbaum & Oltmanns, 1992; for similar null findings using film stimuli, see Rottenberg, Kasch, Gross, & Gotlib, 2002). Finally, there were no-depression related differences in negative emotion expression in response to slides intended to elicit the negative expressions of fear, disgust, and sadness (Sloan et al., 2001).

One explanation for these null findings is that experimental procedures rarely evoke strong forms of negative emotion. A study conducted in our laboratory addressed this issue by examining crying (Rottenberg, Gross, et al., 2002), a strong behavioral form of sadness that many clinical observers believe is potentiated by depression (American Psychiatric Association, 2000). Depressed and nondepressed participants viewed a neutral video clip followed by a sad film clip while observable facial expressions were coded. Surprisingly, and contrary to clinical lore, depressed and nondepressed participants were equally likely to visibly cry during the sad film clip. Additionally, and also contrary to clinical intuition, nondepressed participants who cried tended to exhibit greater changes in observable sadness than did depressed individuals (Rottenberg, Gross, et al., 2002). In other words, potentiation of negative emotion expression was not evident even for a negative behavior that is strongly associated with depression.

Studies of corrugator EMG activity have also undercut the idea of potentiated negative emotion expression in depression. An investigation employing self-generated happy, sad, and "typical day" imagery found that normal controls evidenced appropriate corrugator reactivity to negative stimuli, exhibiting significant increases between baseline and the sad imagery conditions. By contrast, depressed patients exhibited no significant differences in corrugator activity between baseline and any of the imagery conditions (Greden et al., 1986). Another study of self-generated imagery instructed depressed and nondepressed psychiatric patients to envision themselves in hypothetical scenarios that differed in emotional valence (Gehricke & Shapiro, 2000). Again, contrary to the potentiation hypothesis, depressed individuals had lower levels of corrugator activity across all scenarios than did nondepressed individuals and exhibited a non-significant trend toward lower, rather than higher, levels of corrugator activity than nondepressed participants when responding to negative scenarios. Finally, during exposure to emotional face stimuli, only nondepressed individuals demonstrated appropriate corrugator reactivity to changes in face valence; again, depressed individuals displayed an absence of reactivity to changes in face valence (Wexler et al., 1993).

In a novel experimental paradigm, two studies have examined depression-related differences in startle modulation (a defensive reflex to aversive stimulation). In this paradigm, individuals are startled (typically with a loud noise) while they view pictorial stimuli, and the magnitude of each startle eye blink is measured via facial EMG. Among healthy nondepressed individuals, it is well established that the magnitude of blinks increases as the valence of stimuli becomes increasingly negative (reviewed in Patrick et al., 1994). In strong contrast to nondepressed individuals, depressed individuals' blink magnitude is unaffected by changes in picture valence (Allen, Trinder, & Brennan, 1999; Dichter, Tomarken, Shelton, & Sutton, 2004). The loss of appropriate startle modulation is consistent with the body of evidence we have reviewed suggesting depressed persons are behaviorally insensitive to changes in the emotional environment.

Summary of Empirical Findings

Naturalistic studies indicate that when assessed in their everyday environments, depressed individuals exhibit lesser positive emotion expression and greater negative emotion expression than healthy individuals. At the same time, most naturalistic studies assess only a single context and do not impose control over this context. Interestingly, when the environment is carefully controlled in experimental studies, fewer differences in the overall level of negative emotion expression emerge between depressed and nondepressed individuals. More importantly, when emotion is assessed in multiple experimental contexts, data often indicate that depressed individuals exhibit a lack of behavioral responsiveness to changes in the emotional environment. In this light, depressed persons' negative expressivity and lack of positive expressivity appears to be a relatively invariant response set. We now discuss this stereotyped pattern of emotional response in greater detail and consider its implications for social functioning

Toward Integration: Emotion Context-Insensitivity of Behavior in Depression

Depression persons are often less behaviorally reactive to positive emotion cues—so much so that it is regarded by some as the "affective signature" of depression (e.g., Davidson, 1998). However, as we have reviewed, an impressive amount of evidence suggests that depressed persons exhibit constricted emotion-expressive behavior *across* both positive and negative emotional contexts. Though deficits in positive expression have received the bulk of the attention, depressed persons often exhibit a broad behavioral insensitivity that is independent of valence. We thus recommend the term *emotion context-insensitivity* as a parsimonious way to characterize depressed persons' expressive behavior (ECI; Rottenberg & Gotlib, 2004; Rottenberg, Gross, & Gotlib, 2005). In the remainder of this chapter, we discuss the theme of emotion context-insensitivity, highlighting its potential utility for understanding the relationship between emotion expression and social impairment in depression.

Depressed persons experience social dysfunctions that range from rejection, marital difficulties, social isolation, and lack of social support to poor relationship quality with parents, spouses, and friends (for reviews, see Rottenberg & Gotlib, 2004; Segrin & Abramson, 1994). Few empirical links currently exist between these social deficits and patterns of emotion expression such as ECI. If emotion-expressive behavior typically performs *informative* and *evocative* functions that guide social interactions (as is suggested by basic research), it is logical that the absence of dynamic expressive behavior would be socially impairing. Our remaining discussion is intended to underscore the plausibility and potential importance of this hypothesis.

Emotion Context-Insensitivity in Depression and the Informative Functions of Emotion

What information is conveyed by emotion-expressive behaviors in depression? Although expressive displays are typically open to many interpretations, it is plausible that some common interpretations of ECI in depression impair social functioning. For example, an unchanging behavioral display may be construed to mean that the displayer is disengaged and uninterested in the social interaction. Depressed individuals demonstrate a number of other behaviors that are consistent with social withdrawal (e.g., do not answer the telephone) and often report a reduced interest in other people (American Psychiatric Association, 2000). In this way, ECI in depression may powerfully reinforce other signals of social withdrawal.

In addition, depressed individuals' lack of dynamic expressive behavior may render depressed persons "difficult to read," an opacity that presumably impedes social communication. Moreover, in many contexts, depressed persons' expressive displays—to the extent that they are informationally impoverished—may violate others' expectations about interaction. Indeed, theorists have observed that most communicative behaviors carry an implicit demand for an appropriately elaborate and relevant response (e.g., Davis, 1982). For example, during many interactions, people mirror one another's emotional expression (e.g., Provine, 1992), and individuals who engage in high levels of interpersonal mirroring are judged as being more likeable (Chartrand & Bargh, 1999). An individual whose behavior is rigid and unchanging over the course of one or more interactions would naturally frustrate their partners' desire for dynamic feedback both about their own performance and about the state of their relationship. In sum, the lack of emotion-expressive reciprocity inherent in ECI may be one of several routes whereby ECI disrupts depressed persons' interpersonal coordination and erodes relationship quality.

Emotion Context-Insensitivity in Depression and the Evocative Functions of Emotion

We know relatively little concerning the precise evocative effects of emotion expression in depression. One complexity in considering this issue is that depressed people produce such a wide range of effects upon other people. For example, depressed people can elicit both care and rejection even from the same interaction partner (Coyne, 1976). Granting that depressed individuals evoke a multitude of effects upon others, ECI may be implicated in depressed persons' problematic social interactions.

For example, lack of dynamic behavior in ECI may signal to others that the displayer is "out of action" and thus induce others (particularly intimates) to de-escalate conflict and recruit support. This is consistent with recent theories that have highlighted the importance of appeasement and de-escalation in depressive behaviors (Price, Gardner, & Erickson, 2004; Allen & Badcock, 2003). Consistent with this interpretation, Biglan et al. (1985) have shown that depressive behavior can reduce the likelihood of hostile responses from family members. In this respect, depressive displays may be similar to displays of distress in nondepressed individuals, which have the capacity to elicit from others signs of distress, concern, and overt attempts at helping (e.g., Batson & Shaw, 1991).

On the other hand, ECI is also likely to be implicated in the rejection of depressed individuals. Interestingly, we know from "still face" paradigms that infants clearly find a lack of expressive behavior to be aversive and respond to these displays with increased irritability (see Field, 1984). Indirect evidence suggests that this pattern of aversive responses to inexpressive partners may persist into adulthood (Butler, Egloff, Wilhelm, Smith, Erickson, & Gross, 2003). Moreover, as ECI describes emotional behaviors that are emitted without respect for the immediate audience or social context, these behaviors may be judged as being socially inappropriate and lead to rejection, an insight that has been incorporated into social skills treatments for depression (Becker, Heimberg, & Bellack, 1987). Our suggestive remarks indicate a clear need for additional research to document the evocative effects of ECI, particularly the extent to which factors such as the audience, social context, and accompanying verbal behavior modify the evocative effects of expressive behaviors in depression (see also Allen & Badcock, 2003).

Future Research

We are confident that the integration of basic emotion science with psychopathology research will continue to bear important, and sometimes surprising, insights regarding the ways in which emotion-related processes are affected by depression (and other forms of disorder). Further descriptions of emotion-expressive patterns (such as ECI) are needed to integrate our knowledge of social and emotional dysfunction in depression. We close by highlighting three directions critical to this effort.

1. Expressive behavior is one important aspect of a dynamically changing social interaction. Isolating the effects of behavioral patterns such as ECI on social functioning will require methods to disentangle the effects of expressive behavior from other aspects of the social interactions (e.g., verbal content). Although this is a formidable methodological issue, it is not insuperable (e.g., time-series analysis).
2. It is unclear how changes in expressive behavior such as ECI relate to the depressed state. The overwhelming majority of studies of emotional behavior in depression (including those reviewed here) have assessed subjects only when they are acutely ill. It is therefore unclear whether ECI is a correlate of the depressed state, which co-varies with symptoms, or a more trait-like characteristic, which may be related to an enduring vulnerability to depression. Regular inclusion in research studies of asymptomatic individuals who have a history of Major Depressive Disorder is needed to address this important "state-trait" issue.
3. A final unresolved question concerns the specificity of ECI and other abnormalities in expressive behavior to depression. Until comparisons are routinely made

between depression and other psychiatric conditions (such as anxiety disorders), claims about diagnostic specificity must be held in abeyance. We recommend others take a more frankly comparative approach to emotional behavior in psychopathology.

References

Allen, N. B., & Badcock, P. B. T. (2003). The social risk hypothesis of depressed mood: evolutionary, psychosocial, and neurobiological perspectives. *Psychological Bulletin, 129,* 887–913.

Allen, N. B., Trinder, J., & Brennan, C. (1999). Affective startle modulation in clinical depression: preliminary findings. *Biological Psychiatry, 46,* 542–550.

American Psychiatric Association (2000). *Diagnostic and statistical manual of mental disorders* (4th ed,, text revision). Washington, DC: American Psychiatric Association.

Bachorowski, J., & Owren, M. J. (2001). Not all laughs are alike: voiced but not unvoiced laughter readily elicits positive affect. *Psychological Science, 12,* 252–257.

Batson, C. D., & Shaw, L. L. (1991). Evidence for altruism: toward a Pluralism of prosocial motives. *Psychological Inquiry, 2,* 107–122.

Beach, S. R. H., Whisman, M. A., & O'Leary, K. D. (1994). Marital therapy for depression: theoretical foundation, current status, and future directions. *Behavior Therapy, 25,* 345–371.

Beck, A. T. (1967). *Depression: clinical, experimental, and theoretical aspects.* New York: Harper and Row.

Becker, R. E., Heimberg, R. G., & Bellack, A. S. (1987). *Social skills treatment for depression.* New York: Pergamon Press.

Berenbaum, H., & Oltmanns, T. F. (1992). Emotional experience and expression in schizophrenia and depression. *Journal of Abnormal Psychology, 101,* 37–44.

Biglan, A., Hops, H., Sherman, L., Friedman, L. S., Arthur, J., & Osteen, V. (1985). Problem-solving interactions of depressed women and their husbands. *Behavior Therapy, 16,* 431–451.

Bradbury, T. N., Beach, S. R. H., Fincham, F. D., & Nelson, G. M. (1996). Attributions and behavior in functional and dysfunctional marriages. *Journal of Consulting and Clinical Psychology, 64,* 569–576.

Butler, E. A., Egloff, B., Wilhelm, F. W., Smith, N. C., Erickson, E. A., & Gross, J. J. (2003). The social consequences of expressive suppression. *Emotion, 3,* 48–67.

Chartrand, T. L., & Bargh, J. A. (1999). The chameleon effect: the perception-behavior link and social interaction. *Journal of Personality and Social Psychology, 76,* 893–910.

Cohn, J. F., Campbell, S. B., Matias, R., & Hopkins, J. (1990). Face-to-face interactions of postpartum depressed and nondepressed mother-infant pairs at two months. *Developmental Psychology, 26,* 15–23.

Connell, D., & Joint, M. (1996). *Driver aggression.* Washington, DC: AAA Foundation for Traffic Safety.

Coyne, J. C. (1976). Toward an interactional description of depression. *Psychiatry, 39,* 28–40.

Darwin, C. (1872). *The expression of emotions in man and animals.* New York: Philosophical Library.

Davidson, R. J. (1998). Affective style and affective disorders: perspectives from affective neuroscience. *Cognition and Emotion, 12,* 307–330.

Davis, D. (1982). Determinants of responsiveness in dyadic interaction. In W. Ickes & E. S. Knowles (Eds.), *Personality, roles, and social behavior* (pp. 85–139). New York: Springer-Verlag.

Dichter, G. S., Tomarken, A. J., Shelton, R. C., & Sutton, S. K. (2004). Early-and late-onset startle modulation in unipolar depression. *Psychophysiology. 41,* 433–440

Dimberg, U., & Oehman, A. (1996). Behold the wrath: psychophysiological responses to facial stimuli. *Motivation & Emotion, 20,* 149–182.

Ekman, P. (1992). An argument for basic emotions. *Cognition and Emotion, 6*, 169–200.
Ekman, P. (1993). Facial expression and emotion. *American Psychologist, 48*, 384–392.
Ellgring, H. (1989). *Nonverbal communication in depression.* New York: Cambridge University Press.
Field, T. (1984). Early interactions between infants and their postpartum depressed mothers. *Infant Behavior and Development, 7*, 517–522.
Field, T., Healy, B., Goldstein, S., & Guthertz, M. (1990). Behavior-state matching and synchrony in mother-infant interactions of nondepressed versus depressed dyads. *Developmental Psychology, 26*, 7–14.
Fossi, L., Faravelli, C., & Paoli, M. (1984). The ethological approach to the assessment of depressive disorders. *Journal of Mental and Nervous Disease, 172*, 332–341.
Fridlund, A.J. (1992). The behavioral ecology and sociality of human faces. In M. S. Clark (Ed.), *Emotion* (pp. 90–121). Newbury Park, CA: Sage.
Fridlund, A. J., & Cacioppo, J. T. (1986). Guidelines for human electromyographic research. *Psychophysiology, 23*, 567–589.
Frijda, N. (1986). *The emotions.* New York: Cambridge University Press.
Gehricke, J. G., & Shapiro, D. (2000). Reduced facial expression and social context in major depression: discrepancies between facial muscle activity and self-reported emotion. *Psychiatry Research, 95*, 157–167.
Gotlib, I. H., & Robinson, L. A. (1982). Responses to depressed individuals: discrepancies between self-report and observer-rated behavior. *Journal of Abnormal Psychology, 91*, 231–240.
Gray, J. A. (1982). *The neuropsychology of anxiety: an enquiry into the functions of the septo-hippocampal system.* Oxford: Oxford University Press.
Greden, J. F., Genero, N., Price, H. L., Feinberg, M., & Levine, S. (1986). Facial electromyography in depression. *Archives of General Psychiatry, 43*, 269–274.
Hautzinger, M., Linden, M., & Hoffman, N. (1982). Distressed couples with and without a depressed partner: an analysis of their verbal interaction. *Journal of Behavior Therapy and Experimental Psychiatry, 13*, 307–314.
Jaeger, J., Borod, J. C., & Peselow, E. (1986). Facial expression of positive and negative emotions in patients with unipolar depression. *Journal of Affective Disorders, 11*, 43–50.
Jones, I. H., & Pansa, M. (1979). Some nonverbal aspects of depression and schizophrenia occurring during the interview. *Journal of Nervous and Mental Disease, 167*, 402–409.
Keltner, D. & Anderson, C. (2000). Saving face for Darwin: the functions and uses of embarrassment. *Current Directions in Psychological Science, 9*, 187–192.
Keltner, D., & Bonanno, G. A. (1997). A study of laughter and dissociation: distinct correlates of laughter and smiling during bereavement. *Journal of Personality & Social Psychology*, 73, 687–702.
Keltner, D., & Kring, A.M. (1998). Emotion, social function, and psychopathology. *Review of General Psychology, 2*, 320–342.
Keltner, D., Kring, A.M., & Bonanno, G.A. (1999). Fleeting signs of the course of life: facial expression and personal adjustment. *Current Directions in Psychological Science, 8*, 18–22.
Kessler, R. C. (2002). Epidemiology of depression. In I. H Gotlib & C. L. Hammen (Eds.), *Handbook of depression* (pp. 23–42). New York: Guilford Press.
Kring, A. M. (1999). Emotion in schizophrenia: old mystery, new understanding. *Current Directions in Psychological Science, 8*, 160–163.
Lang, P. J. (1978). Anxiety: toward a psychophysiological definition. In H. S. Akiskal & W. L. Webb (Eds.), *Psychiatric diagnosis: exploration of biological criteria* (pp. 265–389). New York: Spectrum.
Mash, E. J., & Foster, S. L. (2001). Exporting analogue behavioral observation from research to clinical practice: useful or cost-defective? *Psychological Assessment, 13*, 86–98.
Nelson, G. M., & Beach, S. R. H. (1990). Sequential interaction in depression: effects of depressive behavior on spousal aggression. *Behavior Therapy, 21*, 167–182.
Patrick, C. J., Cuthbert, B. N., & Lang, P. J. (1994). Emotion in the criminal psychopath: fear image processing. *Journal of Abnormal Psychology, 103*, 523–534.

Provine, R. R. (1992). Contagious laughter: laughter is a sufficient stimulus for laughs and smiles. *Bulletin of the Psychonomic Society, 30,* 1–4.

Price, J. S., Gardner, R., & Erickson, M. (2004). Can depression, anxiety and somatization be understood as appeasement displays? *Journal of Affective Disorders, 79,* 1–11.

Rottenberg, J., & Gotlib, I. H. (2004). Socioemotional functioning in depression. In M. Power (Ed.), *Mood disorders: a handbook of science and practice* (pp. 61–77). New York: Wiley.

Rottenberg, J., & Johnson, S. L. (Eds.) (2007). *Emotion and psychopathology: bridging affective and clinical science.* Washington, DC: APA Books.

Rottenberg, J., Gross, J.J., Wilhelm, F.H., Najmi, S., & Gotlib, I.H. (2002). Crying threshold and intensity in major depressive disorder. *Journal of Abnormal Psychology, 111,* 302–312.

Rottenberg, J., Kasch, K.L., Gross, J.J., & Gotlib, I.H. (2002). Sadness and amusement reactivity differentially predict concurrent and prospective functioning in major depressive disorder. *Emotion, 2,* 135–146.

Rottenberg, J., Gross, J. J., & Gotlib, I. H. (2005). Emotion context insensitivity in major depressive disorder. *Journal of Abnormal Psychology,* 114, 627–639.

Russell, J. A., Bachorowski, J., & Fernandez-Dols, J. (2003). Facial and vocal expressions of emotion. *Annual Review of Psychology, 54,* 329–349.

Ruscher, S. M., & Gotlib, I. H. (1988). Marital interaction patterns of couples with and without a depressed partner. *Behavior Therapy, 19,* 455–470.

Segrin, C., & Abramson, L. Y. (1994). Negative reactions to depressive behaviors: a communication theories analysis. *Journal of Abnormal Psychology, 103,* 655–668.

Sloan, D. M., Strauss, M. E., Quirk, S. W., Sajatovic, M. (1997). Subjective and expressive emotional responses in depression. *Journal of Affective Disorders, 46,* 135–141.

Sloan, D. M., Strauss, M. E., & Wisner, K. L. (2001). Diminished response to pleasant stimuli in depressed women. *Journal of Abnormal Psychology, 110,* 488–493.

Troisi, A., & Moles, A. (1999). Gender differences in depression: an ethological study of nonverbal behavior during interviews. *Journal of Psychiatric Research, 33,* 243–250.

Wexler, B. E., Levenson, L., Warrenburg, S., & Price, L. H. (1993). Decreased perceptual sensitivity to emotion-evoking stimuli in depression. *Psychiatry Research, 51,* 127–138.

Youngren, M. A., & Lewinsohn, P. M. (1980). The functional relationship between depression and problematic behavior. *Journal of Abnormal Psychology, 89,* 333–341.

Chapter 9
Emotion Regulation and the Anxiety Disorders: Adopting a Self-Regulation Perspective

Thomas L. Rodebaugh and Richard G. Heimberg

Introduction

Interest in the relation between difficulties in emotion regulation and the anxiety disorders has surged within recent years. For example, a search performed on PsychINFO in April 2005 for the terms *emotion regulation* and *anxiety disorder* produced 20 citations, 18 of which were published in the year 2000 or later. Recent theory and evidence regarding the anxiety disorders suggest that problems in emotion regulation may be a significant factor in these disorders. The purpose of this chapter is to explore the potential basis of a relationship between the anxiety disorders and problems in emotion regulation, as well as how knowledge of this relationship might inform treatment. We use generalized anxiety disorder (GAD) as a primary example.

GAD, Emotion Regulation, and Past Treatments

The primary characteristic of GAD is excessive, uncontrollable worry (American Psychiatric Association [APA], 2000). A recent conceptualization of GAD, based partially on the avoidance theory of worry developed by Borkovec and colleagues (e.g., Borkovec, Alcaine, & Behar, 2004), suggests that worry serves the function of helping people with GAD temporarily avoid aversive emotional experience generated by poor emotion regulation strategies (Mennin, Turk, Heimberg, & Carmin, 2004). Research generated by this model has demonstrated that individuals with GAD report greater intensity of emotional experience and greater fear of depression than nonanxious participants or participants with social anxiety disorder; compared with nonanxious participants, individuals with GAD also report less clarity regarding emotions, more difficulty identifying emotions, and more difficulty describing emotions, as well as more fear of anxiety, anger, and positive emotions (Turk, Heimberg, Luterek, Mennin, & Fresco, 2005). Individuals with GAD have also reported more difficulty repairing negative moods in their daily lives and in response to a negative mood induced in the laboratory (Mennin, Heimberg, Turk, & Fresco, 2005). Such findings are supportive of the general conclusion that people with GAD are motivated to avoid aversive experiences, and, more particularly,

A. Vingerhoets et al., (eds.), *Emotion Regulation.*

aversive emotions. They may turn to worry in an attempt to avoid these experiences. Indeed, participants who, by self-report, meet criteria for GAD are best discriminated from other groups by their endorsement of worry as a strategy for avoiding thinking about more emotional topics (Borkovec & Roemer, 1995). If the avoidance-of-emotion hypothesis is accurate, an understanding of emotion regulation may be helpful in elucidating the processes underlying GAD and other disorders that involve pathologic worry. Further, the same hypothesis suggests that treatment of GAD may be enhanced by attention to emotion regulation problems, as noted by Mennin, Heimberg, Turk, & Fresco, (2002).

Such a view differs from traditional behavioral and cognitive behavioral perspectives, in which emotions have generally been treated as unwanted symptoms that can be alleviated through changes in behavior and cognition. One of the earlier examples of a behavioral technique is systematic desensitization, which Wolpe (1958) developed to reduce anxiety. Similarly, Beck's cognitive therapy, initially applied to the treatment of depression (Beck, Rush, Shaw, & Emery, 1979) and later to the treatment of a variety of disorders, including the anxiety disorders (e.g., Beck & Emery, 1985), seeks to reduce negative affect through changing cognitions (i.e., automatic thoughts and underlying beliefs). Again, the suggestion is that unwanted emotions can be removed through a modification of other psychological processes.

More recently, some theorists have asserted that emotions are best characterized as action tendencies that serve an adaptive function (e.g., Lang, Bradley, & Cuthbert, 1998). However, when faced with psychopathology, these same theorists are left with the task of describing how normally adaptive aspects of human functioning become dysfunctional, producing what is often called *emotion dysregulation*. The concept of emotion dysregulation has been directly invoked to explain some aspects of psychopathology (e.g., borderline personality disorder; Linehan, 1993). However, tracing psychological problems to a failure in the regulation of emotions leaves open the question of how emotions are usually regulated and what leads this process to break down. A social-cognitive perspective on self-regulation provides a useful approach to defining adaptive emotion regulation strategies.

Self-Regulation and Emotion Regulation

Theories of self-regulation suggest that people have goals, that these goals are organized in some fashion, and that human behavior is largely motivated by pursuit of goals and regulated by feedback regarding goal attainment (e.g., Carver and Scheier, 1998). Carver and Scheier's approach to self-regulation, which is further informed by Higgins's (1997) theory of regulatory focus, suggests that two broad affective systems are involved in motivating pursuit of goals. One system is related primarily to approach behavior, involves largely appetitive processes, and is identified with Higgins's *promotion* focus. Generally speaking, this system is involved with making good things happen for the individual. The other system relates to avoidance behavior, defensive processes, and Higgins's *prevention* focus. Generally speaking, this system is involved with keeping bad things from happening to the individual.

According to this general viewpoint, emotions reflect perceived rate of progress toward goals. Although the term *rate of progress* may, for simplicity's sake, be read as *progress*, Carver and Scheier (1998) argue that it is not accomplishment but rather *rate* of progress toward accomplishment that produces affect. For example, people can have negative emotions despite either moving toward a goal or achieving a goal if they believe they should have been able to do so more quickly. Another point to remember in the discussion below is that the goals in question may be goals that individuals have explicitly stated, but, as Carver and Scheier (1998) note, these goals need not be available in the individual's awareness. Moreover, as reviewed by Fitzsimons and Bargh (2004), many, if not all, self-regulatory processes can proceed with little or no awareness, which suggests that emotions can also indicate rate of progress toward implicit goals.

Carver (2004) describes anxiety and fear as relating to a low rate of progress toward attaining goals of preventing negative outcomes, whereas calmness is related to a satisfactory rate of progress in preventing the same; these are the same affective poles described by Higgins (1997) as relating to a prevention regulatory focus. In contrast, sadness is related to a perceived low rate of progress toward achieving positive goals, and happiness to a satisfactory rate of progress in achieving the same; these affective poles also outline the promotion regulatory focus (Higgins, 1997). Carver (2001) suggests that these two basic goal systems are related to the many two-system motive theories that have been previously proposed (e.g., the behavioral approach and inhibition systems, as reviewed by Gray [1994]). It is beyond the scope of this article to review the large variety of psychological theories that have specified different processes or outcomes depending upon whether a goal is being approached or avoided, but we would argue that this general framework unites a variety of otherwise disparate approaches, including evolutionary approaches to social anxiety (e.g., the defense versus safety systems; Trower, Gilbert, & Sherling, 1990) and the differentiation made in Acceptance and Commitment Therapy between attempts to control unwanted emotions (i.e., avoid them) versus being willing to have them (i.e., approach them; Hayes, Strosahl, & Wilson [1999]; see also below).

The vast body of research concerning emotion, approach and inhibition systems, and prevention and promotion focus suggest that these systems are complex and interactive. Further, as suggested by Carver (2001), examination of the consequences of success and failure in everyday life suggests that goals are often interrelated in complex ways. For example, although anxiety may result from perceived difficulty in preventing negative outcomes, our clinical experience suggests that sadness and depression often also result.

This observation that anxiety often leads to depression may initially appear counterintuitive given the self-regulation theory described above. However, this sequence is explainable if failure to prevent a negative outcome is perceived as blocking one's ability to achieve positive outcomes at a satisfactory rate. For example, consider a person who struggles with social anxiety and consistently perceives social failures that lead to humiliation and embarrassment. An obvious strategy for preventing perceived social failures in the future is to no longer try to interact with people but instead actively avoid being around people. In turn, this strategy interferes with the person's ability to develop intimate relationships with others. Given that intimate relationships are a source of important rewards for many people, difficulty developing or maintaining these relationships would lead the person to perceive a lack of rewards. Indeed, when much of a person's activity is devoted to preventing harm, it is difficult to exert sustained efforts toward obtaining rewards. Thus, upon the adoption of a self-regulatory framework, it appears inevitable that high comorbidity between anxiety and depression should occur. In addition to the reasons given above, we would also expect that a perceived inability to achieve positive outcomes, leading to depression, may lead to concerns about one's ability to do anything at all, including keeping oneself safe from harm (e.g., because the person believes *I cannot do anything right*), which should increase his or her perception that prevention of negative outcomes will be more difficult in the future, leading to an increase in anxiety.

Self-Regulation and the Anxiety Disorders

From a self-regulation viewpoint, disorders primarily characterized by aversive affect (including the anxiety disorders) are, by definition, disorders of self- and emotion-regulation; thus, all anxiety disorders involve failures in emotion regulation. Anxiety disorders may be best described as syndromes that occur when excessive attempts to prevent undesired outcomes lead to impairment in pursuing desired outcomes. For the sake of brevity, we will use the terms *prevention system* and *promotion system.* By *prevention system*, we mean the behavioral framework that consists of the thoughts, behaviors, affect, and the biological underpinnings of these factors, which are all organized around the pursuit of safety or the avoidance of unwanted outcomes. We mean this system to be associated with the pursuit of avoidance goals and the regulatory focus on prevention described above. By *promotion system*, we mean the behavioral framework that is organized around the pursuit of positive goals or the approach of desired outcomes. Accordingly, we mean this system to be associated with the pursuit of approach goals or the regulatory focus on promotion described above. Basically, the implication of these definitions is that people who have anxiety disorders not only have difficulty managing an overactive prevention system, but they also have difficulty engaging their promotion systems effectively, because the prevention system is overactive and demanding of their attentional resources. The two parts of this definition, excessive efforts to prevent undesired outcomes and impairment in approach-related behaviors, are further explicated below.

People with anxiety disorders have a tendency to engage in prevention behavior when none (or at least less) is needed. In part, this statement is simply a reformulation of the evidence that people with anxiety disorders display biases in attention and interpretation that may lead to or amplify the perception of danger (e.g., in social anxiety disorder as described and reviewed by Rapee & Heimberg [1997] and Clark & Wells [1995]), as well as significant avoidance behaviors designed to reduce distress or keep the person safe. For example, people who have panic disorder with agoraphobia often display safety behaviors that are designed to prevent a feared catastrophe that might result from panic (e.g., clinging to objects in order to prevent oneself from fainting and falling), and reduction of such safety behaviors has been found to improve the effects of exposure treatment (e.g., Salkovskis, Clark, Hackmann, Wells, & Gelder, 1999), indicating that such prevention strategies are a key aspect of the disorder. It is beyond the scope of this chapter to specify how a person typically develops a tendency to engage in unnecessary prevention behavior. It is more pressing, here, to explain what we mean by *unnecessary*. The prevention system appears designed to fend off threats, maintain security, and prevent the individual's death. Indeed, all anxiety disorders, on either an individual or evolutionary basis, involve stimuli that, in different contexts, could have posed a real possibility of death (e.g., the stimuli that provoke anxiety in post-traumatic stress disorder are directly associated with an event that either caused or threatened to cause physical harm to oneself or others; APA, 2000). The prevention-related behaviors involved in anxiety disorders are considered unnecessary because they are not required to produce safety in the person's current circumstances and, indeed, tend to produce more distress over the long-term than would less prevention-related behavior.

Although a large research literature supports the relationship between anxiety disorders and excessive prevention-related behaviors, impaired promotion-related behaviors have been highlighted less directly. One strand of evidence that has received more attention lately has been the issue of quality of life, including such constructs as satisfaction with one's job and relationships. Studies have generally, and perhaps unsurprisingly, found that anxiety disorders tend to decrease quality of life (e.g., people with GAD report lower marital satisfaction and are more likely to report having no close friends; Whisman, Sheldon, & Goering, 2000). Indeed, the criteria for the diagnosis of all anxiety disorders require not only some form of excessive anxiety but also a perceived or actual interference in goal-directed behavior in life domains that are typically sources of successful approach behavior for most people (e.g., work, school, and social relationships; APA, 2000).

Perceived excessive emotion (e.g., anxiety) and related thoughts, physiologic responses, and behaviors are the symptoms of the anxiety disorders that are the most obvious. For example, in GAD, anxious apprehension about a number of topics (characterized by worry) and symptoms of excessive central nervous system activation are required for diagnosis (APA, 2000). In self-regulatory theory, emotions act as specific forms of feedback regarding goal pursuit; accepting emotions as action tendencies further implies that specific emotions call for specific types of action. In this sense, excessive experience of emotions is a symptom but not the root of the problem. Because emotions contain information about the person's rate of progress toward particular self-relevant goals, it is more properly the person's inability to effectively use this information to begin an investigation of his or her current situation that constitutes a disorder. That is, the activation of the prevention system implies a threat, and when a threat fails to materialize, the person would be better off beginning to reassess the input that triggered the alarm and quite possibly the tendencies of the alarm system as a whole. Difficulty initiating this self-corrective process may stem from several sources, but the most readily apparent is the tendency to try to prevent the very experience of anxiety (see below). Whatever the source, the person's failure to respond to this information in a self-correcting manner involves a problem not only of self-regulation but also of emotion regulation.

Perhaps the clearest and most common example of anxiety disorders as problems of emotion and self-regulation involves people who attempt to prevent themselves from experiencing one or more forms of negative affect. The concept of avoidance of negative affect as the primary problem in psychological disorders has been proposed, in some form, by multiple theorists (e.g., fear of fear in panic disorder, Goldstein & Chambless [1978]; experiential avoidance, Hayes et al. [1999]). In this circumstance, the person has adopted a goal of directly changing the feedback of the goal-attainment system (e.g., by attempting to reduce anxiety) without actually modifying the system's input in an effective way.[1] Again, the proposition that attempts to directly manage affect without reference to its source is counterproductive is not new; Chambless, Goldstein, Gallagher, and Bright (1986), in discussing the underlying causes of agoraphobia, note that clients often have a tendency of "misattribution of anxiety and other affect, such that effective problem-solving to reduce stress does not occur, and instead the somatic symptoms of anxiety become the focus of attention" (p. 151).

An extended example may be useful in fleshing out this basic problem. A person who is anxious about aversive affect is motivated to prevent such affect, which often includes the experience of fear, sadness, and anger. However, aversive affect is unavoidably triggered, from time to time, by perceptions regarding one's rate of progress toward goal attainment. For example, the person may perceive that her relationship with her husband has become less close than she would like, leading to a degree of sadness as a result of perceiving a meaningful change in position regarding this positive goal. The input, or source for those perceptions (e.g., she and her husband are spending less time together or there is less exchange of expressions of warmth and affection between them), can only be lastingly changed either through changing those perceptions, for example, through cognitive-behavioral techniques or through untrained cognitive reappraisal (e.g., Gross, 1998), giving up the goal (for a review, see Wrosch, Scheier, Carver, & Schultz, 2003), or taking steps to move toward the valued goal.

Attempts to avoid the aversive affect without addressing its relation to a goal produces no change in input and, therefore, generally fails to work. In the example given above, no matter how good the person is at temporarily suppressing sadness, the cues related to that sadness remain. This failure tends to produce further negative affect (because the apparent probability of achieving another goal is decreasing: *Not only is my marriage a shambles, but I cry too much, too [which means I am not as nice to be around as I would like]*). This escalation in affect occurs because the person has adopted a goal that she will find impossible to move toward in an

---

[1] People with anxiety disorders typically use a variety of avoidance behaviors that have the temporary capacity to change the input to the system. Avoidance is, indeed, a very effective strategy for dealing with temporary or spatially limited situations, but this is not the case for situations of concern for a person experiencing an anxiety disorder, at least in the sense that the person does not experience enough time or space to have a field of safety from which to pursue positive goals. When aversive affect itself is the feared situation, the person literally carries his feared situation through life with himself.

acceptable way (preventing negative affect) unless attention is paid to self-regulation regarding the triggering goal (cf. the "clean" vs. "dirty" distress metaphor discussed by Hayes et al. [1999, p. 136]). Such attempts to avoid negative affect constitute a form of emotion dysregulation that will lead to further negative affect as the goal of preventing negative affect is consistently not reached, because progress toward goals is neither reassessed nor adequately mobilized.

GAD: An Example of Self-Regulation Problems in the Anxiety Disorders

The above outline, although brief and relatively general, fits well with current thinking about GAD (Borkovec et al., 2004; Mennin et al., 2004). Above, we suggested that people with anxiety disorders generally attempt to avoid aversive affect without adequately addressing the implicit or explicit goals that trigger this affect. In GAD, the motivation to avoid affect is hypothesized to be answered by worry, which tends to flatten affective response as assessed through physiologic measures (e.g., Borkovec & Hu, 1990). We suggest that worry may, in fact, flatten affective response because it resembles problem-solving; thus, in pathologic worry, the person is acting *as if* goal attainment is being pursued or reevaluated, although it is not. Thus, emotions relating to avoiding (e.g., anxiety) should occur with reduced strength.[2] In other words, worry acts as a trick the person is playing on himself or herself to provide the illusion of action, when useful action seems impossible. However, failure to attend to the original aversive affect and its related goals leads to an inability to skillfully approach, avoid, or reevaluate those goals, full knowledge of which the person has avoided along with the affect. Because the importance of the goal has not changed (because the goal itself has not been reassessed), its influence on affect should periodically resurface.

The above line of reasoning further suggests how attention to emotion regulation processes may improve treatment of GAD. First, it should be noted that cognitive behavioral treatments have actually always addressed emotion regulation in some form. Such techniques implicitly address goals, the stimuli the person associates with success or failure in regard to goals, reevaluation of goals, giving up impractical or unwanted goals, and choice of behaviors to pursue goals. Cognitive restructuring techniques, although not explicitly described as addressing goals, nearly always do, in our experience. For example, Wells (1997) describes using the *vertical* (or *downward*) *arrow* technique (as first described by Burns [1980]) to guide a client from a concern (*What if I babble or talk funny?*) to feared consequences (*People will think I am [and, in fact, I am] stupid*; pp. 87–89). Although described as a method of eliciting assumptions (which will later be challenged), this technique may be

[2] Borkovec and Hu provide a similar explanation, speculating that worry may inhibit affective reaction by reducing the mismatch the behavioral inhibition system perceives between expectation and perception. In a sense, then, they appear to suggest that the behavioral inhibition system may not regard information about an aversive event to be worth reacting to because a reaction has already been ongoing (e.g., the system's output does not call for more action because the process of worry appears to constitute action).

equally well described as a means of eliciting goals and strategies for obtaining them. In the given example, the person wishes to avoid appearing to be (or actually being) stupid and takes babbling or talking funny as input indicating a widening discrepancy between current state and goal. The purpose of challenging this assumption may therefore be described as challenging the validity of *babbling and talking funny* as input in reference to an avoidance goal. We would submit that most, if not all, cognitive therapy techniques encourage more effective self-regulation and, by extension, more effective emotion regulation.

Further, behavioral techniques, such as exposure, prescribe actions that run counter to attempts to prevent negative affect. Exposure should therefore encourage clients to experience, tolerate, and learn from their affect and its relationship to their perceived and actual position relative to valued goals. As suggested by a self-regulation model, any regulation of goal-pursuit is also an emotion-regulation strategy; the fact that cognitive behavioral therapy does not contain the word *emotion* in its name does not mean that emotions are not addressed. Indeed, the fact that cognitive behavioral therapy is effective in reducing symptoms of excessive anxiety provides evidence that emotions are addressed. Further, emotions need not always be addressed explicitly in a treatment for more functional emotion regulation to result.

Direct address of emotions and their informative value, however, is specifically implicated in GAD because it appears likely that avoidance of affect is the implicit goal that drives worry and produces a recursive program of behavior leading to suffering (as suggested by the model proposed by Mennin et al. [2004]). Previously, GAD was a difficult disorder for behaviorally oriented clinicians to treat, given that the anxiety involved in the disorder is typically not tied to any specific, obvious, external situation that could be used for exposure (Borkovec & Newman, 1998). If the hypothesis that people with GAD are motivated to avoid negative affect is accurate, then it may actually be the experience of this affect that constitutes the feared stimulus. Thus, whereas exposure to particular situations is a key component of cognitive behavioral therapies for other anxiety disorders, exposure to affect itself may be the key component in treatment for GAD (Mennin et al., 2002). Again, established treatments already include some exposure to affect, but a formal, defined process of creating such an exposure could help clarify for both client and therapist what the process of change involves (see Mennin [2004] for an example of this approach). Whereas social anxiety disorder, for example, must involve exposure to feared social situations such that the person can begin to adjust her perception of her ability to prevent feared outcomes and achieve positive social interactions, treatment of GAD must include exposure to feared affective states such that the person can begin to adjust her perceived ability to act along with emotions in order to pursue or avoid valued goals, rather than attempt the impossible operation of permanently avoiding the output of the system that, by definition, helps make life meaningful, the system that engages in goal pursuit.[3]

---

[3] It should be noted it remains plausible to us that, despite the obvious external situation inherent in most of the anxiety disorders, avoidance of aversive affect, as well as avoidance of a particular situation, may play a key role for many individuals.

In conclusion, both theory and research suggest that a variety of disorders characterized by unwanted aversive affect, and especially the anxiety disorders, involve problems in emotion regulation. Specific studies have demonstrated relationships between emotion dysregulation and specific anxiety disorders (e.g., Mennin et al., 2005; Turk et al., 2005), but we suggest that it will be difficult to find an anxiety disorder that is completely unassociated with difficulties in emotion regulation (as also implied by Gross [1998]). Self-regulation theories, particularly those detailed by Carver and Scheier (1998), explicitly depict how these problems in emotion regulation relate to cognition, behavior, and difficulties with goal attainment. Therefore, although cognitive behavioral therapy has always implicitly addressed both self-regulation and emotion regulation, an explicit focus on emotion and self-regulation may be helpful for the anxiety disorders, in general, and perhaps GAD, in particular.

References

American Psychiatric Association (2000). *Diagnostic and statistical manual of mental disorders* (4th ed., text revision). Washington, DC: American Psychiatric Association.

Beck, A. T., & Emery, G. (1985). *Anxiety disorders and phobias: a cognitive perspective.* New York: Basic Books.

Beck, A. T., Rush, A. J., Shaw, B. F., & Emery, G. (1979). *Cognitive therapy of depression.* New York: Guilford.

Borkovec, T. D., & Hu, S. (1990). The effect of worry on cardiovascular response to phobic imagery. *Behaviour Research and Therapy, 28,* 69–73.

Borkovec, T. D., & Newman, M. G. (1998). Worry and generalized anxiety disorder. In P. Salkovskis, A. S. Bellack, & M. Hersen (Eds.), *Comprehensive clinical psychology, Vol. 6: adults: clinical formulation and treatment* (pp. 439–459). New York: Pergamon Press.

Borkovec, T. D., & Roemer, L. (1995). Perceived functions of worry among generalized anxiety disorder subjects: distraction from more emotionally distressing topics? *Journal of Behavior Therapy and Experimental Psychiatry, 26,* 25–30.

Borkovec, T. D., Alcaine, O., & Behar, E. (2004). Avoidance theory of worry and generalized anxiety disorder. In R. G. Heimberg, C. L. Turk, & D. S. Mennin (Eds.), *Generalized anxiety disorder: advances in research and practice* (pp. 77–108). New York: Guilford Press.

Burns, D. D. (1980). *Feeling good: the new mood therapy.* New York: William Morrow and Company.

Carver, C. S. (2001). Affect and the functional bases of behavior: on the dimensional structure of affective experience. *Personality and Social Psychology Review, 5,* 345–356.

Carver, C. S. (2004). Self-regulation of action and affect. In R. F. Baumeister & K. D. Vohs (Eds.), *Handbook of self-regulation: research, theory, and applications* (pp. 13–39). New York: Guilford Press.

Carver, C. S., & Scheier, M. F. (1998). *On the self-regulation of behavior.* New York: Cambridge University Press.

Chambless, D. L., Goldstein, A. J., Gallagher, R., & Bright, P. (1986). Integrating behavior therapy and psychotherapy in the treatment of agoraphobia. *Psychotherapy, 23,* 150–159.

Clark, D. M., & Wells, A. (1995). A cognitive model of social phobia. In R. G. Heimberg, M. R. Liebowitz, D. A. Hope, & F. R. Schneier (Eds.), *Social phobia: diagnosis, assessment, and treatment* (pp. 69–93). New York: Guilford Press.

Fitzsimons, G. M., & Bargh, J. A. (2004). Automatic self-regulation. In R. F. Baumeister & K. D. Vohs (Eds.), *Handbook of self-regulation: research, theory, and applications* (pp. 151–170). New York: Guilford Press.

Goldstein, A. J., & Chambless, D. L. (1978). A reanalysis of agoraphobia. *Behavior Therapy, 9,* 47–59.
Gray, J. A. (1994). Three fundamental emotion systems. In P. Ekman & R. J. Davidson (Eds.), *The nature of emotion: fundamental questions* (pp. 243–247). New York: Oxford University Press.
Gross, J. J. (1998). The emerging field of emotion regulation: an integrative review. *Review of General Psychology, 2,* 271–299.
Hayes, S. C., Strosahl, K. D., & Wilson, K. D. (1999). *Acceptance and commitment therapy: an experiential approach to behavior change.* New York: Guilford Press.
Higgins, E. T. (1997). Beyond pleasure and pain. *American Psychologist, 52,* 1280–1300.
Lang, P. J., Bradley, M. M., & Cuthbert, B. N. (1998). Emotion, motivation, and anxiety: Brain mechanisms and psychophysiology. *Biological Psychiatry, 44,* 1248–1263.
Linehan, M. M. (1993). *Cognitive-behavioral treatment of borderline personality disorder.* New York: Guilford Press.
Mennin, D. S. (2004). Emotion regulation treatment for generalized anxiety disorder. *Clinical Psychology and Psychotherapy, 11,* 17–29.
Mennin, D. S., Heimberg, R. G., Turk, C. L., & Fresco, D. M. (2002). Applying an emotion regulation framework to integrative approaches to generalized anxiety disorder. *Clinical Psychology Science and Practice, 9,* 85–90.
Mennin, D. S., Heimberg, R. G., Turk, C. L., & Fresco, D. M. (2005). Preliminary evidence for an emotion dysregulation model of generalized anxiety disorder. *Behaviour Research and Therapy. 43,* 1281–1310.
Mennin, D. S., Turk, C. L., Heimberg, R. G., & Carmin, C. N. (2004). Regulation of emotion in generalized anxiety disorder. In M. A. Reinecke & D. A. Clark (Eds.), *Cognitive therapy across the lifespan: evidence and practice* (pp. 60–89). New York: Cambridge University Press.
Rapee, R. M., & Heimberg, R. G. (1997). A cognitive-behavioral model of anxiety in social phobia. *Behaviour Research and Therapy, 35,* 741–756.
Salkovskis, P. M., Clark, D. M., Hackmann, A., Wells, A., & Gelder, M. G. (1999). An experimental investigation of the role of safety-seeking behaviours in the maintenance of panic disorder with agoraphobia. *Behaviour Research and Therapy, 37,* 559–574.
Trower, P., Gilbert, P., & Sherling, G. (1990). Social anxiety, evolution, and self-presentation: An interdisciplinary perspective. In H. Leitenberg (Ed.), *Handbook of social and evaluation anxiety* (pp. 11–45). New York: Plenum Press.
Turk, C. L., Heimberg, R. G., Luterek, J. A., Mennin, D. S., & Fresco, D. M. (2005). Emotion dysregulation in generalized anxiety disorder: a comparison with social anxiety disorder. *Cognitive Therapy and Research, 29,* 89–106.
Wells, A. (1997). *Cognitive therapy of anxiety disorders.* New York: Wiley.
Whisman, M. A., Sheldon, T. C., & Goering, P. (2000). Psychiatric disorders and dissatisfaction with social relationships: does type of relationship matter? *Journal of Abnormal Psychology, 109,* 803–808.
Wolpe, J. (1958). *Psychotherapy by reciprocal inhibition.* Standorf, CA: Stanford University Press; 1958.
Wrosch, C., Scheier, M. F., Carver, C. S., & Schultz, C. S. (2003). The importance of goal disengagement in adaptive self-regulation: when giving up is beneficial. *Self and Identity, 2,* 1–20.

Chapter 10
The Clinical Assessment and Treatment of Trauma-Related Self and Affect Dysregulation

Annemiek van Dijke

> *... traumatized people are frequently misdiagnosed and mistreated in the mental health system. Because of the number and complexity of their symptoms, their treatment is often fragmented and incomplete. Because of their characteristic difficulties with close relationships, they are vulnerable to become re-victimized by caregivers. They may become engaged in ongoing, destructive interactions, in which the medical ... system replicates the behavior of the abusive family. (Herman, 1992a, p. 123)*

Introduction

Exposure to extreme stressors affects people in many ways, with a strong negative impact on all levels of functioning: emotional, cognitive, behavioral, somatic, and characterological (Allen, 2001; Van der Kolk, McFarlane, & Weisaeth, 1996). However, despite a vast amount of literature on the aftermath of trauma, the long-term sequelae of attachment trauma and the complexity of adaptation to attachment trauma are still to be elaborated. Moreover, Van der Kolk (1996) cautions that one-to-one notions about causal relationships between reported trauma features and the presence of psychiatric disorders in adulthood are an oversimplification of the problem. Partially related to this issue, it appears that traumatized people are frequently misdiagnosed and treated incorrectly by clinicians. Because of the number and complexity of their symptoms, their treatment is often fragmented or incomplete (Herman, 1992a).

The aim of this chapter is to discuss the nature and significance of affect dysregulation[1] in complex and chronic psychiatric patients. In addition, an experimental assessment and treatment protocol for self and affect dysregulation will be described for patients suffering from a combination of trauma-related psychiatric disorders (mood disorders, anxiety disorders, [psycho]somatic disorders, somatoform disorders and personality disorders) and symptoms associated with posttraumatic stress disorder (PTSD). Affect dysregulation is considered a characteristic feature in

[1] Although some authors emphasize possible differences, *affect* and *emotion* are used as synonyms.

A. Vingerhoets et al., (eds.), *Emotion Regulation.*

complex trauma-related psychopathology as defined in *PTSD-associated symptoms,* also known as complex PTSD or DESNOS (Disorders of Extreme Stress Not Otherwise Specified; Herman, 1992b; e.g., Schore, 2002; Zlotnick, & Pearlstein, 1997). Especially in complex psychopathology patients, standard psychiatric classification and assessment procedures seem to be inadequate and treatment-as-usual or diagnosis-specific treatment protocols seem to be ineffective.

The presented assessment and treatment protocol is not intended to be a gold standard but should rather be considered as "work in progress." The assessment and treatment protocol encompasses lessons learned from working with traumatized patients suffering from affect dysregulation, elaborations on theoretical perspectives, and implementations of research findings.

The Theoretical and Clinical Relevance of Affect Dysregulation

According to Zajonc (1984), the initial processing of stimuli implies the appraisal of the affective tone of a stimulus as "positive or negative," or "safe or threatening." This implies that affects are most important because they contain information about our reactions to life experiences, both to the outer world and one's inner world (Schore, 2001a). As such, affects are facts in the way, which give meaning to our experiences (McCullough, Kuhn, Andrews, Kaplan, Wolf, & Hurley, 2003).

Given the importance of affect in human functioning, one would expect affect to have been at the center of attention in therapy development and therapy-effect studies. However, in recent decades, most therapies and therapy-effect studies have rather focused on cognitions and behavior avoidance, whereas the attention to affect for patients' therapeutic changes has moved to the background.

Recently, affect seems to receive more appropriate attention due to new developments in theory, assessment, and therapy (McCullough et al., 2003). Given the close interconnections with cognition, affects are fundamental forces in the development and changes of the self. Mikulincer, Shaver, and Pereg, (2003) come to conclude that since the publication of Bowlby's trilogy *Attachment and Loss* (Bowlby, 1982/1969, 1973, 1980), it has been established that attachment theory has become one of the most important conceptual frameworks for understanding the development of the self, maintaining proximity to significant others and maintaining intimate relations, and the process of affect regulation and self regulation. According to McCullough et al. (2003), profound and early affective experiences need to be taken into account when indicating psychotherapy. Working with strictly cognitive-behavioral techniques will not suffice in cases of complex trauma-related psychopathology.

Despite the increasing interest in affect, the importance of fully experiencing emotions in more complex psychopathology psychiatric patients remains unclear. Experiencing emotions, without being overwhelmed with emotions or being numbed, influences current and future behavior. The role of experiencing emotions while maintaining a sense of agency is to give meaning (Fonagy, Gergely, Jurist, & Target, 2002). The full experience of emotions makes us wonder why situations elicit emotions and why they incite us to reevaluate the situation. It is this emotion-driven reevaluation of cognitions, behaviors, and interactions (and not just through logic without reference to non-or preverbal information) that results in changes in the therapeutic process (McCullough et al., 2003).

To experience emotions while maintaining a sense of agency, one needs to be able to regulate affect in different situations (Fonagy et al., 2002).

Development and Affect

Our cognitive, emotional, behavioral, and social development occurs in an interpersonal context (Bowlby, 1982/1969, 1973, 1980; Gillath, Bunge, Shaver, Wendelken, & Mikulincer, 2005; Schore, 2001a; Siegel, 1999). The expression of emotions is important in the interaction with (significant) others and for establishing and maintaining (emotional) contact or relationships with them. The benefits of expressing emotions for our mental and somatic well-being have been investigated in various ways and in various populations (e.g., Nyklíček, Temoshok, & Vingerhoets, 2004). Nevertheless, despite a vast amount of research, the precise significance of the (non)expression of emotions for psychiatric patients remains unclear. However, it has been established that there is a relation between early adverse experiences and the development of affect dysregulation or cognitive emotional dysfunction and there is substantial evidence that affect dysregulation is involved in the etiology of psychiatric pathology (Bradley, 2000; Schore, 2001b; 2002).

In order to learn and develop strategies to express and experience emotions adequately, one needs to interact from the beginning in an attuned way with significant others. In humans, the main significant other is normally one's caregiver. This early process of interaction is well-known as attachment, and it encompasses the development of social and emotional functioning. Particularly, the process of interaction with the caregiver is critical for the healthy development of emotion recognition and expression of emotions.

Attachment stimulates the brain and thereby seems to improve the quality of the functions of the brain (Bateman & Fonagy, 2004; Siegel, 1999). Positive early human interactions appear to be crucial for the development of neural connections and neural networks necessary for adequate emotional information processing. Moreover, during the first years of life, psychophysiologic homeostasis and hormone balance are established, and attachment may be a main stimulating factor. These early developmental processes of the brain underline the importance of attachment and attuned emotional relationships. The ability to fully experience emotions also implies adequate affect regulation. But, what if something went wrong in one's early social emotional development? What if there was not a secure holding environment available? What if one failed to develop a secure attachment with caregivers? What if human connections were poor and the development of emotional information processing was disturbed? What if patients suffer from affect dysregulation? How do we go from there?

The Nature of Affect Dysregulation and the Emotional Reflective Function

The concept of affect dysregulation has never been well defined, and little research has focused on the nature of affect regulation and dysregulation (e.g., Gross 1998, 1999; Koenigsberg et al., 2002; Zittel Conklin, Bradley, & Westen, 2006). For some theorists, affect regulation denotes a process wherein the object of regulation is the affect itself (Van der Kolk et al., 1996).

For attachment theorists and psychodynamic theorists, the object of regulation is more complex: the regulation of affects is strongly linked to the regulation of the self and affective mentalization[2] (Fonagy et al., 2002). Self regulation encompasses regulation of affect, soma, cognition, behavior, and interaction (Van der Kolk, 1996). Mentalization is not just a cognitive concept, but a concept of the reflective function that encompasses cognitions, affects, and behavior as in affective reciprocity. It requires the capacity to envision mental states in self and others. Mentalized affectivity is a sophisticated kind of affect regulation that denotes how affects are experienced through the lens of emotional self-reflexivity, which can be enhanced in psychotherapy (Fonagy et al., 2002).

In the current contribution, affect dysregulation encompasses (1) the inability to regulate and modulate affective experience; this may keep the person unaware of the affective experience as either being numb or overwhelmed; (2) the incapacity to experience all aspects of affect, due to lack of the specific orienting information associated with each emotion; (3) the inadequate communication of emotion (due to being overwhelmed) or the nonexperiencing and/or nonexpression of affect (numbness), which increases the likelihood that one's needs will not be responded to by others. Consequently, this may increase the likelihood of social isolation and/or a pattern of quickly changing and emotionally instable social contacts (Gross, 1999).

Paivio and Laurent (2001) describe two manifestations of affect dysregulation that are of practical relevance for psychodiagnostic assessment and psychotherapy: *underregulation of affect* and *overregulation of affect*.

Underregulation of Affect

Underregulation of affect could be operationalized as being overaroused and overwhelmed by emotion and not being able to modulate these emotions.

Patients manifesting underregulation of affect may be characterized by either of the following: (1) being overwhelmed by emotions; (2) being overaroused; (3) having difficulty handling aggression; (4) having difficulty handling self-destructive impulses; (5) suicidal preoccupation; (6) provocative sexual behavior.

---

[2] *Affective Mentalization* is also referred to as *Emotional Reflective Function*; both terms are used as synonyms.

The above symptoms of underregulation are characteristic of patients with borderline personality disorder (Linehan, 1993), PTSD, and complex PTSD or DESNOS (Ford & Kidd, 1998; Pelcovitz, Van der Kolk, Roth, Mandel, & Resick, 1997; Roth, Newman, Pelcovitz, Van der Kolk, & Mandel, 1997; Van der Kolk, Pelcovitz, Roth, Mandel, McFarlane, & Herman, 1996; Wolfsdorf & Zlotnick, 2001; Zlotnick, Zakriski, Shea, Costello, Begin, Pearlstein, & Simpson, 1996).

Vignette
Diana, aged 36 years, was admitted to a mental hospital with various complaints: (1) being off-and-on depressed for several years, (2) accident-proneness (several incidents including a recent severe car crash), (3) enmeshed and poor relationships over the years (e.g., "forced" to prostitution), and (4) impulse control problems such as eating problems (lost 40 lb of overweight in 2 years). She had engaged in several psychotherapies that seemed to work out well for her, but as soon as she quit therapy, the benefits seemed to vanish. In daily life situations, she easily became very emotional over small things; it could take her more than 24 hours to get over things. She was not able to soothe herself and instead she had to get drunk and to vomit severely in order to deal with her emotions. At other times, she got so mad over small issues that she was not able to do what she planned to do. When in such a state, she had the strong urge to hurt someone, and it took almost everything in her not to give in to that impulse, but rather to yell at someone close instead. Sometimes, she acted really dangerously and hoped she would get hurt or killed while doing it.

Overregulation of Affect

Overregulation of affect can be described as being afraid to feel or experience emotions. Krystal (1988) referred to this "affect phobia" as "affect intolerance"; the inability to tolerate or experience emotions. In an attempt to ward off the emotions and to protect oneself, the emotional system becomes numb.

Patients suffering from overregulation may be characterized by the following features: (1) being numb or inhibited; (2) suffering from impairments in insight into emotions; (3) having difficulty verbalizing emotions; and (4) having difficulty analyzing emotions. These features form the core of the alexithymia concept (Taylor, Bagby, & Parker, 1997) and have also been described in patients with medically unexplained physical complaints (Kooiman, Bolk, Brand, Trijsburg, & Rooijmans, 2000), with somatization disorder, chronic pain disorder, conversion and undifferentiated somatoform disorder (see the chapter by Lumley et al., this volume).

Vignette
Miranda, 33 years old, presented with dysthymic complaints, physical pains, and interpersonal problems with her family and colleagues. A remarkable feature was her severe nail biting and her frequent up-and-down pacing. In dealing with everyday problems, she did not have any clue about her emotions, but she had headaches instead. Emotional experiencing seemed lacking, only cognitions and physical pains appeared to play a role in her life. During group therapy, she did not know what to tell about herself to group members and stuck to factual information of her experiences. She rarely talked about relations between her behavior and emotions, and she found it extremely difficult to elaborate on emotions when explicitly asked for. She often did not understand why people got so angry at her: "I did not do anything, what did you want from me?" After several weeks, group members and staff became frustrated with her.

Affective Reciprocity

Reciprocity requires a finely tuned give-and-take between individuals. Senders must adjust their messages to what they infer to be the receivers' level of comprehension, while receivers must be able to grasp the message that has been sent. Affective reciprocity requires attuned empathy, the process by which a person responds affectively to another as if she or he is experiencing the same affect (Baron-Cohen, 1988).

For many psychiatric patients, it is difficult to recognize others' facial affective expressions accompanying the emotional experiences (Baron-Cohen, 1991; 1995; Baron-Cohen, Leslie, & Frith, 1985). In addition, patients suffering from affect dysregulation have difficulty analyzing other people's emotions or to elaborate on them, as the emotional signals keep them preoccupied with their own experiences of inhibition or hyperarousal. This leads to a disturbed interpersonal emotional functioning and diminished empathic functioning. In addition, they seem to have a diminished emotional "mind sight," a reduced ability to understand the content and function of other peoples' emotional mental life.

Fonagy and Target (1996) use the term *Theory of Mind* to refer to the capacity to understand mental states in the self and others. This capacity is deficient in patients whose parents lacked empathy and emotional responsiveness. Infants view their physical and social environment in terms of the self, a phenomenon called *egocentrism*. Gradually, however, the developing child is able to view the environment from the perspective of others, to see the world through other people's eyes. This ability also includes perspective taking and is crucial for the ability to communicate and engage in reciprocal social interactions (Wenar & Kerig, 2000).

Vignette
Ann, aged 46 years, was presented to the clinical psychotherapy department by her partner. She was diagnosed with dysthymic disorder and complained of physical pains. The partner reported also interpersonal problems, in particular enmeshed (family) relations. Ann suffered from emotional numbness, lacked the capacity of empathy, and her recognition of emotional facial expressions was poor. She had several quickly changing relationships that usually ended with fierce arguments. During group therapy, she was unable to attune emotionally to others and showed little empathy toward others in emotional situations. She failed to understand what other people experienced and seemed to stick to externally oriented thinking. Others considered her as being blunt and confronting. She risks becoming the scapegoat in groups.

Attachment Trauma-Related Self-Regulation Strategies

The clinical need to diagnose patients' affective styles makes especial sense when treating patients who failed to respond to regular treatment protocols, dropped out of these kinds of treatments, or who suffered from complex and recurrent psychopathology that current treatment protocols do not apply for.

In this contribution, affect dysregulation is not only considered a factor in the development of psychopathology; it is also considered to be an important factor in pertaining, recidivist, or chronic psychopathology.

Elaborating on Mikulincers' attachment-based hyperactivating and deactivating affect regulation strategies (Mikulincer et al., 2003), two distinct insecure attachment-based self-regulation strategies are proposed, namely *Deactivating Self-Regulation Strategies* and *Hyperactivating Self-Regulation Strategies*.

Deactivating Self-Regulation Strategies encompass overregulation of affect, negative psychoform dissociation, negative somatoform dissociation, and a dismissing adult attachment style characterized by interpersonal *avoidant and dismissing* or *avoidant and fearful* behavior, which in turn conditions and upholds the insecure attachment representation. This consequently leads to an "insecure cognitive emotional information processing and insecure attachment-based Deactivating Self-Regulation Strategies" vicious circle.

In contrast, features of Hyperactivating Self-Regulation Strategies are underregulation of affect, positive psychoform dissociation, positive somatoform dissociation, and an *anxious and preoccupied* adult attachment style characterized by interpersonal clinging behavior, which in turn conditions and upholds the insecure attachment representation. This generally results in an "insecure cognitive emotional information processing and insecure attachment-based Hyperactivating Self-Regulation Strategies" vicious circle.

Moreover, when confronted with internal or external adverse events, insecurely regulated persons will never meet the sense of personal efficacy, resilience, and optimism (Mikulincer & Shaver, 2004).

These insecure attachment-based self-regulation strategies are an important factor in the explanation (1) why psychopathology and psychiatric disorders can develop and may become chronic, and (2) why current treatment protocols seem ineffective as they do not consider the impact of insecure cognitive emotional information processing and insecure attachment-based self-regulation strategies.

Traditional Assessment and Treatment of Affect Dysregulation

Well-validated instruments to measure affect dysregulation as a specific syndrome are currently lacking. Anamnesis and heteroanamnesis are useful when attempting to assess (changed) emotional behavior, but patients generally are reluctant to disclose this information. Often, these disturbed patterns of affect regulation or affective styles have been established early in life and consequently often mistaken as temperament or personality traits.

Frequently applied instruments for the assessment of affective pathology such as the Symptom Checklist (SCL-90-R; Derogatis, 1994), the Beck Depression Inventory (BDI; Beck, Rush, Shaw, & Emery, 1979), the Positive And Negative Affect Scale (PANAS, Watson, Clark, & Tellegen, 1988), the State-Trait Anxiety Inventory (STAI; Spielberger, Gorsuch, & Lushene, 1970) all fail to capture the regulatory aspects of emotional experiencing.

The concept of alexithymia can be measured with a well-validated self-report instrument: the Toronto Alexithymia Scale (TAS; Bagby, Parker, & Taylor, 1994). However, this instrument measures only the cognitive aspects of emotional dysfunctioning. The concept of alexithymia and emotional functioning can be more fully assessed with the Bermond-Vorst Alexithymia Questionnaire (BVAQ; Vorst & Bermond, 2001) and the EMOtional development Questionnaire (EMOQ; Vorst & Bermond, 2004). These instruments measure the cognitive aspects of emotional dysfunctioning (alexithymia or overregulation) and the emotional factors (impairments in emotionality and impairments in fantasizing) and social aspects (impairments in insight into other's emotions and impairments in analyzing other's emotions) of emotional (dys)functioning. Although these instruments make it possible to differentiate between subtypes of alexithymia, neither of these instruments do assess affect dysregulation as a two-dimensional phenomenon.

Currently, most affect-focused therapies focus on just one side of affect dysregulation, in particular underregulation. Examples are the Skills Training for Treating Borderline Personality Disorder (Linehan, 1993), Managing Intense Emotions and Overcoming Self-Destructive habits (Bell, 2003), Affect Management group therapy for PTSD (Wolfsdorf & Zlotnick, 2001), and the Sensimotor Therapy for Processing Traumatic Memory (Ogden, 2000). These treatment approaches focus mainly on handling affect and managing emotional behavior.

The aspect of overregulation of affect or alexithymia is often underdiagnosed or neglected. Moreover, specific treatment protocols for the treatment of affect dysregulation are scarce (Greenberg & Borger, 2001).

Preliminary Experiences with Assessing Affect Dysregulation

Given the lack of adequate instruments to assess the nature of affect dysregulation, we have introduced a clinical observation period. The pure individual and "intrapsychic" view on psychopathology and self and affect regulation has been criticized for its neglect of the importance of social and environmental factors in the etiology and maintenance of psychopathology (e.g., Teasdale & Barnard, 1993). Elaborating on that criticism, we emphasize the observation of the quantity and quality of interactions with the staff and other group members. The advantages of a clinical monitoring system for assessing emotional functioning include a prolonged monitoring of emotional behavior in interpersonal situations. During a 6-week period, emotional functioning is observed and assessed by a multidisciplinary clinical team. Each discipline has developed its own emotional functioning assessment instrument, focusing on their specific target of emotional dysfunction (Table 10.1).

Table 10.1 The multidisciplinary therapy indication forms

Discipline	Instrument
Sociotherapist	Social functioning observation form
Psychomotor therapist	"Emotional body" scale
Music therapist	Music therapy emotion scale
Creative therapist	Color emotion observation scale
Psychotherapist	Emotional functioning and group-psychotherapy indication form

To capture the nature and scope of affect dysregulation, recent insights in the fields of affective neuroscience, attachment theory, and mother-infant interaction have been integrated in an assessment procedure (e.g., Cassidy & Shaver, 1999; Griffin & Bartholomew, 1994a; 1994b; Schore, 1994; 2001a; 2001b; 2002; Siegel, 1999; Solomon & Siegel, 2003).

The assessment procedure encompasses (1) a psychodiagnostic therapy-oriented assessment procedure (quantitative assessment), consisting of clinical structured interviews, self-reports, and computerized cognitive-emotional information processing tasks (e.g., facial affect recognition; Ekman, 2003) as well as (2) a pretherapy observation procedure (qualitative assessment), applying specific observation rating scales for each discipline (Table 10.1). These rating scales have been designed to give a more objective description of what, until now, has been a clinical impression based on findings during pretherapy observation sessions. These rating scales reflect the collective sense of the different professions, and they were constructed by collaborative actions (Smeijsters, 2005).

In the pretherapy observation period, information about intrapsychic and interpersonal functioning is obtained on three aspects of affective functioning: recognition, expression, and experiencing affects. Within the experience of affects, the following three dimensions can be discerned and assessed: (1) validation of emotions, ranging from comfortable (positive) to indifference or unwanted (negative); (2) interpersonal affective behavior, all interpersonal actions between withdrawal and approach; and (3) arousability and control concerning expressed emotions, the capacity to find a balance between control over emotional behavior and arousal/excitement accompanying emotions. Below we elaborate on these dimensions.

Validation of Emotions

During patient-staff meetings, the staff can observe emotional expression, interpersonal emotional behavior, and verbalized “hot cognitions” (Teasdale & Barnard, 1993) representing mood congruent memory and context-specific encoding and retrieval of autobiographical events that are involved in coping with current personal problems and dealing with emotions in relation to other group members. During psychomotor therapy, the physical manifestations of emotions during interpersonal encounters and the (in)ability to “read” these manifestations (recognition of affect) are the main focus of attention (Taylor, Bagby, & Parker, 1997). This part of the assessment focuses on the ability to regulate the arousal levels and the ability to physically recuperate from emotions.

In addition, the ability to recognize the physical manifestations of emotions is evaluated (Rothschild, 2000). Patients are invited to experience links between these physical cues and specific emotions and/or accompanying cognitions. Often patients are afraid to experience these physical manifestations of emotions, because they may be overwhelming. Instead, psychological defense mechanisms (e.g., numbing) and attachment-based maladaptive affect regulatory mechanisms (e.g., dissociation) are activated.

During creative therapy, the capacity of identifying emotions, differentiating between emotions, analyzing emotions, and the capacity to express oneself in form and color is observed and explored. Moreover, a color calendar is drawn every week and analyzed by means of a color evaluation system. Each color stands for a particular emotion. In this way, the patient's capacity to reflect on her or his emotions and autobiographical situations is assessed through nonverbal cues, while at the same time the capacity to identify emotions and to differentiate between emotional states (Smeijsters, 2005) is evaluated.

During psychotherapy sessions, the patient's capacity to integrate experiences and to verbalize emotions in relation to other group members' and/or shared experiences is measured. To stimulate the process of validation of emotions, the focus is on interpersonal similarities and differentiation in affect regulation (Linehan, 1993). This approach is developed to assess the quality of the process of mentalized affectivity, emotional reciprocity, and emotional self-reflexivity while maintaining a sense of agency.

Emotional reciprocity involves listening to other people's stories and being able to react empathically toward group members' experiences or "emotional blind sight." In addition, it may encompass sharing stories while experiencing the accompanying feelings without being overwhelmed or being numb in interaction with other group members. Emotional self-reflexivity includes, for example, putting emotional experiences in a time-perspective. Relevant questions include: What preceded and/or what caused the situation or feeling? How does it manifest itself to the patient? How do others comprehend this situation? How do they react to the situation and/or how do they feel? How do they relate to others in the situation? What are the consequences of all these aspects for the near future? and so on (Fonagy et al., 2002).

Interpersonal Affective Behavior

Psychotherapists assess adult attachment style as described by Griffin and Bartholomew (1994a; 1994b) and Bowlby (1988) by interpreting patient's interpersonal behavior in terms of secure or insecure attachment behavior. Attachment clinging behavior and attachment avoidant behavior are typical examples of insecure attachment. This insecure attachment behavior, in combination with the patient's positive or negative verbalizations about the self in relation to the other, helps unraveling the patient's core beliefs if "help" or "harm" can be expected from the other in times of distress or danger. Attachment avoidance behavior is typically accompanied by "fear of closeness" and "a desire for independence," whereas attachment clinging behavior is associated with "fear of abandonment." In both cases, there is a "lack of interpersonal trust" (Griffin & Batholomew, 1994b).

The (inter)personal emotional functioning is described on the basis of observation of the patient's capacity of affective reflective function, emotional perspective taking, and empathy (Fonagy et al., 2002).

Maladaptive affective behavior (such as the incapacity in an interpersonal context to modulate and regulate emotions) is explained in terms of attachment-based affect regulation strategies. These strategies encompass hyperactivating strategies or deactivating strategies of affect regulation, resulting in interpersonal withdrawal (avoidance) or approach (clinging) (Mikulincer et al., 2003).

Concerning the relationship with other group members, patients are asked to reflect on the different positions they take in Leary's Rose of Interpersonal Functioning (Leary, 1957). In addition, patients are requested to reflect on questions such as: Where do they fit in? Which group member can be of help in overcoming their difficulties? Which group member can be an obstacle in meeting therapy goals? How to cope with that? and so forth. This interpersonal position awareness serves the function of reflection and affective mentalizing.

Arousability and Control Over Expressed Emotions

In music therapy, attention is directed toward the (in)capacity or blockage of the expression of emotions in vocal sounds and/or by means of musical instruments. First, patients are invited to choose an ego-matching instrument and play it or make sounds as in a small orchestra. The instruction is to start all at the same moment and after approximately 20 minutes to stop simultaneously. Next, patients are invited to switch instruments and choose the one with opposite or incompatible characteristics. Again, they are encouraged to play the instruments or to make sounds as in a small orchestra and the instruction is repeated. Often, this second part proves to be a difficult task to perform. Emotional blockages and incapacity to make sounds are common reactions for these patients (Smeijsters, 2005). It is often observed that their emotional behavior is disturbed in some ways, either because of underregulation (*hyper*activation of affect and emotions) or due to overregulation (*de*activation of affect and emotions) (Mikulincer et al., 2003).

Sociotherapists observe the patients' affect regulation–related behavior in between therapy sessions and during their everyday activities. They have access to information concerning daily pathologic and normal behavior and interactions. Between therapies, it is observed how the patients try to regulate emotions by interpersonal withdrawal or approach, both attachment-based affect regulation strategies (Mikulincer et al., 2003). It appears that several behaviors, such as skating, engagement in computer games, cigarette smoking, and automutilation all are utilized as affect regulation strategies or mood management.

Finally, the patient's motivation for treatment and engagement is challenged and assessed. In order to improve compliance to psychotherapy, patients are asked to prepare their personal evaluation of the "Pretherapy/Observation and Orientation period." Patients orient themselves in which way inpatient therapy at this particular ward might be "of use" to them. Moreover, the patients have to write a "motivation-for-treatment" paper in order to be admitted in the clinic or day-clinic. Finally, the patient has to write down realistic therapy goals that will be focussed on during psychotherapy and that are sufficiently objective to be used as outcome measures.

The following aspects are integrated in a psychotherapy-oriented assessment procedure at the department of (neuro)psychological assessment for therapy indication at our clinical psychotherapy ward: (1) the validation of emotions, ranging from comfortable (positive) to indifference or unwanted (negative); (2) interpersonal affective behavior, all interpersonal actions between withdrawal and approach; and (3) arousability and control over expressed emotions, the capacity to find a balance between control over emotional behavior and arousal/excitement accompanying emotions.

The DSM-IV-TR disorders (American Psychiatric Association, 1994) are assessed using standardized clinical interviews; the Structured Clinical Interview for DSM IV axis I disorders (SCID-I; First, Spitzer, Gibbon, & Williams, 1997) and the International Personality Disorder Examination (IPDE, World Health Organization, 1993) for DSM-IV-TR axis II disorder.

In addition the following self-report measures tapping signs and symptoms of self dysregulation are administered:

- Affect dysregulation and interpersonal emotional functioning is assessed by the EMOtional functioning Questionnaire-56 items (EMOQ-56; Bermond & Vorst, 2005) measuring the cognitive, affective, and social aspects of emotional functioning and the Dutch self-report version of the Structured Interview for Disorders of Extreme Stress (SIDES-r-nl; Van Dijke & Van der Hart, 2002).
- The concept of somatoform dissociation is measured using the Somatoform Dissociation Questionnaire (SDQ-20; Nijenhuis, Spinhoven, Van Dyck, Van der Hart, & Van der Linden, 1999), and the concept of psychoform dissociation is measured by the Dissociative Experiences Scale (DES; Bernstein & Putnam, 1986).
- The determination of the interaction style is based on adult attachment styles using the Relationship Styles Questionnaire (RSQ; Griffin & Bartholomew, 1994a).
- Traumatic events and their impact on current functioning are evaluated using the Traumatic Events Checklist (TEC; Nijenhuis, Van der Hart, & Kruger, 2002).

Preliminary Experiences with the Affect Dysregulation Treatment Program

Characteristic for these complex pathology patients are the very different disorders on the DSM-IV-TR axis I and axis II and the malign interpersonal patterns on DSM-IV-TR axis IV. The goals of the treatment program focus at changing affect regulation styles and adult attachment styles that negatively influence interaction with significant others. To this end, we designed an inpatient program, followed by a 4-daytime or 3-daytime program, resulting in an outpatient group therapy program. All involved therapists are part of a multidisciplinary team, consisting of a psychiatrist, a clinical psychologist, psychotherapists, a music creative therapist, a psychomotor therapist, a creative therapist, a social worker, and ward nurses.

Characteristic for the therapeutic environment the patients live in are clear therapy goals and boundaries, reflecting a balance between structure and flexibility. To stimulate metacognitive processing, keeping notes of therapeutic impressions and progress and the evaluation of therapy process are important instruments.

Intensive inpatient group therapy seems to be the best setting to learn from own observations of other patients and to learn how one's (emotional) actions elicit reactions in the others and vice versa (social learning). Moreover, information is provided about other people's emotional perspectives.

Important therapeutic techniques are psychoeducation on affect regulation styles, modeling, affect mirroring, and "passing the silver butler tray" (i.e., to give meaning to behavior and to suggest alternative thoughts and feelings, e.g., "I could imagine that you would not only feel mad about this but also disappointed or even sad") all aimed to facilitate new insights in a gentle way. The reflective function is stimulated by inviting the patients to actively mentalize one's own and the others' state of mind and by (emotional) perspective taking. In the beginning of therapy, the therapist reflects more actively the patients' perspective.

An important technique is the stop-rule. Affect regulative interventions concern both overregulation as in "stop thinking . . . and focus on the emotion and experience your emotion instead!" and underregulation as in "stop acting . . . and focus on the emotion and experience your emotion instead!"

Another important aspect of our interventions concerns pointing out interpersonal misinterpretations based on insecure attachment cognitive emotional information processing such as "You think you have everything under control, but your mind tricks you! The therapist is reaching you a hand to help you . . ..However, you interpret this offer for help as a threat, as a hand with a knife in it, pointing at you! Where help is offered, you anticipate harm!"

The psychotherapist's style can best be characterized as active and interactive; he is supportive and not neutral toward the patients in complex interpersonal conflicts. Transference and countertransference are both exploited in the sense that the therapist interprets and explains these interpersonal dynamics in terms of interpersonal or dyadic affect regulatory phenomena to the patients and the accompanying cognitions.

Before entering the program, relevant information about the patient is collected during the intake procedure. Information about previous therapies and therapy-effect or dropout, as well as about the quality of the therapeutic relation from previous therapists is collected after signed informed consent is obtained.

The following phases can be distinguished in our program:

Phase 1

Patients engage in a 6-week "Observation and Orientation" (O&O) period at our ward. They also take part in an extended assessment procedure. The multidisciplinary team members motivate patients to formulate therapy goals in terms of affect dysregulation (Paivio & Laurent, 2001), adult attachment style (Griffin et al., 1994), and consequences for current interaction patterns (Leary, 1957).

Through psychoeducation, the concept of affect dysregulation is explained. Moreover, signs and symptoms of both under- and overregulation of affect are discussed. The concept of affect dysregulation is focused on as a provoking and/or maintenance factor in chronic and complex anxiety and/or affective and/or somatization disorders. Patients learn that "affect dysregulation is not a fixed way of life" (Chefetz, 2000), but a syndrome that can be treated. Behaviors such as drug abuse, alcohol abuse, automutilation, and engaging in unsafe sex are considered as signs of malign affect dysregulation (Linehan, 1993).

At the end of this O&O period, the multidisciplinary team, the patient, and a family member/partner evaluate their experiences and findings during this O&O period. Together with the patient, a conclusion is reached: staying for treatment or referral to another facility. Both parties make up a therapy contract and sign it.

Phase 2

During this first "therapy" phase, patients join the therapy groups they are assigned to. They are invited to explain their symptoms from an interpersonal developmental perspective and to share their (new) treatment goals with the group. In other words, they are verbalizing and explaining their personal therapy rationale to the other group members. All other group members also present and explain their therapy goals and describe their therapeutic developmental process and therapy progress. Group interactions in the here and now are elaborated on in terms of affect dysregulation, attachment representation, and adult attachment style. The motto "attachment is the dyadic interactive regulation of emotions..." is held (Sroufe, 1996). The therapist and group members each have their contribution to the Interpersonal Interpretative Function of group therapy (Fonagy et al., 2002).

Phase 3

The focus is on recognizing and discerning one's own dysregulation of affect styles in different situations. Subsequently, they are expected to be able to distinguish over- and underregulation of affects in self and others. By emotional perspective taking and shared mentalized affectivity (Fonagy et al., 2002), knowledge about one's emotions and cognitions can be improved. In order to understand themselves, patients learn to relate affect dysregulation styles to early adverse interpersonal experiences, such as attachment trauma. Such early adverse interpersonal experiences may explain why the dyadic relation with the attachment figure is frustrated and why the Interpersonal Interpretative Function is ill-developed (Fonagy et al., 2002), possibly resulting in the development of maladaptive cognitive-emotional information processing and maladaptive emotion regulation strategies. Through the dyadic relation with the therapist and the triadic relation with the therapy group and the psychotherapist, the Interpersonal Interpretative Function in the here and now might be reestablished, resulting in improved cognitive-emotional information processing and improved emotion regulation strategies. Mindfulness-based techniques are useful to accept recurrent feelings of rage and anger, and "to let the anger come and go," followed by new more adequate self-regulation behavior (take a walk, listen to calming or playful music, etc.). Mourning about missed feelings of love and secure attachment relationships earlier in life is addressed and processed.

Phase 4

After the mourning has been processed adequately, the focus is on the here and now. New perspectives are visualized and verbalized as metaphors. A self-regulation training based on affect tolerance is the new focus for therapy. When affect regulation and self regulation have improved, an exposure program to potentially affect dysregulative situations in and around the clinic is carried out. The aim is to engage in these situations while maintaining the reflective function. Affect regulation is a process of crafting mental states in accordance with a sense of agency (Fonagy et al., 2002). At the end of this phase, patients should have found a new balance in affect regulation and interaction; they understand that affect dysregulation is indeed not a fixed way of life; there are alternatives!

Phase 5

At this point, an evaluation of the therapy process and progress by the multidisciplinary team and the fellow group members takes place. To this end, the multidisciplinary therapy scales to monitor therapy progress and effect are applied. A therapy effect evaluation and a therapy session with the partner or the parents is arranged in order to obtain additional relevant information. If improvement and therapy progress is clear and significant, the treatment program has been successful, and referral to our daytime clinic or outpatient therapy is appropriate. When there is no significant improvement and therapy progress, losses are counted and it is evaluated what went wrong. Consequently, the patient is either referred to another clinic or together with the therapist new therapy goals are formulated and the therapy process is continued and reevaluated 1 month later.

Phase 6

During outpatient therapy, the focus is on reintegration in the patient's home environment. This phase seems easy but often proves to be very difficult. The more the patient spends time at home, the more the home environment provides cues to relapse into old habits. The family and social network are not familiar with the new representation of the patient's self and interact with the patient and appeal to the patient as if changes in personality have never occurred. Therefore, in order to stick to the new representation of the patient's self, there is attention for the improvement of self regulation by counterconditioning old beliefs about the self in relation to others. After new cognitions and emotions have been integrated into the representation of the self, exposure therapy to potential affect dysregulative situations in the home environment takes place. The aim is to maintain the reflective functions according to the new representation of the self while experiencing a sense of agency. At the end of this phase, patients are supposed to be ready to "find a new, alternative way of life".

Phase 7

During this phase, therapy process and progress are evaluated. Dependent on the outcome, patients subsequently might be referred to either maintenance therapy or relapse prevention therapy. In addition, patients are incited to contact their therapist annually to monitor affect regulation skills and to assess the long-term psychotherapy effect.

Conclusion

In this contribution, the concept of affect dysregulation has been redefined. In addition, the relevance of clinical assessment and treatment of self dysregulation and affect dysregulation in a psychiatric hospital was discussed. After having outlined the theoretical background and the rationale of our assessment procedures and treatment program, some typical cases were presented. Our approach has a multidisciplinary background. Therapists of different disciplines collaborate in inpatient therapy sessions in order to assess signs and symptoms associated with affect dysregulation, more specifically under- and overregulation of affect and treatment possibilities. The assessment program has proved to be successful and helpful in indicating patients for treatment and in evaluating treatment progress and treatment effect. Finally, an integrative psychotherapy program encompassing a multidisciplinary therapy program in clinic, day-clinic, and outpatient setting was outlined. Until now, a well-designed systematic evaluation study has not yet been conducted, but we are currently preparing this important, critical next step.

Acknowledgment The author wishes to acknowledge the multidisciplinary team from "de Waard" Centre for Multidisciplinary Inpatient Psychotherapy at Delta Psychiatric Hospital, Poortugaal, The Netherlands, in particular Annelies Plekker and Sandra Visser, and "Eikenboom" Centre for Psychosomatic Medicine at Altrecht/Zeist, The Netherlands, in particular Martina Bühring, for their collaboration and contributions to the development of the assessment and treatment procedures presented herein. The author also wishes to acknowledge Ad Vingerhoets for his valuable comments on a previous version of this chapter.

References

Allen, J. G. (2001). *Traumatic relationships and serious mental disorders*. London: John Wiley and Sons, Ltd.

American Psychiatric Association (1994). *Diagnostic and Statistical manual of Mental Disorders* (4th ed.). Washington, DC: American Psychiatric Association.

Bagby, R. M., Parker, J. D. A., & Taylor, G. J. (1994). The Twenty-Item Toronto Alexithymia Scale – I. Item selection and cross-validation of the factor structure. *Journal of Psychosomatic Research, 38*, 23–32.

Baron–Cohen, S. (1988). Social and pragmatic deficits in autism: cognitive or affective? *Journal of Autism and Developmental Disorders, 18*, 379–401.

Baron-Cohen, S. (1991). Do people with autism understand what causes emotion? *Child Development, 62*, 385–395.

Baron-Cohen, S. (1995). Theory of Mind and face-processing: how do they interact in development and psychopathology? In D. Cicchetti & D. J. Cohen (Eds.), *Developmental psychopathology, Vol. I: theory and methods* (pp. 343–356). New York: John Wiley & Sons.

Baron-Cohen, S., Leslie, A. M., & Frith, U. (1985). Does the autistic child have a "theory of mind"? *Cognition, 21*, 37–46.

Bateman, A., & Fonagy, P. (2004). *Psychotherapy for borderline personality disorder: mentalization-based treatment.* Oxford: Oxford University Press.

Beck, A. T., Rush, A. J., Shaw, B .F., & Emery, G. (1979). *Cognitive therapy of depression* (pp. 389–399). New York: John Wiley & Sons.

Bell, L. (2003). *Managing intense emotions and overcoming self-destructive habits: a self-help manual*. New York: Brunner-Routledge.

Bermond, B., & Vorst, H.C.M. (2005). Emotional Intelligence Questionnaire: Manual. Amsterdam, The Netherlands: Amsterdam University Press.

Bernstein, E. M., & Putnam, F. W. (1986). Development, reliability, and validity of a dissociation scale. *Journal of Nervous and Mental Disease, 174*, 727–735.

Bowlby, J. (1973). *Attachment and loss. Vol. II: separation: anxiety and anger*. New York: Basic Books.

Bowlby, J. (1980). *Attachment and loss. Vol. III: attachment: sadness and depression.* New York: Basic Books.

Bowlby, J. (1982). *Attachment and loss. Vol. I: attachment* (2nd ed.). New York: Basic Books [original edition 1969].

Bowlby, J. (1988). *A secure base: clinical applications of attachment theory*. London: Routledge.

Bradley, S. J. (2000). *Affect dysregulation and the development of psychopathology*. New York: The Guilford Press.

Cassidy, J., & Shaver, P. (Eds), (1999). *Handbook of attachment*. New York: Guilford Press.

Chefetz, R.A. (2000). Affect dysregulation as a way of life. *Journal of American Academy of Psychoanalysis, 28*, 89–303.

Derogatis, L. R. (1994). *SCL-90-R: administration, coring and procedures manual* (3rd ed.). Minneapolis, MN: National Computer Systems.

Ekman, P (2003). *Emotions revealed. Recognizing face and feelings to improve communication and emotional life.* New York: Times Books Henry Bolt and Company.

First, M. D., Spitzer, R. L., Gibbon, M., & Williams, J. B. W. (1997). *User's guide for the Structured Clinical Interview for DSM-IV Axis I Disorders (SCID-I).* Washington, DC: American Psychiatric Press.

Fonagy, P., & Target, M. (1996). A contemporary psychoanalytical perspective: psychodynamic developmental therapy. In E. D. Hibbs & P. S. Jensen (Eds.), *Psychosocial treatments for child and adolescent disorders: empirically based strategies for clinical practice* (pp. 619–638). Washington, DC: American Psychological Association.

Fonagy, P., Gergely, G., Jurist, E., & Target, M. (2002). *Affect regulation, mentalization and the development of the self.* New York: Other Press.

Ford, J. D., & Kidd, P. (1998). Early childhood trauma and disorders of extreme stress as predictors of treatment outcome with chronic posttraumatic stress disorder. *Journal of Traumatic Stress, 11*, 743–761.

Gillath, O., Bunge, S. A., Shaver, P. R., Wendelken, C., & Mikulincer, M. (2005). Attachment-style differences in the ability to suppress negative thoughts: exploring the neural correlates. *NeuroImage, 28*, 835–847.

Greenberg, L., & Borger, L. (2001). An emotion-focused approach to the over-regulation of emotion and emotional pain. *Journal of Clinical Psychology, 57,* 197–211.

Griffin, D., & Bartholomew, K. (1994a). The metaphysics of measurement: the case of adult attachment. In K. Bartholomew & D. Perlman (Eds.), *Advances in relationships. Vol. 5, Attachment processes in adulthood* (pp. 17–52). London: Jessica Kingsley Publishers.

Griffin, D., & Batholomew, K. (1994b). Models of the self and other: fundamental dimensions underlying measures of adult attachment. *Journal of Personality and Social Psychology, 3*, 430–445.

Gross, J. J. (1998). The emerging field of emotion regulation: an integrative view. *Review of General Psychology*, *3*, 271–299.

Gross, J. J. (1999). Emotion regulation: past, present and future. *Cognition and Emotion, 13*, 551–573.

Herman, J. L. (1992a). *Trauma and recovery*. New York: Basic Books.

Herman, J. L. (1992b). Complex PTSD: a syndrome in survivors of prolonged and repeated trauma. *Journal of Traumatic Stress, 5*, 377–391.

Koenigsberg, H. W., Harvey, P. D., Mitropoulou, V., Schmeidler, J., New, A. S., Goodman, M., Silverman, J. M., Serby, M., Schopick, F., & Siever, L. J. (2002). Characterizing affective instability in Borderline Personality Disorder. *American Journal of Psychiatry, 159*, 784–788.

Krystal, H. (1988). *Integration & self-healing: affect, trauma, alexithymia*. Hillsdale, NJ: The Analytic Press.

Kooiman, C. G., Bolk, J. H., Brand, R., Trijsburg, R. W., & Rooijmans, H. G. (2000). Is alexithymia a risk factor for unexplained physical symptoms in general medical outpatients? *Psychosomatic Medicine, 62*, 768–778.

Leary, T (1957). *Interpersonal diagnosis of personality*. New York: Ronald.

Linehan, M. M. (1993). *Cognitive-behavioral treatment of Borderline Personality Disorder.* New York: Guilford Press.

McCullough, L., Kuhn, N., Andrews, S., Kaplan, A., Wolf, J., & Hurley, C. L. (2003). *Treating affect phobia: a manual for short-term dynamic psychotherapy*. New York: Guilford Press.

Mikulincer, M, & Shaver, P. R. (2004). Security-based self-representations in adulthood: contents and processes. In W. S. Rholes & J. A. Simpson (Eds.), *Adult attachment: theory, research, and clinical implications* (pp.159–195). New York: Guilford Press.

Mikulincer, M., Shaver, P. R., & Pereg, D. (2003). Attachment theory and affect regulation: the dynamics, development, and cognitive consequences of attachment-related strategies. *Motivation and Emotion, 27,* 77–102.

Nijenhuis, E. R. S., Spinhoven, P., Van Dyck, R., Van der Hart, O., & Van der Linden, J. (1996). The development and psychometric characteristics of the Somatoform Dissociation Questionnaire (SDQ-20). *Journal of Nervous and Mental Disease, 184*, 688–694.

Nijenhuis, E. R. S., Van der Hart, O., & Kruger, K. (2002). The psychometric characteristics of the traumatic Experiences Checklist (TEC): first findings among psychiatric outpatients. *Clinical Psychology and Psychotherapy, 9*, 200–210.

Nyklíček, I., Temoshok, L., & Vingerhoets, A. (Eds.). (2004). *Emotional expression and health: advances in theory, assessment and clinical applications*. New York: Brunner-Routledge.

Ogden, P., Minton, K., & Pain, C. (2006). A sensimotor approach to psychotherapy. New York: Norton.

Paivio, S. C., & Laurent, C. (2001). Empathy and emotion regulation: reprocessing memories of childhood abuse. *Psychotherapy in Practice, 57*, 213–226.

Pelcovitz, D., Van der Kolk, B., Roth, S., Mandel, F., & Resick, P. (1997). Development of a criteria set and a Structured Interview for Disorders of Extreme Stress (SIDES). *Journal of Traumatic Stress, 10*, 3–16.

Roth, S., Newman, E., Pelcovitz, D., Van der Kolk, B., & Mandel, F. S. (1997). Complex PTSD in victims exposed to sexual and physical abuse: results from the DSM-IV field trial for Posttraumatic Stress Disorder. *Journal of Traumatic Stress, 10,* 539–555.

Rothschild, B. (2000). *The body remembers: the psychophysiology of trauma and trauma treatment.* New York: Norton.

Schore, A. N. (1994). *Affect regulation and the origin of the self: the neurobiology of emotional development.* Hillsdale, NJ: Erlbaum.

Schore, A. N. (2001a). The effects of secure attachment relationships on right brain development, affect regulation and infant mental health. *Infant Journal of Mental Health, 22*, 201–269.

Schore, A. N. (2001b). The effects of early relational trauma on right brain development, affect regulation and infant mental health. *Infant Journal of Mental Health, 22*, 201–269.

Schore, A. N. (2002). Dysregulation of the right brain: a fundamental mechanism of traumatic attachment and the prognosis of Post Traumatic Stress Disorder. *Australian and New Zealand Journal of Psychiatry, 36*, 9–22.

Siegel, D. J. (1999). *The developing mind: toward a neurobiology of interpersonal experience.* New York: Guilford.

Smeijsters, H. (2005). *Sounding the self: analogy in improvisational music therapy*. Gilsum, NH: Barcelona Publishers.

Solomon, M. F., & Siegel, D. J. (Eds). (2003). *Healing trauma: attachment, mind, body, and brain.* New York: W.W. Norton.

Spielberger, C. D., Gorsuch, R. L., & Lushene, R. E. (1970). *Manual for the State-Trait Anxiety Inventory.* Palo Alto, CA: Consulting Psychologists Press.

Sroufe, L. A. (1996). *Emotional development: the organization of emotional life in the early years.* New York: Cambridge University Press.

Teasdale, J. D., & Barnard, P. J. (1993). *Affect, cognition, and change: re-modelling depressive thought.* Hove, UK: Lawrence Erlbaum Associates.

Taylor, G. K., Bagby, R. M., & Parker, J. D. A. (1997). *Disorders of affect regulation: alexithymia in medical and psychiatric illness.* New York: Cambridge University Press.

Van der Kolk, B. A. (1996). The complexity of adaptation to trauma: self-regulation, stimulus discrimination, and characterological development. In B. A. Van der Kolk, A. C. McFarlane, & L.Weisaeth (Eds.), *Traumatic stress: the effects of overwhelming experience on mind, body, and society* (pp. 182–213). New York: Guilford Press.

Van der Kolk, B. A., McFarlane, A. C., & Weisaeth, L. (Eds.). (1996). *Traumatic stress: the effects of overwhelming experience on mind, body, and society.* New York: Guilford Press.

Van der Kolk, B. A., Pelcovitz, M. D., Roth, S., Mandel, F. S., McFarlane, A., & Herman, J. L. (1996). Dissociation, somatization and affect dysregulation: the complexity of adaptation to trauma. *American Journal of Psychiatry, 153*, 83–93.

Van Dijke, A. (2002). Dutch translation of the Relationship Styles Questionnaire (RSQ). Unpublished manual. Poortugaal, The Netherlands: Delta Psychiatric Hospital.

Van Dijke, A., & Van der Hart, O. (2002). *The Dutch self report version of the Structured Interview for Disorders of Extreme Stress (SIDES-r-nl).* Unpublished manual. Utrecht, The Netherlands: Utrecht University.

Vorst, H.. C. M., & Bermond, B. (2004). *EMOtional development Questionnaire (EMOQ).* Unpublished manual.

Vorst, H. C. M., & Bermond, B. (2001). Validity and reliability of the Bermond-Vorst Alexithymia Questionnaire. *Personality and Individual Differences, 30*, 413–434.

Watson, D., Clark, L. A., & Tellegen, A. (1988). Development and validation of brief measures of positive and negative affect: the PANAS scales. *Journal of Personality and Social Psychology, 54*, 1063–1070.

Wellman, H. M. (1993). Early understanding of the mind: the normal case. In S. Baron-Cohen, H. Tager-Flusberg, & D. J. Cohen (Eds.), *Understanding others minds: perspectives from autism* (pp. 10–39). Oxford: Oxford University Press.

Wenar, C., & Kerig, P. (2000). *Developmental psychopathology: from infancy through adolescence* (4th ed.). Singapore: McGraw-Hill International Editions.

Wolfsdorf, B. A., & Zlotnick, C. (2001). Affect management in group therapy for women with post traumatic stress disorder and histories of childhood sexual abuse. *Journal of Clinical Psychology, 15*, 60–71.

World Health Organization. (1993). *The International Personality Disorder Examination (IPDE): version 1.1-july 1993*. Geneva: WHO, Division of Mental Health.

Zajonc, R. D. (1984). On the primacy of emotion. *American Psychologist, 39,* 117–123.

Zittel Conklin, C., Bradley, R., & Westen, D. (2006). Affect regulation in borderline personality disorder. *Journal of Nervous and Mental Disease, 194*, 69–77.

Zlotnick, C., & Pearlstein, T. (1997). Validation of the structured interview for disdorders of extreme stress. *Comprehensive Psychiatry, 38*, 243–247.

Zlotnick, C., Zakriski, A. L., Shea, M. T., Costello, E., Begin, A., Pearlstein, T., & Simpson, E. (1996). The long-term sequelae of sexual abuse: support for a complex posttraumatic stress disorder. *International Society for Traumatic Stress Studies, 9*, 195–205.

Chapter 11
Emotional Inhibition, Health, Gender, and Eating Disorders: The Role of (Over) Sensitivity to Others

Marrie H.J. Bekker and Sonja T.P. Spoor

Introduction

Of all mental disorders listed in DSM-IV (APA, 2000), eating disorders stand out as the category with the most unequal sex ratios. Anorexia nervosa occurs almost exclusively in women (more than 90% of the cases are women), and the same holds for bulimia nervosa: at least 90% of the patients are women for both clinical and population samples. Not surprisingly, the majority of explanations of eating disorders explicitly or implicitly refer to this unequal sex ratio. This is done by either emphasizing the importance of stressors that affect women more exclusively or more seriously than men, or by stressing vulnerability factors that more typically characterize women than men. One example concerns the impressive body of studies following from the restrained eating theory that all point to the importance of dieting for women due to the Western ideal of feminine slenderness (e.g., Huon & Brown, 1989; Stice, 1998; Stice, Presnell, & Spangler, 2002). Another illustration concerns the emphasis on low self-esteem that also might be more related to the female than to the male sex (e.g., Silberstein, Striegel-Moore, Timko, & Rodin, 1988).

Simultaneously, eating-disordered behavior has repeatedly been considered from the perspective of affect regulation (e.g., Hawkins & Clement, 1984; McCarthy, 1990), and therewith related to inhibition of emotions. Particularly binge eating, which is typical for specific types of anorexia and bulimia as well as for eating disorders not otherwise specified (APA, 2000), has often been associated with (releasing) negative affect. Emotional eating, which substantially overlaps with binge eating, refers to eating in response to negative emotions (Bruch, 1973). It is regarded as coping behavior that makes individuals feel better and serves as a distraction from negative affect (e.g., Elmore & De Castro, 1990). In other words, it can be viewed as a form of avoidant coping, namely avoidance of feeling and expressing negative emotions (e.g., Bekker & Boselie, 2002; Neckowitz & Morrison, 1991; Soukup, Beiler, & Terrell, 1990; Troop, Holbrey, Trowler, & Treasure, 1994; Wardle, Steptoe, Olliver, & Lipsey, 1999).

However, inhibition of emotions as an etiologically relevant factor for eating disorders differs from the aforementioned explanations (referring to the importance of slenderness and to low self-esteem) in its association with gender. Whereas

A. Vingerhoets et al., (eds.), *Emotion Regulation.*

emotional inhibition is usually associated with the male sex and with masculinity (e.g., Eisler & Blalock, 1991), vulnerability to the norm of slenderness and low self-esteem are generally seen as typical female and feminine characteristics. Various authors have argued that, in search for the sources of gender-specific pathology, one should primarily focus on risk factors that are more typically related to the sex in which the pathology occurs most frequently (e.g., Bekker, 2003; Rutter, Caspi, & Moffitt, 2003). It is an intriguing issue how strong the explanatory power is of a risk factor (in this case inhibition of negative emotions) that is more strongly related with men than with women, for pathology with a higher prevalence in women than in men (here: eating disorders).

We will examine this paradoxical issue by first taking a closer look upon the prevalence of eating disorders in both sexes. Second, we will summarize the literature on sex differences in emotional expression and briefly discuss its relationship with (somatic as well as mental) health problems in general. Third, we will present the empirical evidence available for relations between eating disorders and emotional inhibition. Finally, we will conclude which type of emotional inhibition is likely relevant for eating disorders and which pathways might plausibly be operative in their relationship. In addition, the strategy of using sex differences as a source of selection of relevant risk factors for various health problems will be evaluated.

Sex Ratios of Prevalence of Eating Disorders

From several sources (Hoek & van Hoeken, 2003; Lucas, Beard, O'Fallon, & Kurland, 1991), it is clear that the incidence of anorexia nervosa among males is below 1.0 and probably even below 0.5 per 100,000 population per year; the female-to-male ratio being more than 10:1 (Hoek & van Hoeken, 2003). In most cases, the disorder begins between mid and late adolescence (ages 14–18) (APA, 2000). Regarding bulimia nervosa, both Soundy, Lucas, Suman, & Melton, (1995) and Hoek & van Hoeken (2003) reported an incidence of 0.8 for males per 100,000 person-years. Its general prevalence is about 1%, with the similar, very marked female preponderance of about 10:1 in community samples (Garfinkel, Lin, Goering, & Spegg, 1995). Bulimia nervosa usually starts in late adolescence or early adulthood (APA, 2000). Although its course is often chronic, many individuals' symptoms diminish over longer-term follow-up. In summary, the literature is remarkably consistent in the sex-rates presented for eating disorders corresponding with the APA figures, namely on average 10:1 (Rutter, Caspi, & Moffitt, 2003).

Emotional Expression: Sex Differences and Health Implications

Despite cross-cultural variation in sex differences regarding emotional expressiveness, numerous studies have confirmed that, in general, women are more emotionally expressive than men (e.g., Balswick & Avertt, 1977; Brebner, 2003; Brehm,

1992; Brody, 1997; Brody & Hall, 1993; Dindia & Allen, 1992; Fischer, 2000; Gross & John, 1998; Hall, 1984; Kring & Gordon, 1998; Kring, Smith, & Neale, 1994; Mirowsky & Ross, 1995; Timmers, Fischer, & Manstead, 1998). For example, observational studies of nonverbal expressions found females to be considerably more expressive overall. Women smile and laugh more than men do, except in childhood. Also, women cry more frequently, longer, and more intensely than men (Vingerhoets, Cornelius, Van Heck, & Becht 2000; Bekker & Vingerhoets, 1999; 2001). According to Brody & Hall (1993) and Brody (2000), women in general also report to be more emotionally expressive than do men.

Although at first glance anger might appear an exception—with men being more expressive—there is little empirical support for the existence of sex differences with respect to anger expression. In a study by Averill (1983), for example, women compared with men reported a similar frequency of becoming angry. In addition, their anger was as intense, for the same reasons, and expressed as openly as men's anger. A difference was found regarding women reporting crying when angry more often than men. Also, many other studies failed to find sex differences for outwardly expressed anger (e.g., Balswick, 1988; Balswick & Avertt, 1977; Fischer, 2000; Fischer, Smith, Leonard, Fuqua, Campbell, & Masters, 1993; Spielberger, Johnson, Russell, Crane, Jacobs, & Worden, 1985). As far as is known, only Mirowsky and Ross (1995) showed that women could become angrier than men and were more likely to express their anger by yelling. Thus, although there is a general impression of more anger inhibition in women than in men, most empirical studies do not support the claim that women are less expressive of anger or that they suppress their anger more (for a discussion, see Kring, 2000).

What are the health implications of emotional expression? Much research indicates that expressing feelings, especially "negative" ones accompanying traumatic experiences, such as fear, sadness, and depression, is related to better mental and physical health, including better immune functioning (Nyklíček, Vingerhoets, & Denollet, 2002). The long tradition of psychoanalytic theory and practice is even based on the idea that repressed emotions cause psychosomatic and neurotic problems and that awareness raising of and working through these repressed feelings are necessary conditions for recovery. According to Peters (as cited in Brody, 1985, p. 103), "... psychopathology is often defined as the inability to cope with emotions and/or as the expression or experience of inappropriately frequent or intense emotions" (see also Brody, 1999; Pennebaker, 1985). However, various authors critically warned that few studies in the field adopted appropriate designs for examining causal relationships (e.g., Nykliček et al., 2002). In studies by Berenbaum and Oltmanns (1992) and Kring, Kerr, Smith, and Neale, (1993), support was obtained for a generalized expressiveness deficit across both positive and negative emotions in schizophrenia, but also here, conclusions regarding causal relations cannot be drawn. Another line of evidence concerns gender role stress that is claimed to contribute to diseases and disorders with an unequal prevalence in both sexes. In the current context, it is relevant that masculine gender role stress is conceptualized, among other elements, in terms of fear of emotional expressiveness (e.g., Eisler & Blalock, 1991). More in general, the inhibition of particularly negative emotional responses has been associated with increased autonomic activity (e.g., Gross &

Levenson, 1993; Gross, 1998) and increased risk of several diseases (e.g., Berry & Pennebaker, 1993; Denollet, 2000; Eisenberger, Kenemy, & Wyatt, 2003; Friedman & Booth-Kewley, 1987).

However, not all available evidence fits into the picture that emotional expressiveness is associated with better mental and physical health. For example, Mirowsky and Ross (1995), referring to the generally accepted idea that women are more emotionally expressive compared with men, argued that these differences cannot account for the sex differences in depression. Also, data regarding crying do not univocally support the idea that expressing emotions is advantageous for health (Vingerhoets & Scheirs, 2001). For example, in a study by Labott, Ahleman, Wolever, and Martin (1990), contrary to expectations, weeping failed to buffer the effects of life stress upon mood disturbances. On the contrary, compared with infrequent criers, frequent criers were more vulnerable to mood disturbances. Moreover, high levels of weeping were associated with increased mood disturbance as negative life events increased. In addition, crying was found to be immunosuppressive. On the other hand, in self-reports among 30 countries, Becht and Vingerhoets (2002) found a positive self-reported mood change after crying (see also Cornelius [1997] and Vingerhoets, Cornelius, Van Heck, & Becht [2000] for a discussion on the issue).

Data with respect to expressing anger as related to health are also inconclusive and contradictory. Expressing anger in a fashion consistent with male stereotypes, that is, in a loud and fast speech style, has been shown to elevate the risk of cardiovascular disease (Siegman, Anderson, & Berger, 1990). This is in line with findings showing that individuals who frequently express anger eventually may suffer from adverse health consequences (e.g., Schwartz, Weinberger, & Singer, 1981). Thomas and Williams (1991) have described ways in which anger might be related to diseases such as hypertension, coronary heart disease, cancer (see also Appel, Holroyd, & Gorkin, 1983), arthritis, and asthma (e.g., Friedman & Booth-Kewley, 1987; Hockemeyer & Smyth, 2002). Additionally, a study by Gidron, Davidson, and Ilia (2000) showed a positive relation between cardiovascular disease and hostility (defined as verbal or physical expression of anger) for men younger than 60 years old, whereas this association was not found among older men and women. Also, the ways in which emotions are experienced and expressed (e.g., during psychotherapeutic sessions) matter; expression in an unstructured fashion has proved to be potentially harmful (for a review, see Littrell, 1998). Thus, physiologic and psychological effects of anger expression and inhibition are not always easily interpretable. In general, suppressed anger is claimed to have a worse effect on health than the expression of it, but expressing anger has also been shown to have damaging health consequences (see also Brody, 1999; Panagopulou, Kersbergen & Maes, 2002).

In summary, although much of the available evidence suggests that expressing emotions is healthy, or rather that inhibition of negative emotions can be health damaging, there are also data suggesting a more complex association. Explanations for contradictory results refer to, first, methodological issues, for example, varying samples, research designs, and definitions of expression and nonexpression (e.g., see Panagopoulou et al., 2002). Second, moderators might play a role, one of them being the feelings one has about expressing emotions. From this perspective, not the expression or inhibition of the emotion per se is the health-relevant factor, but the person's attitudes and feelings concerning (non)expression, such as feelings of ambivalence about expressing emotions (e.g., Emmons & King, 1988; Pennebaker, 1985). Such attitudes might result in antecedent focused emotion regulation, for example, preventing oneself from entering anger-invoking situations, but also response-focused emotion regulation can play a role: considering anger expression as "not done" can lead to withholding oneself from behaving angry (Gross & Mũnoz, 1995; see also Bekker & Vingerhoets, 2001) for an adaptation concerning sex differences in crying). Another moderator might be the context in which emotions are expressed (e.g., Gottman & Levenson, 1986; Mendes, Reis, Seery, & Blascovich, 2003). For example, in a dysfunctional marriage, expressing anger might induce anger or even physical violence, whereas it might be part of a problem-solving interaction in the context of a functional marriage. A third example of a possible moderator concerns individual differences in emotion regulation and coping. Brody (1999) mentioned gender-related individual differences regarding (1) the level of comfort one feels while expressing emotions, (2) ways of appraising circumstances, and (3) the presence or absence of concomitant ways of coping such as rumination.

More in general, the relationship between emotional (non)expression and health may depend upon the (sub)culture, which may imply gender-or occupation-related differences in display rules regarding emotions.

Inhibition of Emotions: Likely to Be a Risk Factor for Eating Disorders?

From the evidence discussed above, we can conclude that (1) eating disorders occur much more frequently in women than in men; (2) expression of emotions is more common for women than it is for men, except possibly for anger expression; and (3) inhibition of emotions can have negative health effects, but these effects may be moderated by factors like context and (gender-related) individual and (sub)cultural differences.

Which hypotheses can be derived from these conclusions regarding the possible role of emotional inhibition in eating disorders? First, we might expect that its role for eating disorders is not likely to be substantial, except with regard to anger inhibition; other factors with stronger links to the female sex are plausibly more promising sources of explanation. Second, assuming that emotional (non)expression could nevertheless be relevant for eating disorders, one would expect that eating disorders occur in a particular subgroup of women (e.g., in a certain age range) for whom the expression of emotions is a problem. However, as we have seen, emotional (non)expression also predicts disorders with a relatively high prevalence in men. Therefore, this factor should be deemed unlikely to be a *specific risk* factor for eating disorders only. Specific moderators might be working in eating disorders that do not substantially play a role in disorders more exclusively linked to men.

The Role of Emotional Inhibition in Eating Disorders

There is much empirical evidence demonstrating that emotional distress leads to changes in eating behavior (for reviews, see Ganley, 1989; Greeno & Wing, 1994). Generally, appetite loss and decreased food intake have been considered natural physiologic responses to negative emotional states, because physiologic reactions to distress mimic the internal sensations associated with feeding-induced satiety. However, some individuals respond to negative affect by increasing their food intake. Several theoretical models have been developed to explain this stress-induced eating behavior.

The "psychosomatic" theory posits that responding to negative affect by increasing food intake might be the result of learning experiences early in life where food was used as a way of coping with stress and psychological problems (Bruch, 1973; Kaplan & Kaplan, 1957). According to the "affect regulation" theory, some individuals binge eat because they believe it provides comfort and distraction from negative emotions (Hawkins & Clement, 1984; McCarthy, 1990). Finally, theorists have also suggested that people with high levels of self-consciousness, the tendency to focus on and analyze the self (Fenigstein, Scheier, & Buss, 1975), sometimes use binge eating to escape from the self (Abramson, Bardone-Cone, Vohs, Joiner, & Heatherton, 2006; Heatherton & Baumeister, 1991; McManus & Waller, 1995). All three theories emphasize the experience of high levels of aversion to negative emotions, as well as the view that one uses binge eating to distract oneself from these emotions. Both emotional eating and binge are thought to be functional, at least temporarily, in providing comfort and distracting from aversive emotions (McManus & Waller, 1995). Possibly, alternative affect regulation skills are lacking or have been experienced to be ineffective.

Several studies have found associations between bulimic behaviors and high levels of suppressing feelings, thoughts, and actions in eating-disordered women (Milligan & Waller, 2000; Waller, Babbs, Milligan, Meyer, Ohanian, & Leung, 2003; Zaitsoff, Geller, & Srikameswaran, 2002). In addition, there is also some preliminary evidence suggesting that the inhibited expression of emotions is related to body dissatisfaction (Geller, Cockell, Hewitt, Goldner, & Flett, 2000; Hayaki, Friedman, & Brownell, 2002). Possibly, suppression of emotions is less likely than expression to lead to a satisfactory resolution of the factors driving the negative mood. The intensity of negative affect does therefore not decrease, leading to the development of other means that provide distraction or comfort, such as binge eating (e.g., Fairburn, Cooper, & Safran, 2003; Milligan & Waller, 2000).

Several researchers have shown that this relation between suppression of emotions and bulimic behaviors is stronger in women than in men (e.g., Meyer, Leung, Waller, Perkins, Paice, & Mitchell, 2005). Smolak and Munstertieger (2002) examined the association between the (non)expression of feelings, thoughts, and actions and eating problems in female and male college students. They found that compared with men, in women inhibition of feelings, thoughts, and actions was consistently more strongly related to higher reports of dietary restraint, binge eating, and emotional eating. This stronger relationship among women than men was not attributable to higher scores of women on inhibition. Furthermore, even though women reported higher levels of depression than men, inhibition scores were somewhat more related to depression in men than in women. These results are comparable with the findings of the study by Meyer et al. (2005) who found that bulimic attitudes were associated with anger suppression in women, but not in men.

The above-mentioned results of the studies of Smolak and Munstertieger (2002) and Meyer and Colleagues (2005) indicate that inhibition of emotions relevant for eating disorders might particularly refer to anger inhibition. In addition, as the sex difference in findings was not influenced by differences in absolute inhibition scores, other variables might possibly explain the differences found. More specifically, certain moderators might affect the relation between inhibition of emotions, particularly anger, and eating pathology in women, whereas these moderators might play a less important role in men.

One of the most robust psychological sex differences is the fact that women are more connectedness-oriented (e.g., Eisenberg, Miller, Shell, McNalley, & Shea, 1991; McGuire & McGuire, 1982; Smolak & Murnen, 2003), as reflected by their consistently higher levels of social support seeking (e.g., Taylor, Klein, Lewis, Gruenewald, Gurung, & Updegraff, 2000), tendency to affiliate under stress (Lengua & Stormshak, 2000), and sensitivity to others (Bekker & Van Assen, 2006; Bekker, Bachrach, & Croon, 2007; Bekker & Van Assen, under review). The feminine tendency to connectedness seems to be attributable to, among other factors, the internalization of gender roles, in particular with regard to social relationships (Striegel-Moore, 1993; Striegel-Moore, Silberstein, & Rodin, 1993). Also biological factors (e.g., see Taylor et al., 2000) and factors related to attachment development (e.g., see Bekker, 1993; Chodorow, 1989) might play a role. A woman's identity is thus more developed in and closely tied to her personal relationships (Chodorow, 1989; Kaplan, 1986; Kaplan & Surrey, 1984; Gilligan, Lyons, & Hammer, 1990). Although relatively high levels of sensitivity to others belong to the normal feminine identity, extremely high sensitivity to others reflecting neediness (Rude & Burnham, 1995) has been identified as a risk factor for psychopathology with a higher prevalence in women than in men, for example, depression and anxiety (Bekker & Belt, 2006), as well as eating disorders (Bekker, Croon, & Bertrand, under review). In such cases, high sensitivity to others coincides with low self-awareness and a vulnerability to others' opinions of them and negative behaviors toward them. As a result, these women are more susceptible to social pressure, have a higher need for social approval (i.e., from family, peers, and media), and are more likely to conform with the norms and expectations of others in order to be accepted, and simultaneously have only a weak contact with their own needs and emotions. Gilligan and Colleagues (Gilligan, 1982; Gilligan, Rogers, & Tolman, 1991; Taylor, Gilligan, & Sullivan, 1995) have posited that this might be especially the case for women who fear rejection and are willing to put the needs, interests, and desires of others above those of themselves. In particular, eating-disordered women have been found to have an unusual sensitivity to the feelings and needs of others and to be particularly prone to suppress negative affect (e.g., Bekker et al., under review; Cockell, Hewitt, Goldner, Srikameswaran, &

Flett, 1997; Geller et al., 2000). However, this suppression of one's own feelings, thoughts, and actions and focusing on others' needs might not resolve the negative moods experienced. Avoiding the expression of negative emotions toward appropriate targets might be redirected to a less threatening target, such as the body (Bruch, 1973; 1978).

Particularly in eating disorders, these underlying processes might be boosted by cultural mechanisms. Notice that nowadays attractiveness in women functions as a prime currency in women's social relationships (e.g., Fredrickson & Roberts, 1997; Rodin, Silberstein, & Striegel-Moore, 1985). As a result, women who are more attuned to and responsive to the needs of others may be especially vulnerable to the comments or actions of others that serve to support and perpetuate the slim ideal body image for women (e.g., criticism regarding weight, encouragement to diet, modeling disordered eating behaviors) (Stice, 1998). Therefore, they may be more compliant with the expectations regarding weight and appearance and may be at risk for the development of disordered eating behavior (Stice, 1998; Striegel-Moore et al., 1993). Empirical evidence indicates that perceived pressure to be slim, thin-ideal internalization, modeling of eating disturbances by family, peers, and media, and body dissatisfaction predict bulimic behaviors in adolescent females (Stice & Agras 1998; Stice et al., 2002). Adolescent females scoring high on difficulty expressing conflict in friendship, heightened fears of negative evaluations, and public self-consciousness were most at risk to develop bulimia (Lieberman, Gauvin, Bukowski, & White, 2001; Pike, 1995).

In sum, it can be concluded that inhibition of emotions, particularly anger, criticism, and conflict, contributes to bulimic behavior in women but not in men. Furthermore, a specific type of connectedness may moderate this relationship; particularly women who are more susceptible to social pressure or have a higher need for social approval by combining an extremely high sensitivity to others with a low level of self-awareness seem to be at risk.

Discussion and Conclusion

In this chapter, we addressed the plausibility that a risk factor that seems more closely related with men, emotional inhibition, contributes substantially to a disorder more strongly associated with women, eating disorders. From our review it became clear, first, that both these presumptions are valid points of departure; the prevalence of eating disorders is indeed much higher in women than in men, and emotional inhibition seems generally more characteristic for men than for women, although here the evidence is more controversial.

Second, the general idea that emotional inhibition is unhealthy (i.e., a risk factor for various diseases and disorders) appeared to be supported by several sources of evidence, although also here the relationship is more complex and may be different for specific health problems.

Third, we found that emotional inhibition relevant for eating disorders concerns mostly inhibition of anger, moderated by a specific type of autonomy-connectedness, namely high sensitivity to others together with low self-awareness. In other words, the chance that emotional inhibition contributes substantially to eating disorders might be dependent on the presence of a high susceptibility to social pressure and need for approval together with low awareness of and assertiveness regarding one's own needs, wishes, and opinions. This may increase a tendency to "silence oneself" by means of emotional eating. From this perspective, inhibition of emotions is not a specific risk factor for eating disorders, but it may interact with other risk factors, particularly with high sensitivity to others, low self-awareness, and the tendency for emotional eating, in predicting eating disorders.

We started the chapter with a paradox. At the end, we conclude that it is fruitful to pay attention to gender issues with respect to possible risk factors; because this may help in examining the effects of risk factors on health problems with unequal sex ratios and sharpens our understanding of common and specific factors and of main and moderating effects. Of course, further empirical studies are needed to examine whether our hypothesized relations, based on preliminary empirical evidence and a gender analysis, are valid.

References

Abramson, L. Y., Bardone-Cone, A. M., Vohs, K. D., Joiner, T. E., Jr., & Heatherton, T. F. (2006). Cognitive vulnerability to bulimia. In L. B. Alloy & J. H. Riskind (Eds.), *Cognitive vulnerability to emotional disorders* (pp. 329–364). Hillsdale, NJ: Erlbaum.

American Psychiatric Association. (APA; 2000). *Diagnostic and statistic manual of mental disorders* (Fourth edition TR). Washington, DC: APA.

Appel, M. S., Holroyd, K., & Gorkin, L. (1983). Anger and the etiology and progression of physical illness. In L. Temoshok, C. Van Dyke, & L. Zegans (Eds.), *Emotions in health and illness; theoretical and research foundations* (pp. 73–85). New York: Grone & Stratton.

Averill, J. R. (1983). Studies on anger and aggression: implications for theories of emotion. *American Psychologist, 38,* 1145–1160.

Balswick, J. (1988). *The inexpressive male.* Lexington, MA: Lexington Books.

Balswick, J., & Avertt, C. (1977). Differences in expressiveness: gender, interpersonal orientation, and perceived parental expressiveness as contributing factors. *Journal of Marriage and the Family, 39,* 121–127.

Becht, M. C., & Vingerhoets, A. J. J. M. (2002). Crying and mood states: a cross-cultural study. *Cognition and Emotion, 16,* 87–101.

Bekker, M. H. J. (1993). The development of an autonomy scale based on recent insights into gender identity. *European Journal of Personality, 7,* 177–194.

Bekker, M. H. J. (2003). Investigating gender within health research is more than sex disaggregation of data; a multi-facet gender & health model. *Psychology, Medicine, and Health, 8,* 231–243.

Bekker, M. H. J., & van Assen, M. A. L. M. (2006). A short form of the autonomy scale: properties of the Autonomy-Connectedness Scale. *Journal of Personality Assessment, 86,* 51–60.

Bekker, M. H. J., & van Assen, M. A. L. M. (submitted). Autonomy-connectedness and gender.

Bekker, M. H. J., & Belt, U. (2006). The role of autonomy-connectedness in anxiety and depression. *Depression and Anxiety, 23,* 274–280

Bekker, M. H. J., & Boselie, A. H. M. (2002). The role of gender and stress in gender role stress; a reexamination of the relationship between feminine gender role stress and eating disorders. *Stress and Health, 18,* 141–149.

Bekker, M. H. J., & Vingerhoets, A. J. J. M. (1999). Adam's tears; the relationship between crying, biological sex and gender. *Psychology, Evolution and Gender, 1*, 11–31.

Bekker, M. H. J., & Vingerhoets, A. J. J. M. (2001). Male and female tears: swallowing versus shedding? The relationship between crying, biological sex and gender. In A. J. J. M. Vingerhoets & R. R. Cornelius (Eds.), *Adult crying: a biopsychosocial approach* (pp. 91–114). Hove, UK: Brunner-Routledge.

Bekker, M. H. J., Bachrach, N., & Croon, M. A. (2007). The relationships of antisocial behavior with attachment styles autonomy-connectedness, and alexithymia. *Journal of Clinical Psychology, 63*, 507–527.

Bekker, M. H. J., Croon, M. A., & Bertrand, I. (under review). The relationship between parental attachment experiences autonomy-connectedness, and eating disorders *Journal of Clinical Psychology*.

Berenbaum, H., & Oltmanns, T. F. (1992). Emotional experience and expression in schizophrenia and depression. *Journal of Abnormal Psychology, 101*, 37–44.

Berry, D. S., & Pennebaker, J. W. (1993). Nonverbal and verbal emotional expression and health. *Psychotherapy & Psychosomatics, 59,* 11–19.

Brebner, J. (2003). Gender and emotions. *Personality and Individual Differences, 34*, 387–394.

Brehm, S. S. (1992). *Intimate relationships* (2nd ed.). New York: McGraw-Hill.

Brody, L. R. (1985). Gender differences in emotional development: a review of theories and research. *Journal of Personality, 53*, 102–149.

Brody, L. R. (1997). Gender and emotion: beyond stereotypes. *Journal of Social Issues, 53*, 369–394.

Brody, L. R. (1999). *Gender, emotion, and the family*. Cambridge, MA: Harvard University Press.

Brody, L. R. (2000). *The socialization of gender differences in emotional expression: display rules, infant termperament, and differentiation*. New York: Cambridge University Press.

Brody, L. R., & Hall, J. A. (1993). Gender and emotion. In M. Lewis & J. M. Haviland (Eds.), *Sex and gender* (Review of Personality and Social Psychology, *7*) (pp. 149–177). Beverly Hills, CA: Sage.

Bruch, H. (1973). *Eating disorders.* New York: Basic Books.

Bruch, H. (1978). The golden cage: the enigma of anorexia nervosa. Cambridge, MA: Harvard University Press.

Chodorow, N. (1989). *Feminism and psychoanalytic theory*. Cambridge, MA: Polity Press.

Cockell, S. J., Hewitt, P. L., Goldner, M. E., Srikameswaran, S., & Flett, G. L. (1997). Trait and self presentation dimensions of perfectionism among women with anorexia nervosa. Paper presented at Eating Disorders April 1997, London, England.

Cornelius, R. R. (1997). Toward a new understanding of weeping and catharsis? In A. J. J. M. Vingerhoets, F. J. Van Bussel & A. J. W. Boelhouwer (Eds.), *The (non)expression of emotions in health and disease* (pp. 303–321). Tilburg, The Netherlands: Tilburg University Press.

Denollet, J. (2000). Type D personality: a potential risk factor refined. *Journal of Psychosomatic Research, 4,* 255–266.

Dindia, K., & Allen, A. (1992). Sex differences in self-disclosure: a meta-analysis. *Psychological Bulletin, 112*, 106–124.

Eisenberger, N. I., Kenemy, M. E., & Wyatt, G. E. (2003). Psychological inhibition and CD4 T-cell levels in HIV-seropositive women. *Journal of Psychosomatic Research, 54*, 213–224.

Eisenberg, N., Miller, P., Shell, R., McNalley, S., & Shea, C. (1991). Prosocial development in adolescence: a longitudinal study. *Developmental Psychology, 27,* 849–857.

Eisler, R. M., & Blalock, J. A. (1991). Masculine gender role stress: implications for the assessment of men. *Clinical Psychology Review, 11,* 45–60.

Elmore, D. K., & De Castro, J. M. (1990). Self-rated moods and hunger in relation to spontaneous eating behavior in bulimics, recovered bulimics, and normals. *International Journal of Eating Disorders, 9,* 179–190.

Emmons, R. A., & King, L. A. (1988). Conflict among personal strivings: immediate and long-term implications for psychological and physical well-being. *Journal of Personality and Social Psychology, 54*, 1040–1048.

Fairburn, C. G., Cooper, Z., & Safran, R. (2003). Cognitive behavior therapy for eating disorders: A "transdiagnostic" theory and treatment. *Behavior Research and Therapy, 41,* 509–528.

Fenigstein, A., Scheier, M. F., & Buss, A. H. (1975). Public and private self-consciousness: assessment and theory. *Journal of Consulting & Clinical Psychology, 43,* 522–527.

Fischer, A. H. (2000). *Gender and emotion: social psychological perspectives.* Cambridge: Cambridge University Press.

Fischer, P. C., Smith, R. J., Leonard, E., Fuqua, D. R., Campbell, J.L., & Masters, M. A. (1993). Sex differences on affective dimensions: continuing examination. *Journal of Counseling and Development, 71,* 440–443.

Fredrickson, B. L., & Roberts, T-A. (1997). Objectification theory. Toward understanding women's lived experiences and mental health risks. *Psychology of Women Quarterly, 21,* 173–206.

Friedman, H. S., & Booth-Kewley, S. (1987). Personality, type A behavior, and coronary heart disease. The role of emotional expression. *Journal of Personality and Social Psychology, 53,* 783–792.

Ganley, R. M. (1989). Emotion and eating in obesity: a review of the literature. *International Journal of Eating Disorders, 8,* 343–361.

Garfinkel, P. E., Lin, E., Goering P., & Spegg, C. (1995). Bulimia nervosa in a Canadian community sample: prevalence and comparison of subgroups. *American Journal of Psychiatry, 152,* 1052–1058.

Geller, J., Cockell, S. J. Hewitt, P. L., Goldner, E. M., & Flett, G. L. (2000). Inhibited expression of negative emotions and interpersonal orientation in anorexia nervosa. *International Journal of Eating Disorders, 28,* 8–19.

Gidron, Y., Davidson, K., & Ilia, R. (2000). Development and cross-cultural and clinical validation of a brief comprehensive scale for assessing hostility in medical settings. *Journal of Behavioral Medicine, 24,* 1–15.

Gilligan, C. (1982). *In a different voice.* Cambridge, MA: Harvard University Press.

Gilligan, C., Lyons, N., & Hammer, T. (Eds.). (1990). *Making connections:the relational worlds of adolescent girls at Emma Willard School.* Cambridge, MA: Harvard University Press.

Gilligan, C., Rogers, A. G., & Tolman, D. L. (1991). *Women, girls, and psychotherapy.* New York: Haworth Press.

Gottman, J., & Levenson, R. (1986). Assessing the role of aggression in marriage. *Behavioral Assessment, 8,* 31–48.

Greeno, C. G., & Wing, R. R. (1994). Stress-induced eating. *Psychological Bulletin, 115,* 444–464.

Gross, J. J. (1998). Antecendent and response-focused emotional regulation: divergent consequences for experience, expression and physiology. *Journal of Personality and Social Psychology, 74,* 224–237.

Gross, J., J. & Levenson, R. W. (1993). Emotional suppression: physiology, self-report, and expressive behavior. *Journal of Personality and Social Psychology, 64,* 970–986.

Gross, J. J., & John, O. P. (1998). Mapping the domain of expressivity: multimethod evidence for a hierarchical model. *Journal of Personality and Social Psychology, 74,* 170–191.

Gross, J. J., & Munoz, R. F. (1995). Emotion regulation and mental health. *Clinical Psychology: Science and Practice, 2,* 426–438.

Hall, J. (1984). *Nonverbal sex differences: communication accuracy and expressive style.* Baltimore, MD: John Hopkins University Press.

Hawkins, R. C. II., & Clement, P. F. (1984). Binge eating: measurement problems and a conceptual model. In R. C. Hawkins, W. J. Fremouw, & P. F. Clement (Eds.), *The binge purge syndrome: diagnosis, treatment, and research* (pp. 229–251). New York: Springer.

Hayaki, J., Friedman, M. A., & Brownell, K. D. (2002). Emotional expression and body dissatisfaction. *International Journal of Eating Disorders, 31,* 57–62.

Heatherton, T. F., & Baumeister, R. F. (1991). Binge-eating as an escape from self-awareness. *Psychological Bulletin, 110,* 86–108.

Hockemeyer, J., & Smyth, J. (2002). Evaluating the feasibility and efficacy of a self-administered manual-based stress management intervention for individuals with asthma: results from a controlled study. *Behavioral Medicine, 27,* 161–172.

Hoek, H. W., & van Hoeken, D. (2003). Review of the prevalence and incidence of eating disorders. *International Journal of Eating Disorders, 34,* 383–396.

Huon, G. F., & Brown, L.B. (1989). Assessing bulimics' dissatisfaction with their body. *British Journal of Clinical Psychology, 28,* 283–284.

Kaplan, A. G. (1986). The "self-in-relation" implications for depression in women. *Psychotherapy: Theory, Research and Practice, 23,* 234–242.

Kaplan, A. G., & Surrey, J. L. (1984). The relational self in women: developmental theory and public policy. In L. Walker (Ed.), *Women and mental health policy* (pp. 79–94). Beverly Hills, CA: Sage.

Kaplan, H. I., & Kaplan, H. S. (1957). The psychosomatic concept of obesity. *The Journal of Nervous and Mental Disease, 125,* 181–201.

Kring, A. M. (2000). Gender and anger. In A. H. Fischer (Ed.),*Gender and emotion* (pp. 211–231). Cambridge: Cambridge University Press.

Kring, A. M., & Gordon, A. H. (1998). Sex differences in emotion: expression, experience and physiology. *Journal of Personality and Social Psychology, 74,* 686–703.

Kring, A. M., Kerr, S., Smith, D.A., & Neale, J. M. (1993). Flat affect in schizophrenia does not reflect diminished subjective experience of emotion. *Journal of Abnormal Psychology, 102,* 507–517.

Kring, A. M., Smith, D.A., & Neale, J. M. (1994). Individual differences in dispositional expressiveness: development and validation of the emotional expressivity scale. *Journal of Personality and Social Psychology, 66,* 934–949.

Labott, S. M., Ahleman, S., Wolever, M. E., & Martin, R. B. (1990). The physiological effects of the expression and inhibition of emotion. *Behavioral Medicine, 16,* 182–189.

Lengua, L. J., & Stormshak, E. A. (2000). Gender, gender roles, and personality: gender differences in the prediction of coping and psychological symptoms. *Sex Roles, 43,* 787–820.

Lieberman, M., Gauvin, L., Bukowski, W. M., & White, D. R. (2001). Interpersonal influence and disordered eating behaviors in adolescent girls: the role of peer modeling, social reinforcement, and body-related teasing. *Eating Behaviors, 2,* 215–236.

Littrell, J. (1998). Is the reexperience of painful emotion therapeutic? *Clinical Psychology Review, 18,* 71–102.

Lucas, A. R., Beard, C. M., O'Fallon, W. M., & Kurland, L. T. (1991). 50-year trends in the incidence of anorexia nervosa in Rochester, Minn.: a population-based study. *American Journal of Psychiatry, 148,* 917–922.

McCarthy, M. (1990). The thin ideal, depression, and eating disorders in women. *Behavioral Research and Therapy, 28,* 205–218.

McGuire, W. J., & McGuire, C. V. (1982). Significant others in self-space: sex differences and devleopmental trends in the social self. In J. Suls (Ed.), *Social psychological perspectives on the self* (pp. 71–96). Hillsdale, NJ: Erlbaum.

McManus, F., & Waller, G. (1995). A functional analysis of binge eating. *Clinical Psychology Review, 15,* 845–864.

Mendes, W. B., Reis, H. T., Seery, M. D., & Blascovich, J. (2003). Cardiovascular correlates of emotional expression and suppression: do content and gender context matter? *Journal of Personality and Social Psychology, 84,* 771–792.

Meyer, C., Leung, N., Waller, G., Perkins, S., Paice, N., & Mitchell, J. (2005). Anger and bulimic psychopathology: gender differences in a nonclinical group. *International Journal of Eating Disorders, 37,* 69–71.

Milligan, R.-J., & Waller, G. (2000). Anger and bulimic psychopathology among nonclinical women. *International Journal of Eating Disorders, 28,* 446–450.

Mirowsky, J. & Ross, C. E. (1995). Sex differences in distress: real or artifact? *American Sociological Review, 60,* 449–468.

Neckowitz, P., & Morrison, T. L. (1991). Interactional coping strategies of normal-weight bulimic women in intimate and nonintimate stressful situations. *Psychological Reports, 69,* 1167–1175.

Nyklíček, I., Vingerhoets, A. J. J. M., & Denollet, J. (2002). Emotional (non)-expression and health: data, questions, and challenges. *Psychology & Health, 17,* 517–528.

Panagopulou, E., Kersbergen, B., & Maes, S. (2002). The effects of emotional (non-expression in (chronic) disease: a meta-analytic review. *Psychology and Health, 17*, 529–545.

Pennebaker, J. W. (1985). Traumatic experience and psychosomatic disease: exploring the roles of behavioral inhibition, obsession, and confiding. *Canadian Psychology, 26*, 82–95.

Pike, K. M. (1995). Bulimic symptomatology in high school girls: toward a model of cumulative risk. *Psychology of Women Quarterly, 19,* 373–396.

Rodin, J., Silberstein, L. R., & Striegel-Moore, R. H. (1985). Women and weight: a normative discontent. In T. B. Sonderegger (Ed.), *Nebraska symposium on motivation* (pp. 267–308). Lincoln, NE: Univeristy of Nebraska Press.

Rude, S. S., & Burnham, B. L. (1995). Connectedness and neediness: factors of the DEQ and SAS Dependency scales. *Cognitive Therapy and Research, 19*, 323–340.

Rutter, M., Caspi, A., & Moffitt, T. E. (2003). Using sex differences in psychopathology to study causal mechanisms: unifying issues and research strategies. *Journal of Child Psychology and Psychiatry, 44,* 1092–1115.

Schwartz, G. E., Weinberger, D. A., & Singer, J. A. (1981). Cardiovascular differentiation of happiness, sadness, anger and fear following imagery and exercise. *Psychosomatic Medicine, 43*, 343–364.

Siegman, A. W., Anderson, R. A., & Berger, T. (1990). The angry voice: its effect on the experience of anger and cardiovascular reactivity. *Psychosomatic Medicine, 52*, 631–643.

Silberstein, L. R., Striegel-Moore, R. H., Timko, C., & Rodin, J. (1988). Behavioral and psychological implications of body dissatisfaction: do men and women differ? *Sex Roles, 19,* 219–232.

Smolak, L. & Murnen, S. K. (2003). A feminist approach to eating disorders. In J. K. Thompson (Ed.), *Handbook of eating disorders and obesity* (pp. 590–591). Hoboken, NJ: Wiley.

Smolak, L., & Munstertieger, B. F. (2002). The relationship of gender and voice to depression and eating disorders.*Psychology of Women Quarterly, 26*, 234–241.

Soukup, V. M., Beiler, M. E., & Terrell, F. (1990). Stress, coping style, and problem solving ability among eating-disordered inpatients. *Journal of Clinical Psychology, 46,* 592–599.

Soundy, T. J., Lucas, A. R., Suman, V. J., & Melton, L. J. (1995). Bulimia nervosa in Rochester, Minnesota from 1980 to 1990. *Psychological Medicine, 25,* 1065–1071.

Spielberger, C. D., Johnson, E., Russell, S., Crane, R., Jacobs, G., & Worden, T. (1985). The experience and expression of anger: construction and validation of an anger expression scale. In M. A. Chesney, & R. H. Roseman (Eds.), *Anger and hostility in cardiovascular and behavioral disorders* (pp 5–30). New York: McGraw-Hill.

Stice, E. (1998). Relations of restraint and negative affect to bulimic pathology: a longitudinal test of three competing models. *International Journal of Eating Disorders, 23,* 243–260.

Stice, E., & Agras, W. S. (1998). Predicting onset and cessation of bulimic behaviors during adolescence: a longitudinal grouping analysis. *Behavior Therapy, 29,* 257–276.

Stice, E., Presnell, K., & Spangler, D. (2002). Risk factors for binge eating onset in adolescent girls: a 2-year prospective investigation. *Health Psychology, 21,* 131–138.

Striegel-Moore, R. (1993). Etiology of binge eating: a developmental perspective. In C. G. Fairburn & G. T. Wilson (Eds.), *Binge eating: nature, assessment, and treatment* (pp. 144–172). New York: Guilford Press.

Striegel-Moore, R. H., Silberstein, L. R., & Rodin, J. (1993). The social self in bulimia nervosa: public self-consciousness, social anxiety, and perceived fraudulence. *Journal of Abnormal Psychology, 102,* 297–303.

Taylor, J., Gilligan, C., & Sullivan, A. (1995). *Between voice and silence: women and girls race and relationship.* Cambridge, MA: Harvard University Press.

Taylor, S. E., Klein, L. C., Lewis, B. P., Gruenewald, T. L., Gurung, R. A. R., & Updegraff, J. A. (2000). Biobehavioral responses to stress in females: tend-and-befriend, not fight-or-flight. *Psychological Review, 107,* 411–429.

Thomas, S., & Williams, R. L. (1991). Perceived stress, trait anger, modes of anger expression, and health status of college men and women. *Nursing Research, 40,* 303–307

Troop, N. A., Holbrey, A., Trowler, R., & Treasure, J. L. (1994). Ways of coping in women with eating disorders. *Journal of Nervous and Mental Disease 182*, 535–540.

Timmers, M., Fischer, A. H., & Manstead, A. S. R. (1998). Gender differences in motives for regulating emotions. *Personality and Social Psychology Bulletin, 9*, 974–985.

Vingerhoets, A. J. J. M., & Scheirs, J. M. G. (2001). Crying and health. In A. J. J. M. Vingerhoets & R. R. Cornelius (Eds.), *Adult crying: a biopsychosocial approach* (pp 143–166). Hove: Brunner-Routledge.

Vingerhoets, A. J. J. M., Cornelius, R. R., Van Heck, G. L., & Becht, M. C. (2000). Adult crying: a model and review of the literature. *Review of General Psychology, 4*, 354–377.

Waller, G., Babbs, M., Milligan, R., Meyer, C., Ohanian, V., & Leung, N. (2003). Anger and core beliefs in the eating disorders. *International Journal of Eating Dsiorders, 34,* 118–124.

Wardle, J., Steptoe, A, Olliver, G., & Lipsey, Z. (1999). Stress, dietary restraint and food intake. *Journal of Psychosomatic Research, 48*, 195–202.

Zaitsoff, S. L., Geller, J., & Srikameswaran, S. (2002). Silencing the self and suppressed anger: relationship to eating disorder symptoms in adolescent females. *European Eating Disorders Review, 101,* 51–60.

Chapter 12
Emotional Competence and Health in Children

Carolien Rieffe, Mark Meerum Terwogt, and Francine C. Jellesma

Introduction

The prevalence of pain complaints in children is a serious problem. Between 8 and 14 years of age, approximately one-third of children report pain at least once a week (Petersen, Bergström, & Brulin, 2003; Roth-Isigkeit, Thyen, Raspe, Stoven, & Schmucker, 2004). Pain complaints that involve the gastrointestinal system are highly prevalent in children (Perquin, Hazebroek-Kampschreur, Hunfeld, Van Suijlekom-Smit, Passchier, & Van der Wouden, 2000; Roth-Isigkeit et al., 2004). Many of these children have to undergo invasive medical testing, whereby they are missing out on school and outside-school activities. Consequently, their social, emotional, and cognitive development is at risk, which can cause even greater problems for their future (Roth-Isigkeit, Thyen, Stoven, Schwarzenberger, & Schmucker, 2005). Moreover, a clear medical cause can only be found in less than 10% of the children who attend the medical circuit (Edwards, Mullins, Johnson, & Bernardy, 1994; Walker et al., 2004). This raises the question whether factors other than those that are purely medical are involved.

Many studies performed in adults have shown a relationship between somatic complaints and impaired emotional functioning. Emotional problems such as increased levels of stress, excessive experience of negative emotions, and symptoms of depression or feelings of fear often co-occur with an increase in somatic complaints. There is strong evidence that these factors are also important in children (Campo et al., 2004; De Waal, Arnold, Eekhof, & Van Hemert, 2004). The basic idea is that this impaired emotional functioning prevents children from dealing effectively with their negative emotions. This inadequacy enhances the probability of high and prolonged stress levels. It is currently widely recognized that severe and chronic stress has a negative effect on people's biological functioning and in the long-term may cause (irreversible) organic damage (Bhatia & Tandon, 2005; Segerstrom & Miller, 2004).

Yet, it is unclear how exactly children with unexplained somatic complaints react on incoming emotion signals and which impairments in their emotional functioning could be held responsible for that reaction pattern. Besides temperamental factors, emotional functioning is based on emotional competence, which involves a wide range of skills including the ability to detect one's own emotional states, an

A. Vingerhoets et al., (eds.), *Emotion Regulation.*

effective analysis of their causes (eliciting situational elements), and consequences (physiologic correlates as well as action tendencies that might or might not ask for regulation) (Meerum Terwogt & Olthof, 1989; Saarni, 1999). We examined two major areas of emotional competence that are likely to be important with respect to somatization: children's emotion awareness and their coping potential. In this chapter, we summarize the results of a number of studies in which we have examined these two factors in relation to children's pain and other somatic complaints.

Research Population

Pain complaints are most frequently reported by 8- to 18-year-old children: A study in The Netherlands that involved data on more than 5,000 respondents showed that more than one-third of children within this age range reported recurrent or continuous pains for more than 3 months; the proportion is somewhat lower in younger children (Perquin, Hazebroek-Kampschreur, Hunfeld, Van Suijlekom-Smit, Passchier, & Van der Wouden, 2000). Most of the samples we used in the studies described in this chapter consisted of Dutch or British primary and secondary school children aged 9 to 13 years. Younger children were excluded for pragmatic reasons: below the age of 9, not all research instruments used can be considered appropriate and reliable.

Pain and other somatic complaints in our studies are based on children's self-reports by means of a Somatic Complaints List (Jellesma, Rieffe, & Meerum Terwogt, in press), which reflects a selection of the most common complaints in children (and corresponds for example with those identified as common by the more exhaustive Children's Somatization Inventory of Garber, Walker, & Zeman [1991]). Children were asked to score each item on a Likert type scale (0 = never, 1 = sometimes, 2 = often). The internal consistency of the scale has been tested on a sample of 740 children and is adequate ($\alpha > .70$) (Jellesma et al., in press; Rieffe, Meerum Terwogt, & Bosch, in press; Rieffe, Oosterveld, & Meerum Terwogt, 2006).

In most of our own studies, the data were collected among children from a normal population. When the data on the emotion indices were only collected by means of questionnaires, we analyzed the data of the total sample and used correlations and regression analyses. In other studies, children were tested individually in a separate room by the experimenter, for example, when children were to read vignettes that described social interactions with peers and asked how they would feel or what they would do. In those studies, we compared children who reported a high level of symptoms (upper 5%) with children who reported no or few somatic complaints (lowest 5%). These groups will be referred to as HSC (high somatic children) and LSC (low somatic children), respectively. In some studies, we also included a third group, a clinical group, consisting of children with abdominal pain who were attending an outpatient clinic. These children had been referred by their general practitioner to the pediatric outpatient clinic of the VU University Medical Centre Amsterdam, with complaints of abdominal pain. This group will be referred to as OPC (outpatient children). When comparing group outcomes, analyses of variance were used to analyze the data.

Emotion Awareness

Negative emotions arise when a change in the situation is perceived as potentially harmful to one's concerns (Frijda, 1986). They are accompanied by more or less notable physical reactions, such as sweating, a faster heartbeat, and tension in the abdominal area. These physical reactions have an important function because they prepare the system to react adaptively to the situation, for example to attack or to get away from the situation as quickly as one can (Frijda, 1986). However, these primitive action tendencies like fleeing or attacking are rarely socially accepted and therefore often suppressed (Gross & Levenson, 1993). Without any alternative action, the now dysfunctional preparation response might become a problem: the prolonged stress might harm the body in the end. When the emotion rises into consciousness (that is, when people have an emotional experience), the cognitive control system usually enables people to revise their perception of the situation or to refine their basic action tendencies (Levenson, 1999). When this analysis, or "reappraisal," indicates that the situation is less harmful than it initially seemed, the emotion and accompanying preparation response diminishes accordingly. When this reappraisal enables the victim to find a more acceptable response pattern to express his emotion, a similar result is achieved.

Although emotional states include physiologic reactions, people usually refer to emotional labels when they describe how they feel (e.g., "I feel scared" or "I am angry"). In other words, people normally process emotional states on a cognitive level although these emotional states consist of a physiologic component as well. This presupposes the acknowledgment of one's own emotions and their causes, but environmental and personal factors may promote a different interpretation of the physiologic reactions during emotional states (Pennebaker & Skelton, 1981). For example, one could misinterpret sweating as a symptom of an oncoming illness instead of linking it to the stressful situation that caused it. Moreover, some people seem to be more prone to physical interpretations than others, especially when they have difficulties in detecting their own emotions or have learned to ignore them (Robbins & Kirmayer, 1991). There is always some rivalry between physical and emotional attributions (Pennebaker, 1984), which is not without consequences. An emotional interpretation will change one's focus to external stimuli. One will try to detect the causes of the emotion that contain the necessary information to find a way out (Frijda, 1986). Yet, if one only focuses on one's physical discomfort, no appropriate action will be taken to solve the stressful situation. For example, one might lie down instead, in order to deal with the physical complaint.

The inability to identify one's own emotions is put forward by some clinicians as the most prominent characteristic of people with psychosomatic complaints (Sifneos, 1996). This incapacity is a central feature of alexithymia (Sifneos, 1973).

A clear distinction has to be made between *moods* (global affective states without a cause, object, or onset) and *emotions* (affective states that are directly linked to a specific event or situation) (Frijda, 1993). Thus, whereas we are, for instance, *in* a bad mood, we are angry *about* a certain event. It is assumed that people with alexithymia can identify their own mood states, but they fail to identify emotions, because they do not link their affective condition to specific situations, memories, or expectations (Bagby & Taylor, 1999). The physical symptoms associated with emotional arousal are also not adequately identified and these physical signals are easily misinterpreted as organic problems. This continuation of negative feelings and the corresponding physical changes explain the predominately negative mood states and somatizing tendencies that characterize alexithymic individuals (Sifneos, 1996). As noted before, chronic negative mood states, such as depression and anxiety, are repeatedly found to be related to somatic complaints in adults and in children. In line with these studies, we also find the expected negative mood states in the groups with more health complaints (both OPC and HSC). These children report less happiness and more depression, anger, sadness, and fear states than their peers who report few or no somatic complaints (Meerum Terwogt, Rieffe, Miers, Jellesma, & Tolland, 2006; Rieffe et al., 2004; 2006).

Emotion-Evoking Situations to Examine the Alexithymia Hypothesis

In our first attempt to examine the alexithymia hypothesis, we presented children with a set of positive and negative emotion-evoking vignettes (Fig. 12.1). After presenting each vignette, children were asked how they would feel. Additionally, they were asked to rate on a thermometer-like scale how strong they would feel the emotion they named ("How [emotion reported by the child] would you feel?") and how often they had experienced this kind of situation ("Did something like this ever happen to you? If yes: "How often has this happened?").

Contrary to the mood state inventory, here we asked for the detection of emotion within a specified situation. Based on the alexithymia hypothesis, one would expect that children with more somatic complaints (OPC and HSC) would fail to identify an emotional state in negative situations. However, emotion responses to vignettes did not differentiate between the groups. Surprisingly, self-reported somatic complaints were unrelated to children's ability to identify their own emotions in negative situations. Instead, the results demonstrated that children who had reported more somatic complaints (OPC and HSC) had more intense negative emotions in emotion-evoking situations than did their peers from the LSC group. They also reported that they had experienced those kinds of negative social situations more often (Rieffe et al., in press).

It could be argued that children with more somatic complaints experience more negative social interactions as a consequence of their poor health status. Frequent somatic complaints could affect children's social development when the complaints lead to missing out on school and peer activities, which are quite common

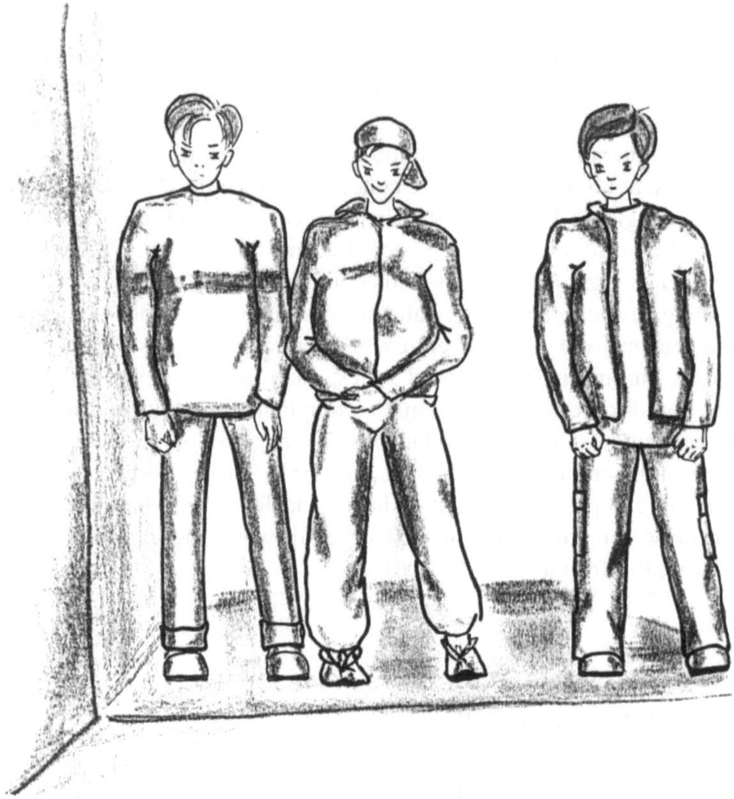

Fig. 12.1 Example of a negative emotion-evoking vignette: "Imagine you have to walk home past another school. Over the past 2 weeks, some boys from the other school have started waiting for you. They stand in your way and will not let you walk past. They are much older and bigger than you. When you try to walk past, they push you and make fun of you."

consequences of somatic complaints in children (Roth-Isigkeit et al., 2005). In order to examine this alternative explanation for our previous findings, we presented LSC and HSC groups ($n = 48$) with three social conflict situations as well as with three nonsocial negative situations. An example of a nonsocial vignette is "Imagine that you get a new Playstation for your birthday. You rush home to play it after school. You are having so much fun that you are still playing when your mum brings your dinner. You pause the game to have a drink, but you accidentally spill your juice on the console. The Playstation stops working. Your mum tells you it is broken and there is nothing one can do." Among other questions (which will be discussed later in the section on coping), children were asked how they would feel and if they had ever experienced a similar situation. Again, there was no difference between the two groups with respect to the initial emotion identification. Almost all children identified a negative emotion for all six vignettes. Consistent with the previous studies, HSC children more often reported to have been in the social conflicting situations they were presented with than the LSC children. However, this difference between the HSC and LSC groups also applied to the nonsocial situations.

Although these outcomes seem to challenge the alexithymia hypothesis, they also give room for another possible alternative explanation. One could argue that because the children in our studies were asked about their emotions, they were focused by these questions on the emotional impact of the situation, which they might fail to do spontaneously. However, the fact that children who report more somatic complaints consistently report more intense emotions and also report to experience these kinds of negative situations more often suggests that these children are well aware of the negative impact of their daily life situations.

Even if children are able to identify their own emotional state, this does not imply that these children are also able to differentiate between specific emotions. Feeling "bad" may mean either of the negative emotions sadness or anger. Whereas feeling bad only implies a general negative feeling, sadness focuses on the loss one experiences and angry focuses on harm that has been done (Stein & Trabasso, 1989). In other words, it is not clear from these experiments whether children who score high on somatic complaints are able to fully analyze the situation and identify the exact causes of their feelings, which would give them the opportunity to identify specific emotions instead of a general negative feeling. This issue was considered in our next set of studies for which we used self-report questionnaires.

Questionnaires to Examine the Alexithymia Hypothesis

Another way to look at the validity of the alexithymia hypothesis is by means of questionnaires, which has frequently been done with adult participants. The most widely used questionnaire for adults is the 20-item Toronto Alexithymia Scale (TAS-20; Bagby, Parker, & Taylor, 1994). This questionnaire consists of three factors that are thought to represent the three core features of the alexithymia concept: (a) Difficulty Identifying Feelings, (b) Difficulty Describing Feelings, and (c) Externally Oriented Thinking, which refers to "a cognitive style that shows a preference for external detail of everyday life rather than thought content related feelings, fantasies and other aspects of a person's inner experiences" (Bagby et al., 1994, p. 31). Numerous studies confirm that the TAS-20 correlates positively with self-reported physical symptoms and negatively with perceived level of health in adult populations (e.g., De Gucht, & Heiser, 2003; Taylor & Bagby, 2000). Also, the predicted positive association between the TAS-20 and negative mood states and a negative correlation with positive mood states is well established (e.g., Bagby & Taylor, 1999; Lundh & Simonsson-Sarnecki, 2001; Suslow & Junghanns, 2002). However, it is argued that the contribution of the third factor to the prediction of somatic complaints should be minimal (Taylor, Bagby, & Luminet, 2000). When investigated separately, the third factor (Externally Oriented Thinking) indeed fails to show the expected associations (De Gucht, Fischler, & Heiser, 2004; Deary, Scott, & Wilson, 1997; Grabe, Spitzer, & Freyberger, 2004; Lumley, Ovies, Stettner, Wehmer, & Lakey, 1996).

With the permission of the authors, we adapted the TAS-20 for children (Rieffe et al., 2006). Seventeen out of 20 items were reformulated to make them more comprehensible for children. For example, the original item "It is difficult for me to find the right words for my feelings" became "I find it difficult to say how I feel inside." When tested among normally developing children and young adolescents ($n = 740$), the results showed that the three-factor structure remained intact and a lower ability to identify and describe their own emotions indeed contributed significantly to the prediction of pain and somatic complaints in children and could account for 25% of the variance of the somatic complaints list in this nonclinical population. However, this was predominately accounted for by the scale Difficulty Identifying Feelings (7 items).

Unfortunately, the scale Difficulty Identifying Feelings contains some items that are directly related to medical problems or that could be interpreted as such; for example, the item "I feel things in my body that even doctors don't understand." This could, of course account for the high contribution of this scale to the prediction of somatization. Although these items do indeed reflect a difficulty identifying feelings, which can include bodily sensations that are not caused by an emotion experience, we wanted to focus more precisely on the ability to identify emotions. Therefore, we developed a more extensive self-report questionnaire that aims to measure a wider variety of emotion awareness aspects (Rieffe, Meerum Terwogt, Petrides, Cowan, Miers, & Tolland, 2007). This Emotion Awareness Questionnaire (EAQ) aims to measure children's and adolescents' understanding of their own emotions and their understanding of the importance of emotions for their daily functioning. We identified six aspects of emotional awareness, which are reflected in six different scales with satisfactory internal consistency (Cronbach's $\alpha > .66$), except for the scale Acting Out Emotions (Cronbach $\alpha = .49$), which needed additional items. Below, example items of the scales can be found. Each scale is represented by approximately five items, and it is expected that a lower ability in these six aspects will cause more somatic complaints.

1. *Differentiating emotions* (six items; Cronbach $\alpha = .77$). The ability to identify how one feels and what kind of emotion one is feeling. An example item is "It is difficult to know whether I feel sad or angry or something else."
2. *Verbally sharing emotions* (five items, Cronbach $\alpha = .71$). The ability to talk about and explain one's own emotions. An example item is "I can easily explain to a friend how I feel inside."
3. *Acting out emotions* (three items, Cronbach $\alpha = .49$). The tendency to bluntly express one's emotions. An example item is "I like to show my feelings as they happen."
4. *Bodily awareness* (five items, Cronbach $\alpha = .74$). The ability to understand the link between emotional arousal and bodily symptoms. An example item is "When I feel upset, I can also feel it in my body."
5. *Others' emotions* (seven items, Cronbach $\alpha = .75$). The tendency to attend to and analyze emotions of others. An example item is "It is important to know how my friends are feeling."
6. *Analyses emotions* (four items, Cronbach $\alpha = .67$). The tendency to attend and analyze one's own emotions. An example item is "My feelings help me to understand what happened to me."

The first scale of the EAQ, Differentiating Emotions, overlaps partially with the factor Difficulty Identifying Feelings. This scale contains three original items from the TAS-20, although they are adapted for children. However, with the formulation of three new items, we emphasize children's ability to differentiate between various emotions and insight into the causes of their affective states. One of those new items is, for example, "Sometimes, I feel upset and I don't know why."[1] The second and the third scales, Verbal Sharing Emotions and Acting Out Emotions, show conceptual overlap with the factor Difficulty Describing Feelings of the TAS-20, but the newly formulated items for Verbal Sharing Emotions are more directed toward talking about one's feelings, whereas the scale Acting Out Emotions is focused on openly showing one's emotions to others.

When tested in a sample of 692 children, most scales showed a moderate to strong relation with somatic complaints, and they accounted for 21% of the variance of somatic complaints in a nonclinical population (Rieffe et al., 2007). Yet, not all scales contributed to this prediction. The scales Verbally Sharing Emotions and Acting Out Emotions failed to contribute to the prediction of somatization, but the other four scales did. As expected, the scales Differentiating Emotions and Analyses Emotions contributed negatively, which means that children with a stronger tendency to analyze their emotions reported fewer somatic complaints. Two of the scales, Bodily Awareness and Others' Emotions, showed a relationship in the opposite direction. The finding that attention to others' emotions is related to more somatic complaints instead of less could be explained by the formulation of the items in this scale. Whereas items in other scales ask for one's abilities and tendencies, the items in this scale ask to what extent one values to understand others' emotions. However, the fact that children think that it is important to know about others' feelings does not necessarily imply that they admit having the capacity. With respect to the scale Bodily Awareness, it was a priori assumed that awareness of bodily symptoms during emotional states would be an indicator of good emotion awareness and therefore would be likely to relate to less somatic complaints. These findings seem to indicate that children who report more somatic complaints indeed report poorer skills in analyzing their emotional states but also have a different understanding of the link between emotional arousal and physical symptoms. This will be further discussed at the end of this chapter.

Summary

In sum, the findings concerning emotional awareness lead to the following conclusions. Children who report frequent somatic complaints—outpatients as well as children who have not yet contacted a clinic—seem to notice their own emotions (linked to a specific situation) as well as their mood states. Both groups report

[1] Note that two separate scales were originally designed that distinguished Differentiating Emotions and Causes of Emotions, but the results of factor analyses in two pilot studies showed that the items from these two scales loaded on the same factor and thus seem to represent only one underlying concept.

negative emotions and negative moods with a higher frequency and a higher intensity than their healthy peers. However, although the group with more somatic complaints seems to be able to identify how they feel affectively, the contribution of two scales in two separate studies (adjusted TAS-20 scale Difficulty Identifying Feelings and EAQ-scale Differentiating Emotions) to the prediction of self-reported somatic complaints suggests that children who report more somatic complaints have less understanding of the causes of their emotional states and find it more difficult to thoroughly analyze their own emotions and differentiate between the various negative emotions.

Emotion differentiation largely depends on processing emotional information (Izard, 2001). It has been shown that the appraisal of emotion is predicted by elements closely related to the *external* emotion eliciting situation, such as who is responsible for the situation, and whether it is possible to influence the event (Sherer, 1997). However, the positive relationship of self-reported somatic complaints and attention to physiologic arousal (EAQ-scale Bodily Awareness) suggests that children reporting more somatic complaints are more attentive to bodily changes than their healthy peers and thus have a stronger *internal* focus on bodily symptoms. This internal focus of children reporting more somatic complaints may result in a decrease of attention to external events and this in turn may cause poor emotion differentiation.

Furthermore, better emotion differentiation in adults is associated with reactions to emotions that are thought to be more efficient (Barrett, Gross, Christensen, & Benvenuto, 2001). Thus, it is likely that the poor emotion differentiation of children reporting more somatic complaints will also affect their coping potential (i.e., their ability to decrease the impact of a negative situation or event).

Coping Strategies

It is not always clear-cut which coping strategies are effective and which ones are not. Different events often call for different approaches. For example, a very common first impulse in reaction to a negative event is the attempt to fix it, to find a solution for the problem in the situation itself. However, an argument with one's best friend could perhaps be solved, but the loss of a beloved pet cannot be "fixed." A so-called problem-focused (Lazarus, 1982) approach is not adequate in this kind of uncontrollable situation. Consequently, an "emotion-focused" strategy that aims to reduce the (negative) emotion without an actual situational change has to be employed.

Four-year-old children acknowledge that emotions are subjected to change. They know that emotions can wane over time (Harris, 1989). Acknowledgement of the link between emotions and cognition appears later in development. The most popular coping strategy at the age of 6 is engagement in some kind of pleasant activity, such as watching a video or playing a game, because this will distract their attention from the negative event at least for a while. It is not before their 10th year that children start to appreciate the role of more complex cognitive processes, such as reevaluating the situation, for example, "I know she is stressed at the moment, she didn't mean it like that" (Band & Weisz, 1988). Ten-year-old children do not switch from problem-focused to emotion-focused, cognitive strategies, but they use them complementarily, and if possible, a problem-focused approach is usually tried initially, even in adults (Meerum Terwogt & Olthof, 1989).

The use of coping strategies related to medical procedures and pain complaints has frequently been studied (e.g., Last & Grootenhuis, 1998), but studies concerning coping strategies related to stressful events in children with more somatic complaints are scarce. Preliminary findings suggest that children with a tendency to somatize have a less advanced coping repertoire in relation to their emotions (Bonner & Finney, 1996). Children with more abdominal pain use fewer or less effective coping strategies to deal with their negative emotions (Walker, Smith, Garber, & Van Slyke, 1997; Wilson Sharrer & Ryan-Wenger, 1991). Rector and Roger (1996) studied a sample of adolescents and found that poor emotion-focused strategies are related to somatic complaints. We have carried out several studies in this area in order to obtain more information about what strategies are related to somatic complaints.

Coping Focus

Before we consider how children deal with the emotional impact of a situation, we first want to examine the coping focus in children with somatic complaints. Possibly, the internally oriented focus of children with more health problems and a possible enhanced sensitivity to internal bodily signals causes them to focus more often on their physical reactions in stressful events. Consequently, these children may rely more often on physical solutions. For example, children could use aspirin in order to relieve a headache that developed during a stressful situation. Yet, the aspirin does not remove the eliciting factors of the emotion that caused the headache. To reach an emotional interpretation, people have to be primarily focused on external information, which reveal the basis for their emotions (Frijda, 1986). However, we have seen already that the capacity to identify detailed information about emotions and their causes seems impaired in children who report many pain complaints. This could result in neglecting the emotional impact of the situation in these children, whereas healthy children might more often deal with their anxiety or other negative emotions through emotion-focused coping styles.

The Coping Focus Questionnaire (Meerum Terwogt et al., 2006) that we designed for this purpose consists of two scales: the Emotional Focus scale (10 items, Cronbach $\alpha = .74$) and the Physiological Focus scale (12 items, Cronbach $\alpha = .82$). Each item gives a short description of a stressful event. The emotional experience and the corresponding physical reaction are explicitly stated. For half of the items in each scale, the emotional experience is anger, for the other half it is fear or nervousness. A possible reaction was then formulated. Following the items in the Emotion Focus scale, children were asked if they would deal with emotion-evoking causes and the emotional impact of the situation. Following the items in the Physiological Focus scale, children were presented with options about how to deal with the physical complaints. An example of a vignette that deals with an emotional problem is "It is your turn today to give a talk in front of your class. Before you start, you feel nervous and you feel nausea coming up." Answer categories are "I would not/maybe/certainly practice in the break, so I'll be less nervous." An example of an item that deals with the physiologic experience is "Today, you are going to have your first tennis lesson. You don't know anyone there. You feel frightened and you get a stomachache" with the following options for answering: "I would not/maybe/certainly take a pill for my stomachache."

The results of this study confirmed that children with more health problems (HSC and OPC) are more likely to act upon physiologic complaints in emotionally stressful situations than their healthy peers. The OPC group, especially, makes frequent use of this strategy to deal with the physical arousal in stressful situations. Unexpectedly, however, this does not cause the two groups with health problems to make less use of emotion-focused strategies. Children from all three groups reported that they would employ the emotion-focused strategies equally often.

Effectiveness of Coping Strategies

Because the findings of the previously described study clearly show that children with more somatic and pain complaints report that they do focus on the emotional impact of the stressful situation, the obvious question now is what kind of emotion-focused strategy they employ and whether those differ from their healthier peers. In order to examine this, we presented 48 participants in our next study with eight emotion-evoking situations as described before (see the example of the Playstation that breaks down because the participant spoiled his juice over the console), and after each vignette, we asked children the following set of questions: (1) How would you feel? (2) How [emotion reported by the child in response to the first question] would you feel? (3) Is there anything you could do to change the way you would feel? Is there anything else you could do? (4) How [emotion reported by the child] would you feel after that? (5) Imagine you are in bed later that night and you think again about what has happened. Would you still feel [emotion reported by the child]? How [emotion reported by the child] would you feel? (6) Has something like this ever happened to you? If yes: How [emotion reported by the child] did you feel?

First of all, note that there are three points in time where we asked children for the intensity of their emotional experience. This is the only study where we did not find a difference between the HSC and LSC on the intensity of their initial emotional reaction, which might have been caused by a ceiling effect (we only used a 5-point scale here instead of the usual thermometer, and children scored near the maximum on this initial question). Both groups reported a decrease when they were asked for the intensity of their emotion the second time, after they had thought of a coping strategy. The LSC group reported an even lower intensity when they would think about the event later that night in bed (time 3), but the emotion between time 2 and time 3 remained equally intense for the HSC group (Fig. 12.2). This finding is in

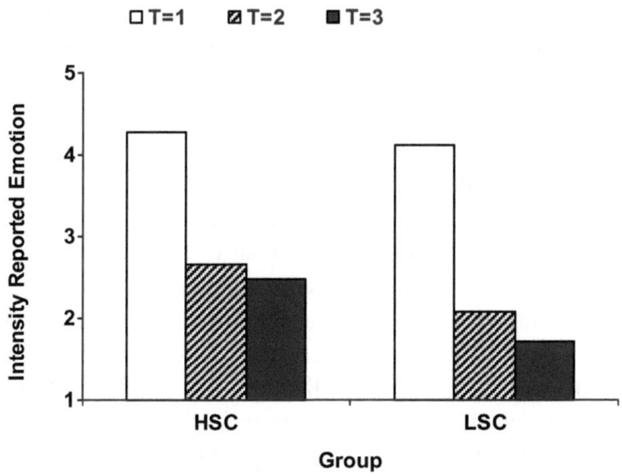

Fig. 12.2 Intensity of the reported emotion at times 1, 2, and 3 after an emotion-evoking event per group.

line with the results of Wilson Sharrer and Ryan-Wenger (1991) that also showed that children with recurrent abdominal pain reported their coping strategies to be less effective.

Children's responses to question 3 ("Is there anything you could do to change the way you would feel?") were tape-recorded and the transcripts that were derived from these recordings were coded by two raters independently (interrater reliability was 92% and differences were solved by discussion). Responses were categorized as *Problem Focused* (direct attempt to solve the problem, e.g., repair or replace the object, ask for social support to solve the problem) or *Emotion Focused* (attempt to change the way the situation is perceived, e.g., reassuring themselves, put situation into perspective). Additionally, *Avoiding strategies* (e.g., doing something else; avoid thinking about the event; thinking about something different, which could be considered as a strategy that is applied by younger children before they have the cognitive abilities to use more sophisticated emotion-focused strategies) and maladaptive strategies, such as *Internalizing* (rumination) and *Externalizing* (slamming a door), were separately categorized.

The results showed no differences between the HSC children and the LSC children in the number of problem- or emotion-focused coping strategies they spontaneously reported in answer to the third question. Nor did the HSC children report more avoiding strategies than the LSC group. Internalizing strategies or externalizing strategies were hardly reported spontaneously by any of the children. The only difference that emerged between the LSC and HSC groups was that children in the HSC group more often failed to think of any strategy at all to make themselves feel better.

Data were also collected by means of the most widely used coping questionnaire for adolescents in The Netherlands: the Utrecht Coping List for Adolescence (UCL-A; Bijstra, Jackson & Bosma, 1994). This questionnaire distinguishes seven reaction patterns: Confrontation (trying to solve the problem), Palliative (distraction),

Avoidance, Social support, Emotion expression, Depressive (being completely occupied by the problem), and Optimism (comforting thoughts). For each scale, a number of items are formulated, which reflect a strategy, and children can report whether they use that strategy rarely or never, sometimes, often, or very often. In a regression analysis, the coping scales accounted for 14% of the variance of somatic complaints in a nonclinical population. Only two scales (Depression and Optimism) contributed significantly to this prediction. They did so in the expected direction: more somatic complaints were related to more depressive and less optimistic thoughts. Additionally, we found a strong positive correlation with a worry questionnaire (Jellesma, Meerum Terwogt, Reijntjes, Rieffe, & Stegge, 2005) and somatic complaints, which further confirms that children with more somatic complaints certainly do not abstain from reflection. Their efforts, however, are maladaptive in the sense that they tend to intensify instead of diminish their negative emotions as was also shown by Rector and Roger (1996).

Summary

Based on these coping studies, we can conclude that children from the groups with more somatic problems (HSC and OPC) indeed report a more frequent use of strategies that deal with the physical symptoms in emotion-evoking situations than LSC children. Yet, they also make use of emotion-focused strategies even though it was expected that their problems with emotion analysis would diminish this. However, note that the Coping Focus Questionnaire explicitly asks children whether they would be inclined to use both coping strategies. If they would think of such a strategy spontaneously is still an open question. Moreover, when considering the effectiveness of their strategies, HSC children do not differ from the LSC children in the kind of strategies they report, but they judged their strategies as being less effective. Thus, it can be concluded that although children with more somatic complaints are willing to use certain strategies to reduce the emotional impact of negative situations, they find it difficult to adaptively apply those strategies. Finally, compared with LSC children, the cognitive activity of the HSC group seems strongly colored by negative thoughts, including ruminative or worrying thoughts. This cognitive process is likely to worsen their negative emotional state even further and potentially also cause more intense physical reactions.

Discussion

At the beginning of this chapter, we postulated that when one focuses on the physical discomfort in an emotion-evoking situation, one will be largely unaware of the emotion experience and fail to deal appropriately with the situation. On the basis of our findings, we have to revise our initial position in two regards.

First, our data strongly support the idea that children who report more somatic complaints indeed give a lot of attention to the physiologic correlates of emotions.

However, the idea put forward by Pennebaker (1984) that people with more somatic complaints attribute these correlates to organic diseases is challenged by the fact that the children in our studies acknowledge the link between emotions and physiologic phenomena even more prominently than other children. This raises the question of why children with few complaints acknowledge the connection between the emotional state and physical phenomena to a lesser extent than their peers with more somatic complaints. Possibly, children with few somatic complaints see bodily reactions as an integral part of the emotion experience, which do not need much attention, because the focus is external, on the emotion-evoking event. For example, in an anger-provoking event with a friend, one might be more focused on the discussion, thereby neglecting the bodily arousal, such as tension in the arms and legs, a faster heart beat and so on. Thus, these children might be less attentive to these physiologic signals. Conversely, children with frequent somatic complaints possibly regard emotions and their physical correlates as separate processes; one causing the other. Moreover, for children experiencing strong emotions more regularly, as appears to be the case in the HSC children, the physiologic symptoms of an emotion experience may also be more obvious. The coping data support this explanation. Whereas children with few somatic complaints seem to feel it is sufficient to tackle the emotional problem and probably trust that the physiologic arousal will disappear as a result (once the argument with the friend is solved, or the emotional impact of the situation decreases, the physiologic response will vanish automatically), the children with more somatic complaints seem to deal with both problems in separate ways. It could be argued that children with more complaints at first take refuge in fighting the somatic symptoms, *because* they are unable to find a sufficiently effective emotional solution. Nevertheless, it is likely that their headaches or stomachaches in time will be regarded as a separate problem.

A second issue that needs reconsideration is the fact that the alexithymia hypothesis seems not to be completely valid. According to the alexithymia questionnaires findings, children with frequent somatic complaints report emotion identification and differentiation problems because they are not aware of their emotional states. However, we found that children with frequent somatic complaints were able to identify and label emotions when presented with scenarios. The results of the Emotion Awareness Questionnaire further illuminate this picture. Not the emotion identification, but rather emotion differentiation seems impaired. In order to deal effectively with a stressful situation, it is important to switch from an internal focus on bodily signals to an external one, including an analysis of the situation in emotional terms and detection of the emotion elicitors. A thorough analysis might lead to different or even multiple emotions, depending on one's focus and interpretation. For example, if your little brother intentionally smashes your portable game computer on the floor and it breaks, you could be angry with your brother for his hostility, and you could feel sad about the loss of your toy. Or if your friend witnessed the event, you could even feel ashamed of your brother's behavior. Although this line of reasoning certainly needs more investigation, there is already clear evidence that children who report more somatic complaints seem to lack a good understanding of the causes for their affective states. Additionally, they do not appreciate the informational value of emotions. In other words, they do not think that it is important to understand why they feel upset about something. As a result, they have problems differentiating between various emotions. Rather than being specific, their emotion awareness will be more global. This combination of factors also prevents them from applying emotion-focused coping strategies successfully, which has become evident from our studies. The inability to deal with negative emotions appropriately could cause their frequently reported more-intense experiences but may also result in longer-lasting arousal.

Finally, we would like to draw attention to the fact that our research included children from a normal population as well as outpatient groups. The latter consulted medical doctors with their pain complaints, which often do not result in finding a medical cause. Previous work indicates that apart from functional conditions such as chronic constipation and irritable bowel syndrome, an organic cause can only be established in less than 10% of the patients (Edwards et al., 1994; Perquin, Hazebroek-Kampschreur, Hunfeld, Bohnen, et al., 2000; Perquin, Hazebroek-Kampschreur, Hunfeld, Van Suijlekom-Smit, Passchier, & Van der Wouden, 2000). More importantly, whether or not an organic cause for the physical complaints can be identified, this appears to have little influence on the strong associations that are found between psychological functioning and pain complaints (Kellner, 1994; Von Baeyer & Walker, 1999). Various studies compared children with medically unexplained symptoms with children for whom an organic problem had been diagnosed (Nygaard, Stordal, & Bentsen, 2004; Walker, Garber, & Greene, 1993). The results of these studies show no differences between the two groups in terms of their psychological functioning. For example, both groups score higher on measures of anxiety, somatization, and internalizing problems and show a lower self-esteem compared with a nonpain group, but the two pain groups do not differ (Sharff, 1997). In this chapter, we have focused uniquely on children's emotional competence as a possible *cause* of somatic complaints. Obviously, both factors have a reciprocal influence: pain also induces negative emotions. Our choice for this approach is based on the fact that unresolved emotional problems imply continuous distress, which can result in bodily dysfunction in the long-term. In this respect, Von Baeyer and Walker (1999) argue that "the old effort to classify pain as either "organic" or "psychogenic" is now gradually laid to rest as we better recognize that pain involves reciprocal relations among biological, cognitive, and situational factors" (p. 308).

The main conclusion that can be made on the basis of the studies on emotion awareness and coping that we described in this chapter is that children with more somatic complaints seem to experience problems in some aspects of their emotional functioning that appear to be caused by a too strong internal focus on bodily symptoms. Although children with more somatic complaints are aware of their general negative feelings, this internal focus might prevent them from a thorough analysis of their emotions. Moreover, less efficient use of coping strategies may be the result of poor emotion differentiation, although more research is needed here. Currently, we are carrying out a longitudinal study among approximately 700 children and their parents in order to further examine these issues.

References

Bagby, R. M., & Taylor, G. J. (1999). Affect dysregulation and alexithymia. In G. J. Taylor, R. M. Bagby, & J. D. A. Parker (Eds), *Disorders of affect regulation* (pp. 26–45). New York: Cambridge University Press.

Bagby, R. M., Parker, J. D. A., & Taylor, G. J. (1994). The 20-Item Toronto-Alexithymia-Scale 1. Item selection and cross-validation of the factor structure. *Journal of Psychosomatic Research, 38*, 23–32.

Band, E. B., & Weisz, J. R. (1988). How to feel better when it feels bad – children's perspectives on coping with everyday stress. *Developmental Psychology, 24*, 247–253.

Barrett, L. F., Gross, J. J., Christensen, T. C., & Benvenuto, M. (2001). Knowing what you're feeling and knowing what to do about it: mapping the relation between emotion differentiation and emotion regulation. *Cognition and Emotion, 15*, 713–724.

Bathia, V., & Tandon, R. K. (2005). Stress and the gastrointestinal tract. *Journal of Gastroenterology and Hepatology, 20*, 332–339.

Bonner, M. J., & Finney, J. W. (1996). A psychosocial model of children's health status. In Th. H. Ollendick & R. J. Prinz (Eds.), *Advances in clinical child psychology* (Vol. 18, pp. 231–282). New York: Plenum Press.

Bijstra, J. O., Jackson, S., & Bosma, H. A. (1994). De Utrechtse coping lijst voor kinderen. [The Utrecht Coping List for Children] *Kind en Adolescent, 15*, 98–109.

Campo, J. V., Bridge, J., Ehmann, M., Altman, S., Lucas, A., Birmaher, B., et al. (2004). Recurrent abdominal pain, anxiety, and depression in primary care. *Pediatrics, 113*, 817–824.

De Gucht, V., Fischler, B., & Heiser, W. (2004). Neuroticism, alexithymia, negative affect, and positive affect as determinants of medically unexplained symptoms. *Personality and Individual Differences, 36*, 1655–1667.

De Gucht, V., & Heiser, W. (2003). Alexithymia and somatisation: a quantitative review of the literature. *Journal of Psychosomatic Research, 54*, 425–434.

Deary, I. J., Scott, S., & Wilson, J. A. (1997). Neuroticism, alexithymia and medically unexplained symptoms. *Personality and Individual Differences, 22*, 551–564.

De Waal, M. W. M., Arnold, I. A., Eekhof, J. A. H., & Van Hemert, A. M. (2004). Somatoform disorders in general practice – prevalence, functional impairment and comorbidity with anxiety and depressive disorders. *British Journal of Psychiatry, 184*, 470–476.

Edwards, M. C., Mullins, L. L., Johnson, J., & Bernardy, N. (1994). Survey of Pediatricians Management-Practices for Recurrent Abdominal-Pain. *Journal of Pediatric Psychology, 19*, 241–253.

Frijda, N. H. (1986). *The emotions*. New York: Cambridge University Press.

Frijda, N. H. (1993). Moods, emotion episodes, and emotions. In J. M. H. M. Lewis & J. M. Haviland (Eds.), *Handbook of emotions* (pp. 381–403). New York: Guilford Press.

Garber, J., Zeman, J. L., & Walker, L. S. (1991). Somatization symptoms in a community sample of children and adolescents: further validation of the children's somatization inventory. *Journal of Consulting and Clinical Psychology*, 588–593.

Grabe, H. J., Spitzer, C., & Freyberger, H. J. (2004). Alexithymia and personality in relation to dimensions of psychopathology. *American Journal of Psychiatry, 161*, 1299–1301.

Gross, J. J., & Levenson, R. W. (1993) Emotional suppression: physiology, self-report and expressive behaviour. *Journal of Personality and Social Psychology, 64*, 970–986.

Harris, P. L. (1989). *Children and emotion*. New York: Cambridge University Press.

Izard, C.E. (2001). Emotional intelligence or adaptive emotions? *Emotion, 1*, 249–257.

Jellesma, F.C., Meerum Terwogt, M., Reijntjes, A., Rieffe, C. & Stegge, H. (2005). De vragenlijst Non-Productieve Denkprocessen voor Kinderen (NPDK): Piekeren en rumineren. [The Non Productive Thinking Questionnaire: Worrying and rumination] *Kind en Adolescent, 26*, 368–378.

Jellesma, F.C., Rieffe, C., & Meerum Terwogt, M. (in press). The Somatic Complaints List: validation of a self-report questionnaire assessing somatic complaints in children. *Journal of Psychosomatic Research*.

Kellner, R. (1994). Psychosomatic syndromes, somatization and somatoform disorders. *Psychotherapy and Psychosomatics, 61*, 4–24.

Last, B. F., & Grootenhuis, M. A. (1998). Emotions, coping and the need for support in families of children with cancer: a model for psychosocial care. *Patient Education and Counseling, 33,* 169–179.

Lazarus, R. S. (1982). Thoughts on the relation between emotion and cognition. *American Psychologist, 37*, 1019–1024.

Levenson, R.W. (1999). The intrapersonal functions of emotions. *Cognition and Emotion, 13,* 481–504.

Lundh, L., & Simonsson-Sarnecki, M. (2001). Alexithymia, emotion and somatic complaints. *Journal of Personality, 69,* 483–510.

Lumley, M. A., Ovies, T., Stettner, L., Wehmer, F., & Lakey, B. (1996). Alexithymia, social support and health problems. *Journal of Psychosomatic Research, 41*, 519–530.

Meerum Terwogt, M., & Olthof, T. (1989). Awareness and self-regulation of emotion in young children. In C. Saarni & P. L. Harris (Eds.), *Children's understanding of emotion* (pp. 209–237). New York: Cambridge University Press.

Meerum Terwogt, M., Rieffe, C., Miers, A. C. Jellesma, F. C., & Tolland, A. (2006). Emotions and self-esteem as indicators of somatic complaints in children. *Infant and Child Development, 15,* 581-592.

Nygaard, E. A., Stordal, K., & Bentsen, B. S. (2004). Recurrent abdominal pain in children revisited: irritable bowel syndrome and psychosomatic aspects. A prospective study. *Scandinavian Journal of Gastroenterology, 39*, 938–940.

Pennebaker, J. W. (1984). The accuracy of symptom perception. In A. Baum, S. E. Taylor, & J. E. Singer (Eds.), *Handbook of psychology and health* (Vol. IV, pp. 189–217). Hillsdale, NJ: Lawrence Erlbaum.

Pennebaker, J. W., & Skelton, J. A. (1981). Selective monitoring of physical sensations. *Journal of Personality and Social Psychology, 41*, 213–223.

Perquin, C. W., Hazebroek-Kampschreur, A. A. J. M., Hunfeld, J. A. M., Bohnen, A. M., Van Suijlekom-Smit, L. W. A., Passchier, J., et al. (2000). Pain in children and adolescents: a common experience. *Pain, 87*, 51–58.

Perquin, C. W., Hazebroek-Kampschreur, A. A. J. M., Hunfeld, J. A. M., Van Suijlekom-Smit, L. W. A., Passchier, J., & Van der Wouden, J. C. (2000). Chronic pain among children and adolescents: physician consultation and medication use. *Clinical Journal of Pain, 16,* 229–235.

Petersen, S., Bergstrom, E., & Brulin, C. (2003). High prevalence of tiredness and pain in young schoolchildren. *Scandinavian Journal of Public Health, 31*, 367–374.

Rector, N. A., & Roger, D. (1996). Cognitive style and well-being: a prospective examination. *Personality and Individual Differences, 21*, 663–674.

Rieffe, C., Meerum Terwogt, M., & Bosch, J. D. (2004). Emotion understanding in children with frequent somatic complaints. *European Journal of Developmental Psychology, 1*, 31–47.

Rieffe, C., Meerum Terwogt, M., Bosch, J. D., Kneepkens, C. M. F., Douwes, A. C., & Jellesma, F. C. (in press). Interaction between emotions and somatic complaints in children that did or did not seek medical care. Cognition and Emotion.

Rieffe, C., Oosterveld, P., & Meerum Terwogt, M. (2006). An alexithymia questionnaire for children: factorial and concurrent validation results. *Personality and Individual Differences, 40,* 123–133.

Rieffe, C., Meerum Terwogt, M., Petrides, K. V., Cowan, R., Miers, A. C. & Tolland, A. (2007). Psychometric properties of the Emotion Awareness Questionnaire for children. *Personality and Individual Differences, 43,* 95–105.

Robbins, J. M., & Kirmayer, L. J. (1991). Attributions of common somatic symptoms. *Psychological Medicine, 21*, 1029–1045.

Roth-Isigkeit, A., Thyen, U., Raspe, H. H., Stoven, H., & Schmucker, P. (2004). Reports of pain among German children and adolescents: an epidemiological study. *Acta Paediatrica, 93,* 258–263.

Roth-Isigkeit, A., Thyen, U., Stoven, H., Schwarzenberger, J., & Schmucker, P. (2005). Pain among children and adolescents: restrictions in daily living and triggering factors. *Pediatrics, 115*, E152–E162.

Saarni, C. (1999). *The development of emotional competence.* New York: Guilford Press.

Segerstrom, S. C., & Miller, G. E. (2004). Psychological stress and the human immune system: a meta-analytic study of 30 years of inquiry. *Psychological Bulletin, 130,* 601–630.

Scherer, K. R. (1997). Profiles of emotion-antecedent appraisal: testing theoretical predictions across cultures. *Cognition and Emotion, 11*, 113–150.

Sifneos, P. E. (1973). Prevalence of alexithymic characteristics in psychosomatic patients. *Psychotherapy and Psychosomatics, 22*, 255–262.

Sifneos, P. E. (1996). Alexithymia: past and present. *American Journal of Psychiatry, 153*, 137–142.

Scharff, L. (1997). Recurrent abdominal pain in children: a review of psychological factors and treatment. *Clinical Psychology Review, 17*, 145–166.

Stein, N. L., & Trabasso, T. (1989). Children's understanding of changing emotional states. In C. Saarni & P. L. Harris (Eds.), *Children's understanding of emotion* (pp. 50–80). New York: Cambridge University Press.

Suslow, T., & Junghanns, K. (2002) Impairments of emotion situation priming in alexithymia. *Personality and Individual Differences, 32*, 541–550.

Taylor, G. J., & Bagby, R. M. (2000). An overview of the alexithymia construct. In R. Bar-On & J. D. A. Parker (Eds.), *Handbook of emotional intelligence* (pp. 40–67). San Francisco: Jossey-Bass.

Taylor, G. J., Bagby, R. M., & Luminet, O. (2000). Assessment of alexithymia: self-report and observer-rated scales. In R. Bar-On & J. D. A. Parker (Eds.), *Handbook of emotional intelligence* (pp. 301–319). San Francisco: Jossey-Bass.

Von Baeyer, C. L., & Walker, L. S. (1999). Children with recurrent abdominal pain: issues in the selection and description of research participants. *Journal of Developmental and Behavioral Pediatrics, 20*, 307–313.

Walker, L. S., Garber, J., & Greene, J. W. (1993). Psychosocial correlates of recurrent childhood pain – a comparison of pediatric-patients with recurrent abdominal-pain, organic illness, and psychiatric-disorders. *Journal of Abnormal Psychology, 102*, 248–258.

Walker, L. S., Smith, C. A., Garber, J., & Van Slyke, D. A. (1997). Development and validation of the Pain Response Inventory for Children. *Psychological Assessment, 9*, 392–405.

Walker, L. S., Garber, J., Smith, C. A., Van Slyke, D. A., & Claar, R. L. (2001). The relation of daily stressors to somatic and emotional symptoms in children with and without recurrent abdominal pain. *Journal of Consulting and Clinical Psychology, 69*, 85–91.

Walker, L. S., Lipani, T. A., Greene, J. W., Caines, K., Stutts, J., Polk, D. B., et al. (2004). Recurrent abdominal pain: symptom subtypes based on the rome ii criteria for pediatric functional gastrointestinal disorders. *Journal of Pediatric Gastroenterology and Nutrition, 38,* 187–191.

Wilson Sharrer, V., & Ryan-Wenger, N. M. (1991). Measurements of stress and coping among school-aged children with and without recurrent abdominal pain. *Journal of School Health, 61*, 86–91.

Chapter 13
Crying in Psychotherapy: Its Meaning, Assessment, and Management Based on Attachment Theory

Judith K. Nelson

Introduction

Although crying is well recognized as a frequent and important part of the therapeutic process, little direct or conscious attention has been paid to it in clinical training programs or in the clinical literature. The few theories that address it directly generally assume that it is a positive therapeutic experience with cathartic value. The most frequently advocated therapeutic technique is to encourage crying and support the crier. Underpinning most of these theories, as well as much popular psychology, is the early Freudian theory of affects as quantitative and in need of expression or release. Breuer and Freud (1895/1968) refer to tears in "Studies on Hysteria" as "involuntary reflexes" that discharge affect so that a "large part of the affect disappears" (p. 8). To describe this process they use the term *sich austoben*, which translates to English as "to cry one-self out."

The absence of crying when it would be expected or appropriate in a particular situation or the absence of the ability or wish to cry as a general life pattern is typically regarded in the clinical literature as defensive (Wallerstein, 1967; Yazmajian, 1966) or symptomatic, especially in association with psychophysiologic disorders (Cappon, 1958; Greenacre, 1945; Lindahl, 1977). The most frequently advocated psychotherapeutic technique for dealing with inhibited crying is a combination of interpreting the defenses and actively encouraging the patient to cry.

Empirical research on crying in psychotherapy is likewise rare. Susan Labott (2001) reported only one study by Trezza and Coworkers (as cited in Labott, 2001) that asked therapists about crying in psychotherapy. It focused on the frequency and intensity of crying and also asked therapists whether they openly encouraged patients to cry (73% said they did) or ever tried to stop a patient from crying (63% said they did not). Labott found no studies on the efficacy of crying in psychotherapy, although she did find several that reported positive outcomes for emotive and/or experiential therapies, which are assumed to emphasize crying.

In the absence of a comprehensive clinical theory of crying or research about crying in psychotherapy, I have turned to attachment theory and research in order to construct a theory of crying in psychotherapy. I will first outline the theory itself and the attachment research and precepts on which it is based and then show how the theory illuminates the meaning of crying in psychotherapy. Finally, I will apply

A. Vingerhoets et al., (eds.), *Emotion Regulation.*

the theory to the clinical assessment of crying, crying in the therapeutic process, and crying in the therapeutic relationship.

Crying as Attachment Behavior

Crying in psychotherapy, as in infancy and throughout life, is part of the inborn attachment system (Bowlby, 1969; Cassidy, 1999). In infancy, crying is a survival behavior designed to signal parental caregivers that their presence and nurturance are needed. According to attachment theory, separation from the caregiver is the prototypical trigger for infant crying. Because crying at the death of a close loved one occurs in every culture in the world (Habenstein & Lamers, 1963) even when it is considered dangerous to the living (Kracke, 1981; 1988), it may be seen as the prototypical trigger for adult crying, paralleling separation from the caregiver in infancy. Physical contact is the most effective means of soothing infant cries (Bowlby, 1969). All other forms of soothing and nurturance also require the physical presence of the caregiver, supporting the attachment view of crying as being an appeal for the presence of the caregiver. Bereaved adults may also be soothed by touch, words, or by the sympathetic presence of another. Many adults, unlike infants, are also able to appeal to symbolic caregivers or to self-soothe in the absence of literal caregiving.

Caregiving Behavior

The recognition that attachment is by definition a two-way process is crucial for the understanding of crying in psychotherapy. Attachment by definition involves an attachment figure or caregiver making it a two-person process (George & Solomon, 1999). Attachment behaviors occur in tandem with caregiving behaviors, and the two systems are reciprocal in nature. Repeated experiences of crying (as well as of the positive attachment behaviors such as smiling, cooing, grasping, and reaching), coupled with the responses of the caregiver, lead to the establishment and maintenance of the attachment bond (Cassidy, 1999). The promptness, consistency, and effectiveness of the caregiving responses over the first 1 to 2 years of life determine the quality (or style) of the infant's—and later the adult's—attachment, whether secure or insecure (Ainsworth, Blehar, Waters, & Wall, 1978; Schore, 1994). Neurobiological attachment research reveals that caregiver responses to the positively valenced attachment behaviors, along with crying, establish a right-brain-to-right-brain connection between caregiver and child that, in addition to the style of attachment, also contributes to the development of the ability to regulate affect throughout life (Schore, 2003).

Early attachment and caregiving experiences are also crucial in determining caregiving styles in later life (George & Solomon, 1999; Hesse, 1999). Effective caregiving requires the ability to apprehend the attachment signals of others and the ability to empathize with their affects (Donovan & Leavitt, 1985; Frodi, Lamb, Leavitt, & Donovan, 1978; Schore, 2003). Although the quality of the caregiving may vary, infant crying is particularly effective in triggering some type of response as parents react viscerally to crying (Boukydis & Burgess, 1982; Donovan & Leavitt, 1985; Weinfeld, Sroufe, Egeland, & Carlson, 1999) more than to smiling infants. Caregivers also do not habituate to the infant crying stimulus. The power of crying to disturb the caregiver is evidenced in the sad fact that 80% of parents who abuse infants cite crying as the provocation (Frodi, 1985).

Crying appears to retain its visceral beckoning power throughout life, and it continues in adulthood to evoke caregiving behavior from others—spouses and partners, family and friends (see Hendriks et al., this volume). Even acquaintances and strangers notice crying behaviors and feel urges, of varying levels of intensity, to respond with offers of help, comfort, or soothing. In a study comparing reactions to photographs of tearful faces and the same photographs with the tears digitally removed, Cornelius and Lubliner (2003) found that 59% of the viewers said they would comfort the person with visible tears while only 19% said they would leave the person alone. Because adult crying is primarily silent, its attachment message is conveyed through a combination of visible tears, red, swollen, or watery eyes, facial expressions, characteristic movements of the shoulders, or changes in respiration.

When adult crying takes place in the presence of others, as it does in psychotherapy, it activates the companion's caregiving behavioral system with varying results depending on the type of cry, the nature of the relationship and its current status, learned behavior, sociocultural values, and the attachment experiences and attachment style of the crier and of the potential caregiver. Distinguishing attachment styles and their characteristic patterns of activating or deactivating attachment behaviors and their characteristic patterns of caregiving and care-receiving is the first step in being able to assess and manage crying in psychotherapy. Identifying different types of crying and the types of caregiving experiences each evokes is the next step necessary for tracking the reciprocal attachment/caregiving cycles that take place with crying in psychotherapy.

Adult Attachment Styles and Crying

An attachment perspective on crying in psychotherapy provides valuable background information for the psychotherapist to use in assessing the quality of the patient's early attachments, current adult bonds, and the here-and-now of the therapeutic connection. The ways in which a person cries or does not cry, and their openness to receiving care and soothing from the therapist—even, at times, their offers of care to the therapist (Bader, 1996)—are related to what Bowlby (1969; 1973; 1980) termed *internal working models* of attachment and what have since been classified and termed *attachment styles* (Ainsworth et al., 1978).

Ainsworth et al. (1978) and others (Solomon & George, 1999), based on extensive research using the Strange Situation research design, have designated three styles of attachment in 12-month-old infants: one secure type and two insecure types (anxious/ambivalent and avoidant). Main and Solomon (1990) later identified a third style of insecure attachment: disorganized/disoriented. Adult attachment styles or states of mind have been identified through use of the Adult Attachment Interview, which initially focused on maternal caregivers in order to match caregiving experiences with attachment styles (Hesse, 1999). Adult attachment styles parallel those of infants, although adult attachments are different in several ways, including the mutuality of attachment and caregiving between adult partners and the additional presence of a sexual bond in romantic relationships, that also function as attachment/caregiving relationships. Adults also have the cognitive ability to withstand prolonged separations and to anticipate reunions, which infants do not have.

Hazan and Shaver (1987), for research purposes, translated Ainsworth's descriptions of infant attachment styles into adult terms in order to study the relationship between attachment and romantic love. The terms they use for adult attachment styles are the same as those used for infants and children: secure, anxious-ambivalent, and avoidant. I have used Hazan and Shaver's basic model to describe adult attachment styles with the addition of crying and caregiving responses to crying. I have also transcribed the disorganized/disoriented attachment style of infancy into adult terms for purposes of clinical conceptualization and comparison. The parallel categories used by Mary Main and others (Hesse, 1999) who use the more complex and lengthy protocol of the Adult Attachment Interview are different though related and are shown in parentheses below.

Secure Attachment Style (Secure-Autonomous)

An adult with a secure style of attachment is confident in the reliability and availability of attachment figures, able to activate attachment behavior (crying) when vulnerable, and capable of intimacy, including being comfortable with the soothing, caregiving behavior evoked in others by his or her crying or evoked internally by the crying of others.

Anxious-Ambivalent Style (Preoccupied)

Individuals with an anxious-ambivalent style are unable to trust in the availability of attachment figures. They demonstrate a desperate desire for connection along with a strong fear of rejection. They are likely to hyperactivate the attachment system (crying) during times of distress and to cling to their attachment figures, showing an anxious, even demanding, need for caregiving and soothing coupled with great difficulty in being soothed. They are prone to compulsive caregiving to others as a way of binding their anxiety and securing the presence and caregiving responses of the attachment object.

Avoidant Style (Dismissing)

A person with an avoidant style is unable to trust in the reliability of attachment figures and defensively attempts to deactivate the attachment system (crying) during times of vulnerability and distress. He or she is typically seen as emotionally distant and compulsively self-reliant and is often intolerant of caregiving from others and uncomfortable with giving care to others when they cry.

Disorganized-Disoriented Style (Unresolved/Disorganized)

Individuals whose attachment style is disorganized/disoriented demonstrate chaotic, confused relationships with attachment figures, unpredictably mixing approach and avoidance. Attachment behavior (crying) occurs at unexpected and often seemingly inappropriate times. Caregiving may be desperately sought and resisted simultaneously, and actual caregiving attempts from others may evoke hostility or fear. Caregiving needs expressed by others may be met inconsistently with expansive, even excessive, soothing or, alternatively, with hostility, fear, and retreat.

A Classification of Types of Crying

Adult crying may be an expression of a wide range of different feelings or mixtures of feelings, including sadness, anger, joy, or fear (Vingerhoets, Boelhouwer, Tilburg, & Van Heck, 2001). Consistent with the prototype of crying in infancy at separation from the caregiver and crying at the death of a close loved one in adulthood, I propose that the vast majority of adult crying is triggered by separations or losses that may be literal, threatened, avoided, symbolic, or imagined. Even tears of joy may represent losses averted or losses mixed with gains.

When the core trigger is loss, crying may be seen as a grief reaction—written large in the case of death or permanent separation or in miniature in the less profound losses of everyday life (Nelson, 1998). An episode of crying—or not crying at a time when it would be expected or appropriate—may then be classified by the stage of the grieving process to which it corresponds. Although there are many schemas for describing stages of grief, John Bowlby's (1961) are particularly relevant because they are rooted in his observations of infants reacting to separations from their primary caregivers and adults reacting to death of a close loved one.

As Bowlby (1961) noted, infants respond to separations first with protest, then with despair, and finally with detachment. Crying during the protest stage is loud and active; during the phase of despair, crying becomes a low wail; in the final stage, detachment, there is a noncrying silence. Bowlby identified parallel responses in bereaved adults. He notes, "... when he weeps the bereaved adult is responding to loss as a child does to the temporary absence of his mother" (p. 15). The difference is that adults are able to proceed from despair to a stage Bowlby called reorganization rather than necessarily ending in the silent, withdrawn detachment of infancy.

Adult crying may then be classified according to the stage of the grieving process to which it corresponds as either protest crying, sad crying of despair, or, in the case of some inhibited crying, detached tearlessness (Nelson, 1979; 1998; 2000; also Hendriks et al., this volume). Based on observation and clinical experience, these three types of (non)crying may be distinguished by their unique characteristics and by the typical caregiving responses they evoke.

Protest Cries

Protest crying in infancy is a loud, active summons for the caregiver to return. Protest crying throughout life has in common a refusal to recognize, accept, or allow the loss or its impact and a demand that caregivers act to undo or redress losses rather than console or comfort. Protest crying has a demanding, harsh, almost angry-sounding force behind it, and the quality it conveys to potential caregivers is often accusatory, demanding, or hostile. Except in the immediate aftermath of a significant or traumatic loss, caregivers often feel irritated, apathetic, or even guilty in response to protest crying, especially if they are being accused of causing or threatening the "loss." This is the type of crying that causes the most interpersonal difficulties and leaves caregivers feeling defensive, devalued, frustrated, or hopeless. Unless the crier succeeds in undoing the loss or potential loss, he or she will not, in all likelihood, feel any relief after the cry.

Sad Cries of Despair

Infants in this stage of reacting to loss of the caregiver appear to give up hope of reunion, and crying becomes a low-energy wail. In adults, this type of crying, usually silent weeping, represents the stage of grief when the reality of the loss is recognized and faced. The crier is no longer resisting or demanding change. Instead, she or he surrenders to the loss and feels despair. This is the type of crying that stirs up great empathy and sympathy in others as it delivers a "come-hither" message to potential caregivers and evokes a powerful urge to offer solace and comfort. This beckoning, interpersonal feature of crying in despair is what I believe provides the healing component in working through grief. This type of crying does what attachment behavior is designed to do: establish and maintain a close bond with others that gives security and a safe haven in times of need. In the face of loss, these tears help to reestablish or affirm a sense of connection with others, thereby bringing hope for a resolution of grief.

Detached Tearlessness

The final stage of reaction to the loss of a primary caregiver in infancy is a life-threatening silent detachment. Not all adult inhibited crying in the aftermath of a profound or significant loss is detached, however. To fit this category, the inhibited crying must isolate the sufferer as he or she withdraws from potential caregivers. Some noncriers find other connected ways to express their sadness and despair and to seek the care and closeness of others. They might, for example, express their feelings of loss in words, music, or painting or seek comfort physically through touch or hugging. Sexual closeness may also stand in for caregiving behavior when other kinds of closeness are not available or cannot be tolerated.

The Assessment of Crying in Psychotherapy

Healthy Crying

Sad cries of despair are the type most frequently associated with healthy crying. People with secure attachment styles are most able to withstand the despair that comes with recognizing losses, great or small. The "letting go" aspect of the descent into despair is best accomplished with a safety net in the form of reliable or available caregivers and by a crier who is able to be soothed and comforted by them. In the absence of literal caregivers, securely attached people are also able to call upon symbolic or internalized caregivers or to assume the caregiving function themselves.

In the course of adult relationships, insecurely attached people may also develop sufficient trust in close caregivers that they, too, may experience the healing potential of crying in despair. For the many people in psychotherapy who are insecurely attached, the therapist as a professional caregiver often serves this function once a sufficiently safe and trusting bond has been established. Not only do these therapeutic crying experiences enable the patient to begin to work through grief, but they may also over time help to reshape the earlier working models of attachment and eventually lead to the development of new internal working models, and to an attachment style that has been termed *earned secure* (Hesse, 1999).

In an earlier article (Nelson, 1998), I describe a patient of mine, Katherine, whose severe early neglect resulted in an avoidant attachment style. Prior to coming to therapy, she had worked diligently to provide her infant son with attachment experiences that were vastly different from her own, thus beginning the long journey toward earning a secure attachment style for herself. At first in therapy she was unable to tolerate any crying and was also unable to take in soothing from me. On one occasion after many years of treatment, however, she began to cry in despair over a debilitating illness. I empathized with her by helping her to identify some of the many losses she suffered because of the illness. It was the first time she was able to allow me to truly be with her in her grief and represented a distinctly positive shift in her ability to accept and benefit from caregiving.

Symptomatic Responses to Healthy Crying

Even healthy, appropriate crying in despair may lead to social awkwardness and discomfort. Such negative feelings about crying may be related to social expectations or embarrassment, the context in which the crying takes place, or early attachment experiences where crying was demeaned by caregivers, siblings, or peers. I am struck by the frequency with which patients, especially in the early hours of treatment, apologize for shedding tears even in a therapist's office. In an initial hour, for example, Bev began to cry as she talked about her husband's plans to move out the following weekend. She shook her head when she started to cry saying, "I'm so sorry. I promised myself I wasn't going to do this." Her misdirected resolve appeared to result from the social dichotomization of the rational and the emotional. She thought that if she cried she would not be able to cover everything and be "wasting" her time and mine.

Symptomatic Crying

The signs that are associated with symptomatic crying are protest crying that elicits irritation or apathy instead of sympathy or empathy; crying accompanied by infantile body movements or sounds; crying in the absence of a clear or appropriate stimulus; prolonged or frequent crying (not associated with grief over a significant loss); and dramatic crying over minor losses or over significant losses but with shallow emotion. I have described the clinical assessment of each of these in an earlier article (Nelson, 2000) with case examples, and in *Seeing Through Tears: Crying and Attachment* (Nelson, 2005). For the sake of brevity, I will summarize three of the key assessment issues and relate them to attachment style.

Protest Crying

Protest crying, except in the immediate aftermath of a significant loss, sidesteps the healing qualities of crying in despair because it refutes and refuses to accept the possibility of loss and because it resists a positive response to caregiving. Protest crying activates caregiving systems but in negative rather than positive ways. Even if it is successful in undoing or preventing a loss, it may leave caregivers feeling resentful, irritated, or guilty. When protest crying occurs in solitude, it is generally unsatisfactory in that it leaves the crier feeling stuck, frustrated, or disturbed.

Protest crying is often associated with the anxious-ambivalent attachment style where attachment behavior is easily activated but difficult to soothe. A person with this attachment style may also find it difficult to tolerate or express feelings of aggression and instead may rely upon protest crying as a substitute, obscuring the anger behind the tears.

Crying in the Absence of a Clear and Appropriate Precipitant

Both unprovoked crying and frequent crying may be symptomatic of physical or psychiatric disorders or a side-effect of certain drugs. Psychotherapists should be certain that somatic disorders are ruled out in cases of chronically unprovoked crying. Green, McAllister, and Bernat (1987) studied a group of medically hospitalized men with prominent crying and found that crying associated with neurologic disorders is disconnected from external or internal stimuli and has an abrupt beginning with each episode being alike rather than varying in quality or intensity. In the absence of physiologic determinants, unprovoked crying may be linked to unacknowledged grief or to unacceptable or unrecognized attachment needs. For example, individuals with avoidant attachment styles during times of loss may be unable to maintain their normal pattern of inhibited crying while remaining in denial about the losses provoking their tears.

Prolonged or Frequent Crying

When evaluating complaints or observations of too much crying, it is essential to gather data about the frequency, duration, and intensity of the crying and compare it to the normal pattern for that individual as there are people, male and female, with no disorder who cry up to several times a day (Frey & Langseth, 1985; Green et al., 1987; Hastrup & Baker, 1986). Notable changes in an individual's usual pattern of crying frequency in the absence of significant personal loss or physical disorder indicate a need for further evaluation for clinical depression. Excessive crying is believed to be associated with depression (though recent research by Rottenberg, Gross, Wilhelm, Najmi, & Gotlib [2002] has called this into question) as is the inability to cry in a person who normally cries (Steer, Beck, Brown, & Berchick, 1987).

Healthy and Symptomatic Inhibited Crying

As mentioned above, healthy inhibited crying includes the ability to acknowledge and express sadness, grief, and despair and the ability to seek, accept, and benefit from caregiving. Many noncriers prefer not to cry, believing that it would increase their distress. People with avoidant styles of attachment, who suppress or repress their vulnerabilities and are compulsively self-reliant, are at greatest risk for symptomatic inhibited crying. Although the avoidant style may cause difficulties in everyday relationships, it becomes clinically problematic in the aftermath of a significant loss when detachment may become life-threatening, leading to suicide, substance abuse, or physical decline.

Crying and the Therapeutic Process

Much of the process of psychotherapy involves working through grief over inadequate, traumatic, threatened, or ruptured attachments. As the therapist listens to the patient's narrative, it is possible to assess early and ongoing losses, vulnerabilities, attachment behaviors, and caregiving responses. Taken together, these provide valuable information about the state of the patient's attachment and caregiving styles and their impact on current feelings and functioning.

From the very beginning of therapy, these observations may serve as a guide in responding to crying or inhibited crying. The therapist as professional caregiver, like early parental caregivers, has two tasks: affect attunement and affect regulation. Both require tremendous empathy and the ability to respond flexibly to different individuals and their crying behaviors rather than a single technique, such as encouraging all crying.

For some people, particularly those with anxious-ambivalent or avoidant attachment styles, crying can be quite threatening. People with an anxious-ambivalent style of attachment cry easily and yet find it difficult to believe and accept that another person is truly "there" for them in a reliable, soothing, and comforting way. Crying and caregiving, in other words, can make them more anxious and so they may resist the therapist's efforts at comfort, empathy, and reassurance.

The therapist, at certain points in the treatment, may feel that the patient's anxiety levels are too great when they cry, and rather than encourage crying or try to force caregiving, may attempt to regulate and reduce the patient's overwhelming affect. One way of doing this might be to ask a soothing question that will help the crier to focus or distract them slightly, thereby diminishing the crying behavior. On the other hand, being empathic at such moments might intensify the anxiety without increasing the person's ability to tolerate or benefit from caregiving.

Crying in the Therapeutic Relationship

In order to respond effectively to crying, it is important for therapists to closely monitor their internal responses to a patient's crying or to inhibited crying. A high degree of self-awareness regarding one's own attachment and caregiving styles is a prerequisite. Given that level of awareness, the therapist's internal responses provide valuable clues about the type of crying the patient is doing, the stage of working through grief their crying represents, and the most effective and appropriate caregiving responses. Self-awareness includes noticing whether the patient's crying arouses empathy (including the urge to cry oneself), sympathy, apathy, irritation, frustration, guilt, inadequacy, or anxiety. Each of these different feelings relates to the attachment style of the patient (in conjunction with that of the therapist) and the openness to caregiving by the patient (also in conjunction with the caregiving style of the therapist).

The therapist's internal responses to crying also provide valuable clues about what the patient is grieving and the stage of the grieving process, whether protest, despair, or detachment. Protest crying in psychotherapy may be in response to grief over past losses or to perceived deficits in the current psychotherapeutic relationship or to both. Protest crying may leave the therapist feeling pushed away, frustrated, or devalued or that the patient is unable to allow the therapist to "be there" for them and with them.

Crying in despair, on the other hand, almost unfailingly elicits deep empathy and a desire to comfort. At times, the therapist may feel so deeply that he or she is near tears or may actually cry. This is a highly individual response and must be carefully attuned to the attachment needs of the patient. When there is a good solid connection with the patient, when the therapist's strength and availability as a caregiver are assured, crying by the therapist may be felt as a deeply empathic response that draws therapist and patient closer together. Several colleagues, however, have shared reports of their patients' experiences with previous therapists whose crying severely damaged the therapeutic relationship. If the patient sees any hint of fragility in the caregiver or if the patient is a compulsive caregiver ever at the ready to look for neediness in another person, the crying of the therapist as professional caregiver may be overwhelming, unsettling, or distancing.

When we feel a patient expending caregiving efforts in our direction, it may be appropriate or it may be burdensome—to them and to us. We are familiar with the dangers and pitfalls of patients who push to be caregivers to the therapist but less familiar with the benefits (Bader, 1996). Because attachment and caregiving in adulthood are mutual and because a successful therapeutic bond requires attachment on both sides, allowing the patient to care for and about the therapist is an important ingredient of the therapeutic relationship, but one that requires a great deal of skill and sensitivity on the part of the therapist. We are the designated caregivers but being open to the healthy concern and interest in us and our well-being is part of what the relationship requires. One of my most thought-disordered, psychiatrically disabled patients grabbed my hand after an appointment when I announced that I had to leave town to attend to my father who was ill. She looked right into my eyes and said, "take care of yourself, too." As she turned away to walk down the hall, tears came to my eyes as I allowed myself to experience the poignancy of her caregiving in the face of my own grief.

Conclusion

Although crying plays a crucial role in the therapeutic dialogue, it has been overlooked in professional training and literature. A theory of crying based on attachment enables the therapist to understand the meaning of crying, to distinguish different types of crying, and to identify the attachment and caregiving styles of each partner in the therapeutic relationship. It also offers new understanding about the therapeutic management of crying and its role in the therapeutic process and the therapeutic relationship.

References

Ainsworth, M. D. S., Blehar, M., Waters, E., & Wall, S. (1978). *Patterns of attachment*. Hillsdale, NJ: Lawrence Erlbaum.

Bader, M. J. (1996). Altruistic love in psychoanalysis: opportunities and resistance. *Psychoanalytic Dialogues, 6,* 741–764.

Boukydis, C. F. Z., & Burgess, R. L. (1982). Adult physiological response to infant cries: effects of temperament of infant, parental status and gender. *Child Development, 53,* 1291–1298.

Bowlby, J. (1961). Processes of mourning. *International Journal of Psycho-analysis, 42,* 317–339.

Bowlby, J. (1969). *Attachment.* New York: Basic Books.

Bowlby, J. (1973). *Separation: anxiety and anger.* New York: Basic Books.

Bowlby, J. (1980). *Loss.* New York: Basic Books.

Breuer, J., & Freud, S. (1895/1968). Studies on hysteria. In *The standard edition of the complete psychological works of Sigmund Freud* (pp. 3–17). London: Hogarth Press.

Cappon, D. (1958). Emotional aspects of the common cold. *Canadian Medical Association Journal, 79,* 173–179.

Cassidy, J. (1999). The nature of the child's ties. In J. Cassidy & P. R. Shaver (Eds.), *Handbook of attachment. Theory, research and clinical applications* (pp. 3–20). New York: The Guilford Press.

Cornelius, R., & Lubliner, E. (2003). The what and why of others' responses to our tears: adult crying as an attachment behavior. Paper presented at the Third International Conference on the (Non) Expression of Emotions in Health and Disease, Tilburg, The Netherlands.

Donovan, W. L., & Leavitt, L. A. (1985). Physiology and behavior: parents' response to the infant cry. In B. M. Lester & C. F. Z. Boukydis (Eds.), *Infant crying: theoretical and research perspectives* (pp. 241–259). New York: Plenum Press.

Frey, W. H. I., & Langseth, M. (1985). *Crying: the mystery of tears*. Minneapolis, MN: Winston Press.

Frodi, A. (1985). When empathy fails: aversive infant crying and child abuse. In B. Lester & C. F. Z. Boukydis (Eds.), *Infant crying: theoretical and research perspectives* (pp. 263–277). New York: Plenum Press.

Frodi, A. M., Lamb, M. E., Leavitt, L. A., & Donovan, W. L. (1978). Fathers and mothers' responses to infant smiles and cries. *Infant Behavior and Development, 1,* 187–198.

George, C., & Solomon, J. (1999). Attachment and caregiving: the caregiving behavioral system. In J. Cassidy & P. R. Shaver (Eds.), *Handbook of attachment: theory, research and clinical applications* (pp. 649–670). New York: The Guilford Press.

Green, R., McAllister, T., & Bernat, J. (1987). A study of crying in medically and surgically hospitalized patients. *American Journal of Psychiatry, 144,* 442–447.

Greenacre, P. (1945). Urination and weeping. *American Journal of Orthopsychiatry, 15,* 81–88.

Habenstein, R., & Lamers, W. (1963). *Funeral customs the world over.* Milwaukee, WI: Bulfin Printers.

Hastrup, J. L., & Baker, J. G. (1986). Crying and depression among older adults. *Gerontologist, 26,* 91–96.

Hazan, C., & Shaver, P. (1987). Romantic love conceptualized as an attachment process. *Journal of Personality and Social Psychology, 52,* 511–524.

Hesse, E. (1999). The Adult Attachment Interview. In J. Cassidy & P. R. Shaver (Eds.), *Handbook of attachment. Theory, research, and clinical applications* (pp. 395–433). New York: The Guilford Press.

Kracke, W. (1981). Kagwahiv mourning. *Ethos, 9,* 258–275.

Kracke, W. (1988). Kagwahiv mourning II. *Ethos, 16,* 209–222.

Labott, S. (2001). Crying in psychotherapy. In A. J. J. M. Vingerhoets & R. R. Cornelius (Eds.), *Adult crying: a biopsychosocial approach* (pp. 213–226). Hove, UK: Brunner-Routledge.

Lindahl, M. (1977). Psychogenic purpura: report of a case. *Psychosomatic Medicine, 39,* 358–368.

Main, M., & Solomon, J. (1990). Procedures for identifying infants as disorganized/disoriented during the Ainsworth strange situation. In M. T. Greenberg, D. Cicchetti, & E. M. Cummings (Eds.), *Attachment in the preschool years* (pp. 121–160). Chicago, IL: University of Chicago Press.

Nelson, J. K. (1979). *An ego psychological and object relations study of crying.* Berkeley, CA: California Institute for Clinical Social Work.

Nelson, J. K. (1998). The meaning of crying based on attachment theory. *Clinical Social Work Journal, 26,* 9–22.

Nelson, J. K. (2000). Clinical assessment of crying and crying inhibition based on attachment theory. *Bulletin of the Menninger Clinic, 64,* 509–529.

Nelson, J. K. (2005). *Seeing through tears: Crying and attachment.* New York: Routledge.

Rottenberg, J. Gross, J. J., Wilhelm, F. H., Najmi, S., & Gotlib, I. H. (2002). Crying threshold and intensity in major depressive disorder. *Journal of Abnormal Psychology, 111,* 302–312.

Schore, A. (1994). *Affect regulation and the origin of the self.* Hillsdale, NJ: Lawrence Erlbaum.

Schore, A. N. (2003). *Affect dysregulation and disorders of the self.* New York: W.W. Norton.

Solomon, J., & George, C. (1999). The measurement of attachment security in infancy and childhood. In J. Cassidy & P. R. Shaver (Eds.), *Handbook of attachment: theory, research, and clinical applications* (pp. 287–316). New York: Guilford Press.

Steer, R., Beck, A.,Brown, G., & Berchick, R. (1987). Self-reported depressive symptoms that differentiate recurrent-episode major depression from dysthymic disorders. *Journal of Clinical Psychology, 43,* 246–250.

Vingerhoets, A. J. J. M., Boelhouwer, A. J. W., Van Tilburg, M. A. L. & Van Heck, G. L. (2001). The situational and emotional context of adult crying. In A. J. J. M. Vingerhoets & R. R. Cornelius (Eds.), *Adult crying: a biopsychosocial approach* (pp. 71–90). Hove, UK: Brunner-Routledge.

Wallerstein, R. (1967). Reconstruction and mastery in the transference psychosis. *Journal of the American Psychoanalytic Association, 15,* 555–583.

Weinfeld, N. S., Sroufe, A., Egeland, B., & Carlson, E. A. (1999). The nature of individual differences in infant-caregiver attachment. In J. Cassidy & P. R. Shaver (Eds.), *Handbook of attachment: theory, research, and clinical applications* (pp. 68–88). New York: Guilford Press.

Yazmajian, R. (1966). Pathological urination and weeping. *Psychoanalytic Quarterly, 35,* 40–46.

Chapter 14
Expressive Writing in the Clinical Context

Joshua M. Smyth, Deborah Nazarian, and Danielle Arigo

Introduction

The use of writing in a therapeutic manner can be traced back to psychotherapeutic traditions that encourage the expression of emotions (see Smyth & Helm, 2003). The majority of psychotherapeutic paradigms, regardless of theoretical orientation, consist of some form of interpersonal disclosure that includes identifying, labeling, and disclosing emotional experiences (Smyth & Helm, 2003). Although individuals may have a desire to disclose their thoughts and emotions about a distressing experience, social constraints may limit such interpersonal disclosure (Lepore, Silver, Wortman, & Wayment, 1996). Some individuals may refrain from discussing negative events due to the social stigma thought to be associated with the experience. Other people may lack a social support system and/or receive insensitive or inappropriate support (Wortman & Silver, 1989). In contrast, written emotional expression offers the opportunity to express one's thoughts and feelings without regard to social constraints or barriers that might accompany interpersonal disclosure and reduces the likelihood of negative interpersonal responses.

Writing has long been a common strategy for expressing strong emotion and has informally been used both personally and in therapeutic settings for a variety of purposes and goals (e.g., Progoff's intensive journaling; see Smyth & Greenberg, 2000). Despite widespread use, such methods have not been extensively studied within the context of therapy. It is only recently that investigators have begun to systemically examine the effects of structured expressive writing on psychological and physical health. Expressive writing has increasingly been applied as a psychosocial intervention across settings and samples and represents an effective supplemental intervention that clinicians can add to their array of therapeutic tools for clients—both within and outside of the therapy session. The goals of this chapter are to provide an overview of the expressive writing literature as it relates to its use in various health care settings, including its effects among medically ill populations as well as purported mechanisms responsible for these effects. This background information will hopefully serve as the foundation for recommendations on how expressive writing may be used by clinicians and health professionals as a supplement or alternative to traditional forms of care.

A. Vingerhoets et al., (eds.), *Emotion Regulation.*

Expressive Writing as an Intervention: An Overview

Participants in expressive writing studies are typically randomly assigned to one of two (or more) conditions or groups. Individuals in both groups are instructed to write without regard to spelling, style, or grammar and are informed that their written narratives will remain confidential. Writing usually takes place over 3–5 days, for 15–30 minutes each day. Although specific procedures may vary across studies, the time and attention is matched for each group to ensure that the experimental manipulation (i.e., writing instructions) is the only difference between the two conditions. Participants in the experimental condition are encouraged to identify and explore their cognitions and emotions about a significant life event or stressor (e.g., Pennebaker & Beall, 1986). Typical instructions are as follows:

> During each of the three writing days, we would like you to write about the most stressful or upsetting experiences of your entire life. You can write on different topics each day or on the same topic for all three days. The important thing is that you write about your deepest thoughts and feelings about the experience. You can write about anything you want, but whatever you choose, it should be something that has affected you very deeply. It is critical, however, that you let yourself go and touch those deepest emotions and thoughts that you have. Some people find this writing upsetting, and may cry or feel sad or depressed afterwards. This is quite normal, and we will allow you as much time as you want when you have finished to compose yourself.

Control participants are instructed to write in an emotionally neutral way about benign topics, such as their plans for the week and upcoming week (often framed as time management). For example, session 1 focuses on strategies used over the previous week; session 2 redirects this topic toward the previous 24 hours, and session 3 asks about plans for the upcoming week. Instructions for the first day of writing are as follows:

> During each of the three writing days, we would like you to write about an assigned topic. You should write about the specific topic in detail without discussing any of your thoughts and feelings surrounding the topic, but rather focus on a factual description. Today we want you to write about your plans for the *previous week*. Again, describe them in detail without referring to your thoughts or feelings associated with them.

Findings from prior studies that have utilized these control instructions suggest that participants report that the exercise is valid and valuable, although no relationship was found between the emotionally neutral (control) writing exercises and mental or physical health outcomes (e.g., Hockemeyer & Smyth, 2002).

An important issue to consider is whether participants asked to write in the manner described above would, in fact, do so, particularly outside of a formal therapy setting. Based on existing evidence, asking people to write about stress, traumatic experiences, or other powerful emotions is something most individuals are willing and able to do. In response to relatively open-ended instructions to write about, for example, the most stressful or traumatic experience in one's life, individuals generally do disclose relatively serious experiences or events. Very few seem unwilling or unable to disclose as requested (although, of course, one cannot ascertain if there are relatively *more* serious topics that were not expressed, few individuals write about topics that appear objectively neutral or trivial). A variety of serious topics are commonly observed when even relatively "healthy" individuals are asked to disclose via writing, including (but not limited to) physical/sexual abuse, the death of a loved one, relationship difficulties, serious personal illness or injury, and thoughts of suicide. Not only are people generally willing to disclose when asked to write, but also the benefits of engaging in this activity have appeared in several groups of participants who do not have specific training in writing. Participant samples have ranged from children to the elderly and have varied across wide education levels. That is, there does not seem to be any special training or even high-level literacy requirements for people to engage in this activity.

Disclosure of strong emotions, whether through talking to another individual or through writing, has been shown to have significant positive effects on health. Structured writing interventions encourage the disclosure of these emotions in a way that is both confidential and anonymous, which allows the individual to freely express his thoughts and feelings without fear of criticism. This method of emotional disclosure has been associated with reductions in health center visits, lower reports of distress, depression, and illness-related behavior, and improved role functioning. The benefits of this intervention have been found across various populations, including college students, community samples, and specific medical and psychiatric patient populations.

It is important to note that the benefits of expressive writing have been studied across a range of research methodologies, each of which generates distinct types of conclusions. Naturalistic studies, which investigate the use of writing in participants' everyday lives, suggest that expression of emotion related to significant life experiences is associated with improved outcomes (Davison & Pennebaker, 1997; Pennebaker & O'Heeron, 1984; Silver, Boon, & Stones, 1983). In an exploration of online newsgroups and mailing lists, Davison and Pennebaker (1997) found that patient groups (including breast cancer, prostate cancer, diabetes, heart disease, arthritis, and chronic fatigue syndrome) differed in their communication styles. Other correlational studies have demonstrated a relationship between increased disclosure and better outcome. Among spouses of accidental death victims, those individuals who reported more discussion and less rumination about the death were less likely to report health problems (Pennebaker & O'Heeron, 1984). Victims of father-daughter incest who did not have someone in whom they could confide were less likely to report coming to a resolution about the experience than those who reported having a confidant (Silver et al., 1983).

Although naturalistic studies have high external validity (i.e., generalizability to real-world settings), they pose a threat to internal validity (i.e., the extent to which results can be attributed to emotional disclosure rather than reflecting other, perhaps preexisting, differences), thereby limiting inferences of causality. Naturalistic studies can thus present evidence for the association between disclosure and mental and/or physical health but cannot lead to the conclusion that disclosure causes these effects. Random assignment to experimental groups is necessary in order to demonstrate a causal relationship between variables. This process reduces the likelihood that these conditions are systematically different from one another prior to experimental manipulation, which increases confidence that results are due to the intervention. Ideally, investigations of expressive writing are based on this design, which randomly assigns participants to different experimental groups. Tests of the influence of expressive writing as an intervention compare the means of these groups on various measures subsequent to their involvement in the study procedure.

Participants involved in the expressive writing condition typically show more improvement relative to neutral writing groups across various outcomes—an effect demonstrated in several cultures and languages (see Smyth & Pennebaker, 1999). The earliest literature on this intervention focused on examining the effect of expressive writing in student samples, typically finding significant improvement in reported anxiety and depression and less frequent health center visits (e.g., Pennebaker & Beall, 1986; Pennebaker, Colder, & Sharp, 1990). More recent work has found improvement in grade point average for students who engaged in the expressive writing intervention (Lumley & Provenzano, 2003) and improved lung function for students with asthma (Hockemeyer & Smyth, 2002). In the interest of extending expressive writing interventions to clinical samples, a number of studies have examined the generalizability of effects to various clinical populations.

Emotional Disclosure and Health in Clinical Settings and Populations

Expressive Writing in Medically Ill Populations

One of the first studies to report significant benefit from expressive writing for medically ill patients was conducted by Smyth, Stone, Hurewitz, & Kaell, (1999). Community samples of patients with chronic asthma or rheumatoid arthritis (RA) were randomly assigned to write about either stressful life events or a neutral topic (time management). Outcome was measured both through self-report as well as objective health assessments (collected at baseline, 2 weeks, 2 months, and 4 months after writing). Health assessments included spirometry (pulmonary function in asthma patients) and clinical examinations conducted by a rheumatologist (RA patients). Four months after treatment, asthma patients in the experimental group showed improvements in lung function, whereas control group patients showed no change. Rheumatoid arthritis patients in the experimental group showed improvements in overall disease activity, whereas control group patients did not change. In fact, across both disease groups, 47% of experimental patients had clinically relevant improvement, whereas 24% of control patients had improvement.

Expressive writing interventions have been tested for other medically ill populations as well, including patients with breast cancer (Stanton, Danoff-Burg, Sworowski, Collins, Branstetter, & Rodriguez-Hanley, 2002; Walker, Nail, & Croyle, 1999), rheumatoid arthritis (Kelley, Lumley, & Leisen, 1997), fibromyalgia (Gillis, Lumley, Mosley-Williams, Leisen, & Roehrs, 2006), HIV (Mann, 2001; Petrie, Fontanilla, Thomas, Booth, & Pennebaker, 2004), renal cell carcinoma (de Moor et al., 2002), men diagnosed with prostate cancer (Rosenberg et al., 2002), women with chronic pelvic pain (Norman, Lumley, Dooley, & Diamond, 2004), patients undergoing bladder papilloma resection (Solano, Donati,

Pecci, Persichetti, & Colaci, 2003), and transurethral prostate resection (Solano, Pepe, Donati, Persichetti, Laudani, & Colaci, 2007). Several of these studies have found significant improvement as the result of expressive writing; however, many have reported either few or no significant findings. Applications of the expressive writing intervention have now also extended beyond medical populations to use in health care settings (often with a more effectiveness based, community implementation), a topic discussed next.

Expressive Writing in Health Care Settings

Expressive writing has been studied in a variety of medical settings, using either the standard or a modified version of the expressive writing protocol. A study on the effectiveness of translating the expressive writing intervention into a community-based intervention presented the writing activity in the form of a videotaped program to patients with rheumatoid arthritis (Broderick, Stone, Smyth, & Kaell, 2004). Although this format (self-administration by patients at their homes via videotaped instructions) differed from traditional efficacy trials, the intervention failed to produce benefit, as no reliable differences were found between the expressive writing and control writing groups.

Several studies have investigated the feasibility of using structured expressive writing in primary care settings. For example, Klapow and colleagues (2001) implemented a standard written self-disclosure protocol in a primary care setting, concluding that this activity can be practically applied as a primary care intervention. Because only descriptive outcomes were reported, however, the implications of these findings remain unclear. Hannay and Bolton (1999) examined the use of therapeutic writing in a primary care setting based on an unstructured variation of the traditional writing paradigm. Specifically, general practitioners provided their patients suffering from anxiety or depression with writing guidelines. Although this study also reported only descriptive data, the authors concluded that therapeutic writing was a viable tool for general practice.

Schilte et al. (2001) investigated the effects of home visits by a trained "disclosure doctor" on patients who frequently attended general practice with somatizing symptoms. Participants in the experimental condition were encouraged to discuss an emotionally significant experience with the visiting doctor, and results for patients who received these visits were compared with a control group that received usual care. This study found no significant differences in outcome measures over a 2-year follow-up between the disclosure and control group. Despite the rigorous methods used in the study, the results suggest that patients may not find benefit from general practitioners who play multiple roles in their lives. In addition, this study employed a modified disclosure intervention that involved talking about a significant emotional experience to an "expert," which differs from traditional disclosure studies that ask participants to write about meaningful or stressful experiences. Taken together, findings from the aforementioned expressive writing studies among medically ill populations and in different health care settings have produced inconsistent results.

One source of potential variation may be the use of widely differing samples. Distinct patient populations possess unique sample characteristics (e.g., different treatment regimens, treatment adherence, etc.) that may contribute to varying results in expressive writing studies. At present, however, it is unclear whether inconsistent findings observed in many recent expressive writing studies are due to little or no efficacy of the expressive writing intervention, variations in contextual variables (e.g., location of writing), changes in sample, or other interstudy differences.

Quantitative Reviews of Expressive Writing

In an attempt to clarify the consistency of results from expressive writing interventions, a number of quantitative reviews have been conducted. Several meta-analyses have been conducted, the purpose of which is to synthesize effect sizes across a number of studies to generate estimates of overall intervention efficacy. The first meta-analysis to examine the effects of the structured writing task (Smyth, 1998) estimated an overall effect size of $d = .47$. The types of outcomes influenced by the intervention, with accompanying effect size, were grouped into the following categories: reported health ($d = .42$), psychological well-being ($d = .66$), physiologic functioning ($d = .68$), general functioning ($d = .33$), and health behaviors ($d = .029$). The last categorical outcome was the only one that did not generate a significant effect size, suggesting that this type of structured writing intervention may have direct, rather than indirect (i.e., through the modification of health-related behaviors), effects on psychological and physical health.

Using a similar framework, Frisina, Borod, and Lepore (2004) performed a meta-analysis on the effects of structured writing in studies that utilized participants from clinical populations. Clinical populations were further conceptualized as either medical or psychiatric. Medical populations included patients suffering from physical disease, such as renal, breast, and prostate cancer, asthma, rheumatoid arthritis, and so forth. Psychiatric populations were those recruited on the basis of psychiatric disorder or dysfunction and included samples such as psychiatric prison inmates, patients with posttraumatic stress disorder (PTSD), and major depressive disorder. The use of expressive writing as an intervention with these clinical patients generated an overall effect size of $d = .19$ (across the two groups). Specific effect sizes were estimated for each clinical subgroup. For patients with medical/physical disorders, a significant benefit was observed ($d = .21$). In contrast, however, there was no reliable benefit observed when utilizing expressive writing as a (standalone) intervention for patients with psychiatric disorders ($d = .07$; not significantly different from zero). Although this overall effect was not significant, further analysis showed that expressive writing produced significant improvement on measures of sleep quality, anxiety, and depression. Frisina and colleagues (2004) thus concluded that structured expressive writing can provide important physical health benefits among patients coping with chronic and/or terminal illness and may produce meaningful psychiatric improvement in certain domains (e.g., depression, anxiety).

Harris (2006) applied a meta-analytic strategy to assess the effects of expressive writing on health care utilization in healthy, medically ill, and "psychologically defined" populations. The effect size of the intervention in healthy individuals was estimated at $d = .16$, suggesting that the expressive writing intervention significantly reduced health care utilization; however, the effects for medical and psychological populations were not significant. The lack of significant health care reductions in clinical samples, however, is difficult to interpret. In particular, it is not clear if reductions in health care utilization should be a desirable outcome of the writing intervention, particularly among those requiring care (i.e., those with medical or psychological needs; Harris, 2006). More fine-grained analyses would be necessary to explore this issue. For example, it would be desirable to reduce visits resulting from injury or illness (presuming that this reflects an underlying reduction in causes, not increased neglect). In contrast, for some clinical samples, an *increase* in health care utilization may be desirable (e.g., if this represents better attention to required self and/or medical management for chronic medical or psychiatric conditions).

The most recent meta-analysis of the effects of expressive writing interventions included 146 randomized trials (Frattaroli, 2006). In general, the evidence suggested that expressive writing was a useful intervention, but one that was associated with fairly modest improvements (although across a very wide array of outcome types). Overall effect size was estimated at $r = .075$, with subtype effect sizes calculated for reported health outcome ($r = .072$), psychological health outcome ($r = .056$), physiologic functioning outcome ($r = .059$), health behaviors ($r = .007$, NS), subjective impact of the intervention ($r = .159$), and general functioning/life outcomes ($r = .036$; all effect sizes unweighted). Consistent with Smyth's (1998) findings, only the effect size for health behaviors failed to reach significance, which the author attributed to a possible need for cognitive restructuring in order to induce behavior change (Frattaroli, 2006).

Although the overall effect sizes were small, a number of conditions were examined to determine if there were optimal settings and processes for expressive writing to produce benefit. To do so, the effects of several moderating variables were examined and divided into five categories: report information variables (e.g., published vs. unpublished studies), setting variables, participant variables, methodological variables, and treatment variables (Frattaroli, 2006). Expressive writing interventions were found to be more helpful (produce more benefit) for some people and under certain circumstances. For example, greater benefit was observed for participants from the general population (as opposed to college students), for those with preexisting health problems, for individuals with a history of trauma, and for males. Several procedural variables were also determined to be important. Greater levels of privacy for those writing, a larger number of writing sessions, longer writing periods, and more detailed disclosure writing instructions also appeared to enhance the benefit of expressive writing interventions. Based on these results, Frattaroli (2006) suggested that future research studies should focus attention on these and related characteristics in order to identify and develop the most effective conditions for administration of a structured writing intervention.

Experimental Context of Expressive Writing Studies

As the quantity of expressive writing studies rapidly increases and uneven quality and procedural variations become prevalent, additional comprehensive reviews may help to summarize and keep up with new research evidence. A systematic review was recently conducted in order to evaluate the design and reporting quality of randomized expressive writing studies (Nazarian & Smyth, 2007). Two independent judges rated 70 studies using a standardized rating scheme that examined the following objective criteria: (1) the extent to which each study met Consolidated Standards of Reporting Trials (CONSORT) checklist items; (2) methodological and statistical reporting quality features (suggested by the American Psychological Association Task Force on Statistical Inference); and (3) alterations in clinically and theoretically relevant parameters of the expressive writing intervention and the reporting of these alterations when they occurred. Findings suggest that, in general, expressive writing studies had mixed methodological reporting quality, suboptimal reporting quality of statistical hypothesis testing, and demonstrated considerable heterogeneity in reporting of treatment fidelity pertaining to the delivery of the intervention (Nazarian & Smyth, 2007).

The latter findings regarding the reporting quality of parameters of the intervention are especially noteworthy. Of particular relevance to the current discussion on the use of expressive writing in the clinical context is the reporting quality of contextual factors, broadly defined as those variables that affect an intervention. For example, 61% of trials failed to report the location of writing sessions (e.g., whether participants wrote in a clinic setting or on their own at home). In addition to information regarding the location of writing, details that pertain to the status of study personnel (i.e., those that had participant contact) also helps to clarify the nature of the experimental (intervention) context. The majority of trials (70%), however, omitted information regarding the status of study personnel. This lack of methodological and reporting quality makes interpretation of interstudy differences in outcomes very difficult to evaluate. Moreover, the suboptimal reporting quality of these common variations in study personnel and location of writing appear to reflect an implicit assumption in the literature that altering contextual variables is inconsequential.

It is important to emphasize that the issue is not whether or not these choices are necessarily appropriate (although evidence suggests that they impact the outcomes of the intervention). Rather, it is incumbent on researchers to carefully describe the context of their studies (e.g., setting and location of writing, the status and training of research staff, etc.) to allow the careful examination (and meta-analytic modeling) of these issues. Recent empirical evidence suggests that the experimental context can affect the results of an expressive writing intervention, and different samples may respond differentially to contextual variables (e.g., location of writing and legitimate authority of investigator; Nazarian & Smyth, 2006). In order to examine the effects of context on an expressive writing intervention, the "legitimate authority" of the investigator (high vs. low authority) and the location of writing (home vs. laboratory) were manipulated in two different samples (college students and high-stress community participants). Overall findings support the hypothesis that context moderates the effects of an expressive writing intervention and different samples appear sensitive to different aspects of the experimental context (Nazarian & Smyth, 2006). These findings have important clinical implications that must be taken into account, particularly if clinicians ask clients to do the intervention in settings that are unsupervised and less structured (e.g., at home) than that of the laboratory and/or clinical setting. The safety and well-being of clients is an issue that must be considered and further evaluated when the intervention is administered in a self-help format outside of the laboratory (Smyth & Helm, 2003).

Proposed Mechanisms

Although the benefits of expressive writing appear to be widespread, much less is certain about the mechanism through which expressive writing exerts its positive effects (despite considerable empirical attention to this issue; see Lepore & Smyth, 2002). Regardless of the specific theoretical model, it is important to keep in mind that the effects of the writing intervention appear to reach beyond the boundaries of the actual writing session. In other words, the thoughts, emotions, and experiences disclosed in writing may remain with participants long after their 20 minutes of writing. This effect makes it difficult to determine exactly which mechanisms are at work and at what point in the process they become relevant. In addition, it is important to differentiate between findings that are *consistent with* a given model (correlational support) and those that are *in support* of the model (experimental support). The models discussed next have varying degrees of each type of empirical support.

The Inhibition Model

Initial work in this area focused on the role of emotional inhibition; typically construed as conscious attempts to inhibit strong emotions (and associated thoughts and behaviors). Active inhibition has been shown to cause autonomic and central nervous system arousal, which may over time function as chronic, low-level stressors. As inhibition is thought to pose a risk of illness and other health-related problems (e.g., Pennebaker, Hughes, & O'Heeron, 1987), disclosing strong thoughts and feelings was thought to reduce this stress and lead to improved outcomes. Although this idea is plausible, experimental investigation of this model has not provided much support of this view. For example, effectiveness of the intervention has not reliably differed between individuals that have previously disclosed versus those that have not (e.g., Greenberg & Stone, 1992), and benefit has been observed when writing about vividly imagined traumas that have not actually been experienced (Greenberg, Wortman, & Stone, 1996). As such, the role of inhibition in the written disclosure process does not appear to be the central mechanism of action.

An Integrated Cognition, Memory, and Emotion Model

Another theory given early attention focused on participants' organization of traumatic or stressful memories. This theory posits that, because emotional memories are typically stored in a sensory or affective format, converting these memories into language promotes the formation of coherent narratives. Although this process typically increases initial distress, it may allow participants to modify their fear surrounding the trauma, leading to integration of the traumatic memory. Integration of these memories should reduce unwanted reexperiencing of the trauma, which can allow for extinction of conditioned fear and other negative emotions and diminish associated autonomic arousal. This process of integration, through lessening negative affect and arousal, was thought to ultimately lead to reductions in psychological and physiologic symptoms (e.g., Smyth, 1999; Smyth & Pennebaker, 1999).

A related but conceptually distinct model is one that argues for a more basic process of exposure and habituation. Partial support for this model has been generated by Sloan and colleagues, who have examined the immediate effects of expressive writing in relation to overall outcome. Sloan and Marx (2004) showed that participants in the experimental condition exhibited physiologic arousal after the first writing session, and this reactivity was correlated with greater improvement in psychological symptoms. In a further investigation of this model, Sloan, Marx and Epstein (2005) found that instructing participants to write about the same topics at each session produced physiologic arousal after session 1 only, but that instructing participants to switch the topics of their writing resulted in arousal at both sessions 1 and 2. Significant improvements on psychological and physical outcome measures were only found for the group that did not switch topics. The authors suggested that these results were evidence that the same-topic group habituated more quickly to their negative emotions, which may have facilitated the positive effects of expressive writing (Sloan et al., 2005).

The Experiential Model

Consistent with an experiential model of emotional disclosure (based on the work of Janet, 1909), some evidence supports the existence of an experiential aspect of writing. According to this model, schematic organization guides the processing of stressful or traumatic events. Relevant schemas may include cognitive representations of these events, affective responses, and specific patterns of autonomic arousal. Failure to resolve powerful emotions surrounding a stressful or traumatic event may therefore be maintained through somatic states (e.g., tension, arousal; Gendlin, 1996; Greenberg & Safran, 1987).

The experiential model suggests that processing these events enables individuals to reexperience related sensations, cognitions, and emotions, resulting in new, less threatening perspectives on the events in question (Lutgendorf & Ullrich, 2002). Empirical investigation has supported the necessity of a combination of cognitive/emotional processing and a moderate level of emotional arousal in producing change (Lutgendorf & Ullrich, 2002). As better psychological and immune functioning are thought to occur through cognitive restructuring and alleviation of physical tension, the degree of processing that occurs through emotional disclosure (expressive writing) remains a critical variable.

Self-Regulation

Written disclosure has also been thought to allow for the regulation of cognitions, behaviors, and (most importantly) affect. Research supports the view that emotional dysregulation (inappropriate levels of control over emotional experience, expression, physiology, or behavior) can have negative effects on physical and psychological health. Expressive writing may help to normalize an individual's capacity to regulate emotion in several ways. This type of writing focuses attention on thoughts and feelings surrounding stressful events, which facilitates habituation to stressful stimuli and to negative emotions, and may lead to the reorganization of thoughts associated with stressful events and resulting emotions (Lepore, Greenberg, Bruno, & Smyth, 2002). Empirically, writing instructions that encourage problem-solving (Cameron & Nicholls, 1998), finding positive aspects of traumatic experiences (King & Miner, 2000), expression of ideas about one's ideal self (King, 2001), and effective goal pursuit (King, 2002) have each generated significant positive effects. Evidence consistent with this theory has also been shown through the moderating effect of respiratory sinus arrhythmia (an indicator of emotion regulation ability) on the relationship between written disclosure and self-reported depression and physical health in college students (Sloan & Epstein, 2005).

Language Use

In an effort to better understand processes of change in response to writing, a number of researchers have attempted to examine the content of the written essays. Rather than qualitatively examine such writings, much of the attention has been paid to automatic linguistic analyses conducted by computer software. The Linguistic Inquiry and Word Count (LIWC) is a computerized program that allows for "low level" examination of language through quantitative analysis of written text (Pennebaker, Mayne, & Francis, 1997). The program quantifies language statistics (e.g., word count, sentence length) and linguistic dimensions (e.g., pronouns) of written text. Additionally, this program can also provide information about psychological processes by summing relevant words in a text. Pertinent information may include the frequency of positive and negative words in each narrative, words that signify causal or insight-oriented processing (e.g., cause, effect, reason, because), and tense-related words (e.g., past, resent, and/or future).

The LIWC has been used to analyze the content of written narratives in several investigations of expressive writing (Pennebaker & Francis, 2005; Pennebaker et al., 1997). These studies have shown that moderate amounts of negative emotion words, as well as increases in causal/insight and positive emotion words as sessions progress, are related to improved health outcomes. It has been noted that participants who showed increases in causal and insight words seemed to be building a narrative framework over the course of writing. This information provides correlational support for the notion that the formation of coherent narratives or stories is an important aspect of expressive writing (Pennebaker et al., 1997), although this finding has not been consistent (Graybeal, Sexton, & Pennebaker, 2002). Smyth and colleagues provided empirical support for the necessity of narrative structure through experimental manipulation of the degree to which participants used narrative techniques, and concluded that positive outcome requires writing to tell stories with a clear start, middle, and end (as opposed to the mere ventilation of thoughts and/or feelings; Smyth, True, & Souto, 2001).

Final Comment on Mechanisms

There is a desire in the research literature and by clinical practitioners for a definitive answer on this matter, and thus there exists a tendency to interpret results in a way that implies a single mechanism is at work. It is possible, however, that the positive effects of expressive writing involve many or all of the pathways and processes reviewed here (and presumably many others not reviewed here). Benefits may be attributable to the cumulative effects of small changes, or different mechanisms may be at work for different people or in different situations. Several studies investigating potential mechanisms have applied only one theory and have reported little or equivocal evidence for that mechanism. Methods that take a pluralistic approach to mediation, assessing multiple mechanisms that may work together within individuals or differently between individuals, may allow researchers to draw more informative conclusions.

Using Writing in the Clinical Context

Expressive writing may serve as a useful and viable supplement to traditional forms of clinical practice in a number of different ways. Written emotional disclosure may improve both the process and outcomes of psychotherapy. The intervention can serve as an adjunct to psychotherapy and may also extend contact between the psychotherapist and client (by expanding the temporal and contextual boundaries of the therapeutic relationship). In addition, the expressive writing activity can be implemented easily and for very low cost to clinicians. Although the majority of writing studies have involved writing longhand about a stressful or traumatic experience, some studies have also demonstrated the efficacy of emotional disclosure through typewritten narratives (Brewin & Lennard, 1999). The use of computerized "written" disclosure may thus be a viable alternative for clinical application of this intervention.

Yet, despite the feasibility and potential benefit of using expressive writing as a treatment tool, certain issues warrant consideration. Assigning expressive writing as between-session "homework" activities can maximize privacy and client control, which has been shown to relate to improved outcome (Frattaroli, 2006). However, engagement in expressive writing typically results in immediate distress and discomfort (Smyth, 1998). As such, clients who experience unpleasant emotions may choose to stop writing in unmonitored settings, which would reduce the effectiveness of the writing activity. For this reason, it is also important to determine how to help clients address their distress when writing on their own. Some evidence also suggests that situations of great distress do not provide optimal conditions for finding benefit from expressive writing. This effect has been demonstrated in patients with PTSD (Gidron, Peri, Connolly, & Shalev, 1996) and in patients about to undergo high-risk prostate surgery (Solano et al., 2007). In addition, some clients may not see the value in writing about upsetting experiences. In such instances, it may be useful for practitioners to emphasize the findings of expressive writing studies and refer patients to lay publications on the benefits of this activity (e.g., Desalvo, 1999; Pennebaker, 1997, 2004).

The outline provided in Table 14.1 highlights general suggestions for applying expressive writing within the clinical context.

In reference to these recommendations, clinicians should keep a few factors in mind. There is no magical number of sessions required for clients to experience the positive effects of expressive writing: some individuals benefit from a single session, whereas others may require more. Optimal session spacing has been inconsistent in the literature, but the most recent research synthesis did not find spacing to moderate the effects of the writing intervention (Frattaroli, 2006). The solitary nature of written disclosure may be advantageous because it provides participants/patients with privacy, confidentiality, and control over their own intervention dosage (Pennebaker, 2002). Clinicians should also consider the "audience" to which the client is directing his or her narratives. Brody and Park (2004) have suggested that some participants in expressive writing studies begin their writing with an implicit audience in mind, which may contribute to the effectiveness of this activity. This audience is made explicit when writing is shared with the client's therapist, but it is unclear if and how this change might influence the process and outcomes of the writing intervention.

Table 14.1 Using writing in the clinical context

- Writing should be completed in a safe, quiet location without disruptions.
- Approximately 30- to 45-minute sessions should be allotted, with the majority of time devoted to writing and a few minutes afterward to compose oneself.
- A comfortable number of sessions should be selected, often three or four.
- Sessions might be conducted daily or spaced out over several weeks (or even months).
- Therapists should encourage the exploration of thoughts and feelings regarding the experiences or thoughts that are important to the client.
- Topics to consider during writing sessions may include: How does the stressful experience relate to the client's current condition/situation? How does it relate to other aspects of life (e.g., relationships, childhood, goals, who the client is, etc.)?
- It is recommended that clients should write continuously for the allotted time without regard to spelling, style, grammar, or "polish" of their writing.

Although the traditional expressive writing instructions ask participants to focus on negative events, improved outcome has also been associated with topics that ask for focus on positive aspects of such events (e.g., future positive goals; King & Miner, 2000). Stanton and colleagues (2002) found that asking patients with breast cancer to explore the potential benefit in their stressful medical experiences through writing led to reductions in both physical symptoms and symptom-related medical visits. Modifying the standard writing instructions to direct written narratives toward "intensely positive experiences" produced health benefits (i.e., fewer health center visits) comparable with writing about negative experiences in a college student sample (Burton & King, 2004). Similarly, Cameron and Nicholls (1998) demonstrated that focusing writing around future coping strategies effectively reduced health center visits and improved reported affect in college students.

However, it would seem that the inclusion of both thoughts and feelings surrounding an experience is necessary for improvement, as including only one has been shown to undermine the benefit of writing (e.g., Pennebaker & Beall, 1986). Efforts to "improve" the expressive writing intervention have added guidelines (such as narrative structure, processing, word use, etc.) to the writing instructions, which have produced mixed results. Specificity of writing instructions has been associated with better outcome (Frattaroli, 2006), but this can also be taken too far—the imposition of too much structure may restrict the client's potential range of emotional expression or willingness to engage in the intervention at all.

A further consideration for clinicians is the individual variability in physical and cognitive ability. Clients may present with disabilities that prevent them from engaging in the traditional expressive writing task, making it essential that practitioners and researchers take these issues into account. Physical disabilities, learning disabilities, and literacy issues may influence clients' willingness and ability to write. One alternative for individuals who are unable to write might be the private disclosure of their experiences into a tape recorder.

The Role of Feedback

In experimental studies, participants are aware that their writing may be viewed by the researchers (although they are assured of confidentiality and anonymity). This aspect of a research setting can imply an audience for the participant, possibly exerting an influence on the way that person expresses himself or herself. Some evidence does indeed suggest that a greater presumed audience will result in increased censorship of disclosure (e.g., Wortman & Silver, 1989). Therefore, when this intervention is used in clinical settings, the nature of writing should be established to allow for clients to decide whether their writing will be private or shared. Although writing interventions are successful in the absence of feedback from therapists, the potential benefit of receiving this feedback has not yet been ruled out.

Individual client and therapist dyads may determine the level of involvement and feedback from a therapist based on the individual case. Many factors may make feedback from a therapist undesirable, such as client self-motivation to improve or a therapist-client mismatch of goals/approaches to treatment. Conversely, some individuals may require more involvement and/or guidance from the therapist. In such cases, "self" administered writing may not always be beneficial, and some evidence suggests there are identifiable subgroups that would benefit from assistance (e.g., alexithymic patients; Lumley, Tojek, & Macklem, 2002). Therapist involvement can focus on clarifying the process and goals of writing, providing appropriate feedback, and regulating the writing "dose," which may increase benefit for certain clients. Therapists may also want to check in with clients after the first writing session is completed in order to address any resulting questions or concerns.

Therapist feedback can take several forms, each of which may prove to be effective with individual clients. Suggested feedback strategies include (adapted from Riordan & Soet, 2000) (a) therapists responding after clients read their writing out loud (particularly parts that are of increased emotional importance to them), (b) therapists reading written narratives during a session and subsequently discussing the writing with the client, and (c) therapists reading the writing samples between sessions and providing feedback during the following session. Deciding on which of these options to use will in part depend on a client's individual desire for therapist feedback and comfort level with sharing his or her writing. Therapists and clients should decide on whether or not to share or discuss writing samples before writing begins (Smyth & Helm, 2003).

New applications

Several studies have tested the effects of the expressive writing intervention in new ways, expanding its utility and broadening its range of application. These studies have demonstrated the effectiveness of distance writing, including workbooks or other alternatives to live psychotherapy (L'Abate & Kern, 2002), across mental and physical health care settings (for a review, see Smyth & L'Abate, 2000). Workbooks may be used as preventive or parapreventive activities in the absence of any additional intervention. A meta-analysis on the effectiveness of workbooks found a medium effect size for these activities for mental health outcomes and a slightly smaller effect size for physical health outcomes (Smyth & L'Abate, 2000).

A recent study examined the use of expressive writing through letters, as applied within treatment for couples who had experienced an extramarital affair (Snyder, Gordon, & Baucom, 2004). The couple's therapist read drafts of the written narratives and provided feedback on the letters before they were shared between partners. This relational model uses letters for different purposes as treatment progresses, emphasizing different content at each stage. The results of this study support the effectiveness of this type of extension of the expressive writing paradigm; however, as these findings were based on case studies, experimental trials of this modified intervention are necessary in order to draw strong conclusions about its benefits.

Lastly, the Internet provides an area of focus for future research on the implementation of expressive writing. Writing naturally occurs in great frequency over the Internet, through mechanisms such as e-mail, blogs (online journals), and instant messaging. Structured writing has been applied on the Internet through a program called Interapy (or Internet therapy), which provides a combination of structured expressive writing with therapist feedback and instructions (Lange, Schoutrop, Schrieken, & Van de Ven, 2002).

Issues for consideration

This chapter has presented several important factors in the transfer of the expressive writing paradigm to the clinical setting. The following questions remain matters of deliberation for clinicians who wish to successfully implement a structured writing intervention. First, how should writing be introduced to the client? Will writing be approached as a primary treatment technique or as a supplement to more traditional methods? For whom will this activity be the most beneficial? Should it be used on an inpatient or outpatient basis? How and how much should the instructions be structured, as opposed to allowing the client to guide the narrative? What are the potential effects of the legitimate authority of a medical setting? Will this intervention be as effective at home as it has been in the laboratory? Most importantly, how can clients' unattended distress be minimized? These questions continue to require purposeful clinical and empirical attention, but the potential for the integration of expressive writing interventions into clinical practice in a wide array of settings remains high.

Acknowledgement Preparation of this chapter was supported in part by grant #R01 HL67990 from the National Heart, Lung, and Blood Institute to Joshua Smyth.

References

Brewin, C. R., & Lennard, H. (1999). Effects of mode of writing on emotional narratives. *Journal of Traumatic Stress, 12*, 355–361.

Broderick, J. E., Stone, A. A., Smyth, J. M., & Kaell, A. T. (2004). The feasibility and effectiveness of an expressive writing intervention for rheumatoid arthritis via home-based videotaped instructions. *Annals of Behavioral Medicine, 27*, 50–59.

Brody, L. R., & Park, S. H. (2004). Narratives, mindfulness, and the implicit audience. *Clinical Psychology: Science and Practice, 11*, 147–154.

Burton, C. M., & King, L. A. (2004). The health benefits of writing about intensely positive experiences. *Journal of Research in Personality, 38*, 150–163.

Cameron, L. D., & Nicholls, G. (1998). Expression of stressful experiences through writing: effects of a self-regulation manipulation for essimists and optimists. *Health Psychology, 17*, 84–92.

Davison, K. P., & Pennebaker, J. W. (1997). Virtual narratives: illness representations in online support groups. In K. J. Petrie & J. A. Weinman (Eds.), *Perceptions of health and illness: current research and applications* (pp. 463–486). Amsterdam, The Netherlands: Harwood Academic Publishers.

de Moor, C., Sterner, J., Hall, M., Warneke, C., Gilani, Z., Amato, R. et al. (2002). A pilot study of the effects of expressive writing on sychological and behavioral adjustment in patients enrolled in a Phase II trial of vaccine therapy for metastatic renal cell carcinoma. *Health Psychology, 21*, 615–619.

Desalvo, L. (1999). *Writing as a way of healing: how telling our stories transforms our lives.* San Francisco, CA: Harper.

Frattaroli, J. (2006). Experimental disclosure and its moderators: a meta-analysis. *Psychological Bulletin, 132*, 823–865.

Frisina, P.G., Borod, J. C., & Lepore, S. J. (2004). A meta-analysis of the effects of written emotional disclosure on the health outcomes of clinical populations. *Journal of Nervous and Mental Disease, 192*, 629–634.

Gendlin, E. T. (1996). *Focusing-oriented psychotherapy: a manual of the experiential method.* New York: Guilford Press.

Gidron, Y., Peri, T., Connolly, J. F., & Shalev, A. Y. (1996). Written disclosure in posttraumatic stress disorder: is it beneficial for the patient? *Journal of Nervous and Mental Disease, 184*, 505–507.

Gillis, M. E., Lumley, M. A., Mosley-Williams, A., Leisen, J. C. C., & Roehrs, T. (2006). The health effects of at-home written emotional disclosure and fibromyalgia: a randomized trial. *Annals of Behavioral Medicine, 32,* 135–146.

Graybeal, A., Sexton, J. D., & Pennebaker, J. W. (2002). The role of story-making in disclosure writing: the psychometrics of narrative. *Psychology and Health, 17*, 571–581.

Greenberg, L. S., & Safran, J. D. (1987). *Emotion in psychotherapy: affect, cognition, and the process of change.* New York: Guilford Press.

Greenberg, M. A., & Stone, A. A. (1992). Emotional disclosure about traumas and its relation to health: effects of previous disclosure and trauma severity. *Journal of Personality and Social Psychology, 63*, 75–84.

Greenberg, M. A., Wortman, C. B., & Stone, A. A. (1996). Emotional expression and physical health: revising traumatic memories or fostering self-regulation? *Journal of Personality and Social Psychology, 71*, 588–602.

Hannay, D., & Bolton, G. (1999). Therapeutic writing in primary care: a feasibility study. *Primary Care Psychiatry, 5*, 157–160.

Harris, A .H. S. (2006). Does expressive writing reduce health care utilization? A meta-analysis of randomized trials. *Journal of Consulting and Clinical Psychology, 74*, 243–252.

Hockemeyer, J., & Smyth, J. (2002). Evaluating the feasibility and efficacy of a self-administered manual-based stress management intervention for individuals with asthma: results from a controlled study. *Behavioral Medicine, 27,* 161–172.

Janet, P. (1909). *Les nervoses*. Paris: Flammarion.

Kelley, J. E., Lumley, M. A., & Leisen, J. C. C. (1997). Health effects of emotional disclosure in rheumatoid arthritis patients. *Health Psychology, 16,* 331–340.

King, L. A. (2001). The health benefits of writing about life goals. *Personality and Social Psychology Bulletin, 27,* 798–807.

King, L. A. (2002). Gain without pain? Expressive writing and self-regulation. In S. J. Lepore & J. M. Smyth (Eds.), *The writing cure: how expressive writing promotes health and emotional well-being* (pp. 119–134). Washington, DC: American Psychological Association.

King, L. A., & Miner, K. N. (2000). Writing about the perceived benefits of traumatic events: implications for physical health. *Personality and Social Psychology Bulletin, 26*, 220–230.

Klapow, J. C., Schmidt, S. M., Taylor, L. A., Roller, P., Li, Q., Calhoun, J. W., et al. (2001). Symptom management in older primary care patients: feasibility of an experimental, written self-disclosure protocol. *Annals of Internal Medicine, 134,* 905–911.

L'Abate, L., & Kern, R. (2002). Workbooks: tools for the expressive writing paradigm. In S. J. Lepore & J. M. Smyth (Eds.), *The writing cure: how expressive writing promotes health and emotional well-being* (pp. 239–255). Washington, DC: American Psychological Association.

Lange, A., Schoutrop, M., Schrieken, & Van de Ven, J. P. (2002). Interapy: a model for therapeutic writing through the internet. In S. J. Lepore & J. M. Smyth (Eds.), *The writing cure: how expressive writing promotes health and emotional well-being* (pp. 215–238). Washington, DC: American sychological Association.

Lepore, S. J., & Smyth, J. M. (Eds.). (2002). *The writing cure: how expressive writing promotes health and emotional well-being.* Washington, DC: American sychological Association.

Lepore, S. J., Silver, R. C., Wortman, C. B., & Wayment, H. A. (1996). Social constraints, intrusive thoughts, and depressive symptoms among bereaved mothers. *Journal of Personality and Social Psychology, 70*, 271–282.

Lepore, S. J., Greenberg, M. A., Bruno, M., & Smyth, J. M. (2002). Expressive writing and health: self-regulation of emotion-related experience, physiology, and behavior. In S. J. Lepore & J. M. Smyth (Eds.), *The writing cure: how expressive writing promotes health and emotional well-being* (pp. 99–117). Washington, DC: American Psychological Association.

Lumley, M. A., & Provenzano, K. M. (2003). Stress management through written emotional disclosure improves academic performance among college students with physical symptoms. *Journal of Educational Psychology, 95*, 641–649.

Lumley, M. A., Tojek, T. M., & Macklem, D. J. (2002). Effects of written emotional disclosure among repressive and alexithymics people. In S. J. Lepore & J. M. Smyth (Eds.), *The writing cure: how expressive writing promotes health and emotional well-being* (pp. 75–95). Washington, DC: American sychological Association.

Lutgendorf, S. K., & Ullrich, P. (2002). Cognitive processing, disclosure, and health: psychological and physiological mechanisms. In S. J. Lepore & J. M. Smyth (Eds.), *The writing cure: how expressive writing promotes health and emotional well-being* (pp. 177–196). Washington, DC: American sychological Association.

Mann, T. (2001). Effects of future writing and optimism on health behaviors in HIV-infected women. *Annals of Behavioral Medicine, 23*, 26–33.

Nazarian, D., & Smyth, J. M. (2006). *Context moderates the effects of an expressive writing intervention: A randomized two-study replication and extension* (manuscript under revision).

Nazarian, D., & Smyth, J. M. (2007). *Randomized trials of expressive writing: An evidence-based evaluation of scientific integrity. Poster presented at the Annual Meeting of the Society of Behavioral medicine, Washington, DC.*

Norman, S. A., Lumley, M. A., Dooley, J. A., & Diamond, M. P. (2004). For whom does it work? Moderators of the effects of written emotional disclosure in a randomized trial among women with chronic pelvic pain. *Psychosomatic Medicine, 66*, 174–183.

Pennebaker, J. W. (1997). *Opening up: the healing power of expressing emotions* (Revised ed.). New York: Guilford Press.

Pennebaker, J. W. (2002). Solitary disclosure allows people to determine their own dose. *British Medical Journal, 324*, 544.

Pennebaker, J. W. (2004). *Writing to heal: a guided journal for recovering from trauma and emotional upheaval.* Oakland, CA: New Harbinger Press.

Pennebaker, J. W., & Beall, S. K. (1986). Confronting a traumatic event: toward an understanding of inhibition and disease. *Journal of Abnormal Psychology, 95*, 274–281.

Pennebaker, J. W., & Francis, M. E. (1996). Cognitive, emotional, and language processes in disclosure. *Cognition and Emotion, 10*, 601–626.

Pennebaker, J. W., & O'Heeron, R. C. (1984). Confiding in others and illness rate among spouses of suicide and accidental-death victims. *Journal of Abnormal Psychology, 93*, 473–476.

Pennebaker, J. W., Hughes, C. F., & O'Heeron, R. C. (1987). The psychophysiology of confession: linking inhibitory and psychosomatic rocesses. *Journal of Personality and Social Psychology, 52*, 781–793.

Pennebaker, J. W., Colder, M., & Sharp, L. K. (1990). Accelerating the coping process. *Journal of Personality and Social Psychology, 58*, 528–537.

Pennebaker, J. W., Mayne, T. J., & Francis, M. E. (1997). Linguistic predictors of adaptive bereavement. *Journal of Personality and Social Psychology, 72*, 863–871.

Petrie, K. J., Fontanilla, I., Thomas, M. G., Booth, R.J., Pennebaker, J. W. (2004). Effect of written emotional expression on immune function in patients with human immunodeficiency virus infection: a randomized trial. *Psychosomatic Medicine, 66*, 272–275.

Riordan, R. J., & Soet, J. E. (2000). Scriptotherapy: therapeutic writing for couples and families. In R. E. Watts (Ed.), *Techniques in marriage and family counseling: volume 1* (pp. 103–110). Alexandria, VA: American Counseling Association.

Rosenberg, H. J., Rosenberg, S. D., Ernstoff, M. S., Wolford, G. L., Amdur, R. J., Elshamy, M. R., et al. (2002). Expressive disclosure and health outcomes in a prostate cancer population. *International Journal of Psychiatry in Medicine, 32*, 37–53.

Schilte, A. F., Portegijs, P. J. M., Blankenstein, A. H., Van der Horst, H. E., Latour, M. B. F., Van Eijk, J. T. M., et al. (2001). Randomised controlled trial of disclosure of emotionally important events in somatisation in primary care. *British Medical Journal, 323*, 1–6.

Silver, R. L., Boon, C., & Stones, M. H. (1983). Searching for meaning in misfortune: making sense of incest. *Journal of Social Issues, 39*, 81–102.

Sloan, D. M., & Epstein, E. M. (2005). Respiratory sinus arrhythmia predicts written disclosure outcome. *Psychophysiology, 42*, 611–615.

Sloan, D. M., & Marx, B. P. (2004). A closer examination of the structured written disclosure procedure. *Journal of Consulting and Clinical Psychology, 72*, 165–175.

Sloan, D. M., Marx, B. P., & Epstein, E. M. (2005). Further examination of the exposure model underlying the efficacy of written emotional disclosure. *Journal of Consulting and Clinical Psychology, 73*, 549–554.

Smyth, J. M. (1998). Written emotional expression: effect size, outcome types, and moderating variables. *Journal of Consulting and Clinical Psychology, 66*, 174–184.

Smyth, J. M., & L'Abate, L. (2000). A meta-analytic evaluation of workbook effectiveness in physical and mental health. In L. L'Abate & M. Torem (Eds.), *Distance writing and computer assisted intervention in psychiatry and mental health* (pp. 239–255). Westport, CT: Ablex.

Smyth, J. M., & Greenberg, M. A. (2000). Scriptotherapy: the effects of writing about traumatic events. In P. R. Duberstein & J. M. Masling (Eds.), *Psychodynamic perspectives on sickness and health* (pp. 121–160). Washington, DC: American Psychological Association.

Smyth, J., & Helm, R. (2003). Focused expressive writing as self-help for stress and trauma. *Journal of Clinical Psychology/In Session: Psychotherapy in Practice, 59*, 227–235.

Smyth, J. M., & Pennebaker, J. W. (1999). Sharing one's story: translating emotional experiences into words as a coping tool. In C. Snyder (Ed.), *Coping: the psychology of what works* (pp. 70–89). New York: Oxford University Press.

Smyth, J. M., Stone, A., Hurewitz, A., & Kaell, A. (1999). Effects of writing about stressful experiences on symptom reduction in patients with asthma and rheumatoid arthritis: a randomized trial. *Journal of the American Medical Association, 281*, 1304–1309.

Smyth, J., True, N., & Souto, J. (2001). Effects of writing about traumatic experiences: the necessity for narrative structuring. *Journal of Social and Clinical Psychology, 20*, 161–172.

Snyder, D.K., Gordon, K. C., & Baucom, D. H. (2004). Treating affair couples: extending the written disclosure paradigm to relationship trauma. *Clinical Psychology: Science and Practice, 11*, 155–159.

Solano, L., Donati, V., Pecci, F., Persichetti, S., & Colaci, A. (2003). Postoperative course after papilloma resection: effects of written disclosure of the experience in subjects with different alexithymia levels. *Psychosomatic Medicine, 65*, 477–484.

Solano, L. S., Pepe, L., Donati, V., Persichetti, S., Laudani, G., & Colaci, A. (2007). *Differential health effects of written processing of the experience of a surgical operation in high and low pre-operative risk conditions. Journal of Clinical Psychology, 63*, 357–369.

Stanton, A. L., Danoff-Burg, S., Sworowski, L. A., Collins, C. A., Branstetter, A. D., Rodriguez-Hanley, A. et al. (2002). Randomized, controlled trial of written emotional expression and benefit finding in breast cancer patients. *Journal of Clinical Oncology, 20*, 4160–4168.

Walker, B. L., Nail, L. M., & Croyle, R. T. (1999). Does emotional expression make a difference in reactions to breast cancer? *Oncology Nursing Forum, 26*, 1025–1032.

Wortman, C. B., & Silver, R. C. (1989). The myths of coping with loss. *Journal of Consulting and Clinical Psychology, 57*, 349–357.

Chapter 15
Writing for All, for Some, or for No One? Some Thoughts on the Applications and Evaluations of the Writing Technique

Luigi Solano, Maria Bonadies, and Michela Di Trani

Introduction

In the past decades, writing about traumatic events or situations has progressively obtained high status as a fast, efficient, and low-cost method of promoting health. It is increasingly being employed in new populations, notably clinical ones. However, recently a review and meta-analysis including 61 studies on different situations (Meads, 2003) challenged the view that this intervention has overall beneficial health effects. This study received some methodological criticism. However, more recent, often considered as more methodologically sound, meta-analyses by Frisina, Borod, and Lepore, (2004) and Frisina, Lepore, and Borod (2005), which focused on nine studies performed on samples with physical or psychiatric disorders, yielded results that also were not very impressive: although the technique was significantly effective, the effect size obtained was only $d = .19$. This is a small effect size and low compared to the $d = .47$ found in a meta-analysis on studies performed in the general population (Smyth, 1998).

Comparing results obtained in somatic patients with findings from patients with psychiatric problems yielded a $d = .21$ for physical disorders and $d = .07$ (non-significant) for psychiatric distress. Concerning the latter finding, it is not surprising that improvement of mental disorders through psychological interventions needs much more effort and a good relationship with the patient. But also the effect on physical symptoms appeared much less impressive when compared to the results obtained in the general population. In our view, this may be due to the same factors as those responsible for the null findings in the Meads (2003) meta-analysis. In both cases, very heterogeneous samples such as terminal renal cancer, prostate cancer, asthma, and rheumatoid arthritis patients were combined.

Before proposing an attempt for a classification of patients into those "for whom it does work" (Norman, Lumley, Dooley, & Diamond, 2004) and those "for whom it does not," it is important to understand the origin of the homogenizing approach, such as used in a meta-analysis, because it refers to a scientific-ideological attitude with a rather long history.

A. Vingerhoets et al., (eds.), *Emotion Regulation.*

Nineteenth Century Positivism and Its Influence on Psychology

Positivism was a prominent philosophical movement whose basic formulations were written down during the second half of the 19th century and which brought us such formidable discoveries as to outsize anything discovered in the preceding 5,000 years in the fields of biology and medicine; for example, bacteriology, vaccines, antibiotics, and anesthesia (which led to an enormous enlargement of the possibilities of surgery) to mention just a few important developments. The effect of these discoveries and of their practical applications on the view of the world, not only by scientists, but by the public in general, was so great that the main foundations and constructions of Positivism, rather than being considered as just one of the possible views, came to be seen as the only true "objective" and "scientific" method.

The currently used classification of diseases, for instance, which has been developed in the late 1800s, was based on the organ, tissue, and cell alterations (anatomopathology) that are present in a specific clinical situation. It is difficult to deny that this kind of classification is superior to its predecessors. We should bear in mind, however, that it remains a *cultural construction*, possibly to be replaced in the future by a better one, that is, capable of explaining more clinical phenomena. We have the impression that both physicians and lay people think that diseases like, for instance, diabetes and peptic ulcers *exist in themselves*, irrespective of the thought that created them, and all that the future may bring is a better knowledge of these entities. As if the truth—at least in this field—had manifested itself for the first time, once and for all, in the late 19th century, whereas anything before should be considered as just obscurantism, while anything afterward may only consist of developments that remain immanent to that framework.

It could be sustained, however, that this very paradigm, so useful in defining and combating diseases for which an etiologic agent external to the organism may be readily identified (more specifically, infectious diseases), is showing strong drawbacks when confronted with diseases that now mainly afflict Western populations: cardiovascular pathology, cancer, degenerative and autoimmune pathology. For none of these, causes or risk factors explaining more than small percentages of variance have been found; correspondingly, no simple causal treatment or prevention (comparable with a vaccine preventing tetanus) is available. Possibly, a model of disease including not only specific alterations in an organ but processes involving the whole organism and its relationships with the environment would be more useful at this point.[1]

Although Positivism largely developed in the specific philosophical domain, residuals of the original propositions subtly, implicitly, and unconsciously continue

---

[1] Traditional Chinese medicine provides an example where pathology is seen as deriving from an imbalance between different trends and forces present in the organism. Although the language in which these formulations are expressed may appear esoteric to Western minds, many formulations appear quite similar to those developed by Western *psychology* (not medicine) in explaining health and disease. For example, "Fire arising from liver or heart" may well be seen as a picture of irritability and impatience which we know as the Type A Behavior Pattern.

to pervade scientific and everyday thinking.[2] We shall therefore try to review (in a rough and general way) the main foundations of 19th century Positivism and discuss whether and to what extent they may be useful in evaluating psychological interventions, particularly in the health field.

a. *Confidence mainly in what can be seen and measured*, directly through the senses or through instruments. The offspring of this attitude in psychology was behaviorism, which in its earlier formulations ended up in discarding the very object of study: the mind. Today, not only psychoanalysts, who have always emphasized the importance of unconscious processes, but many cognitive and system-oriented psychologists have come to recognize that many important things go on in a person's mind that are not directly amenable to direct and "objective" measurement. Planning of studies and analysis of results should avoid implicit acceptation of a stimulus/response framework and therefore consider the presence of such phenomena as more or less conscious expectations, intentions, and so forth. A person with untreatable cancer is very probably in a very different state of mind compared with a person with arthritis, even though this cannot exactly be measured. When a drug-dependent individual scores 30 on the Toronto Alexithymia Scale-20 (TAS-20), for instance, we should ask ourselves whether this is an "objective measurement" of a concept such as alexithymia or whether we are measuring something else.
b. *Refusal of anything that might sense of magic, mysticism, religion or "suggestion."* While we are currently convinced that separating medicine and psychology from magic and religion is useful,[3] the rejection of the importance of "suggestion," which was one of the pillars of pre-Positivist medicine, quickly caused disregard for the relevance of interpersonal relationships—including professional relationships—in health promotion or disruption. While psychology has obviously highlighted the importance of interpersonal relationships, we have the feeling that it has all too readily accepted the possibility of easily separating the effects of "suggestion," the so-called aspecific qualities of relationships among individuals, and more specific interventions, disregarding the risk of throwing away the baby with the bath water. One well-known example of absurd results that can be reached through blindly following this idea concerns the conclusions of the meta-analysis by Hrobjartsson and Gøtzche (2001) on placebo effects, demonstrating that this effect (well-known and experienced daily by every physician) does not actually exist. The problem is that this meta-analysis

---

[2] This is also true, for instance, for naive stimulus-response formulations in behaviorism, or for the concept of energy discharge in psychoanalysis, both of which, though largely superseded in the specific fields, continue to live in the back of many people's minds.

[3] Some psychologists, generally those with a psychoanalytic background, have laid our discipline open to accusations of mysticism by implying that some phenomena, such as unconscious communication between individuals, or the bodily effects of psychic processes, possess some extrasensory or somehow not rationally explainable quality. Some of these phenomena have been given adequate explanations through not previously available techniques, such as single-picture analysis of video recordings of mother-infant interactions; in other cases, we are more inclined to believe that our instruments are not as yet capable of detecting some signals, rather than resort to metaphysics.

was based only on double-blind hospital studies, in which, in the effort to separate suggestion from placebo, the placebo effect itself was totally abolished! If we agree that it is absurd to try and separate "suggestion" from the placebo effect, we might be more alert to the possibility that it may be difficult to separate it from other interventions as well.

In the same vein, the idea of "no-treatment" control groups in our field appears highly problematic if we realize that people have a mind and are influenced by relationships. As pointed out by Lumley (2003), "no-treatment groups" may easily become "frustration groups" if individuals have even the slightest idea that others are exposed to experiences they are not having access to. This may be true, for instance, when people who are asked to write about trivial topics come to learn that someone else is being asked to write about what was possibly the most important, though traumatic, episode of their lives. In other instances, the opposite may happen. In the field of psychotherapy evaluation research, it has been reported that people on a waiting list after some months show *higher* well-being scores than the other half of the sample who was actually having psychotherapy. This can easily be explained in psychodynamic terms as an effect of the idealization of an as yet unknown treatment but fits poorly with the idea of an untreated control group. In fact, the idea of untreated control groups has virtually been abandoned in psychotherapy research and substituted by the comparison of different treatments.

It is not possible, therefore, to define a priori and for all situations the best kind of control group, but we should decide on every occasion whether a control group *adequate for that context* was employed. We might decide in some cases that it is practically impossible to have an adequate, untreated control group, and that other control methods need to be used (such as comparison with other treatments or serial measurements instead of only before/after treatment, etc.).

c. Search for and confidence in *laws and recurrences that hold generally, for the whole of mankind.* Even better is, if it can be demonstrated that the same laws hold transdisciplinarily, such as the idea of "social Darwinism." Statistically speaking, this may be referred to as a "*search for main effects.*"

We believe that this premise has been most devastating for research in psychology. Hundreds of laboratories all over the world have produced thousands of studies on irrelevant and/or artificial psychological phenomena, provided that these could be considered general features of the functioning of the human mind and not peculiarities of a specific population or condition. Neisser (1989) noticed that, of so many studies produced on the functioning of human memory, not one was of any use for a practical problem such as defining the reliability of the report of a witness in a practical court setting.

In fact, when we deal with real-life situations, it is very difficult to obtain laws that can be considered universally valid. In many places, this has divided researchers into those who preferred to investigate functions so simplified as to have little relevance in everyday life and others who have studied the most complex nuances of the individual mind and of interpersonal relationships, but remaining at the level of single-case individual observations. Only occasionally space is given to studies that, on the one hand, are empirically controlled and, on the other hand are performed on real-life situations, in an attempt to provide answers to questions billions of people are asking around the world, such as what causes disease and good health. In order to make this possible, most of us have abandoned the hope for main effects and have adopted the interaction model: what works for whom? Under what circumstances? What are the moderating variables? [4]

In this framework, posing questions such as "Is the writing technique useful to people?" or "Is emotional expression useful to people?" appears senseless. We think it is high time that psychology gives up the false hope of obtaining a degree of certainty and universality comparable with the "hard" sciences, such as physics, or rather abandons the idealized view of these sciences, as in modern physics also the impact of the observer on the observed has long been recognized, such that no observations may be considered "objective" and "universal." Following this path, we might end up by suggesting that the main effects model is unsuited also in other fields, such as medicine (which is certainly not a "hard" science, having to do with people and their relationships, exactly like psychology). The idea that a drug should work for all people with a certain disease, irrespective of any individual differences, in order to be acceptable, probably leads to totally discarding drugs that could be useful to some subjects and to the loss of information about individual features that may be associated with resistance to an accepted drug (see also Koolhaas and De Boer, this volume, who demonstrate differential effects of pathogenic agents and drugs dependent on behavioral characteristics of animals). In this regard, we may note how psychological research always requires (to an extent that sometimes appears extenuating) controlling for biological factors, while no medical research requires controlling for psychological factors.

Applications of the Writing Technique in Different Contexts

Concerning the writing technique, we feel that we should focus explicitly on "What, why, for whom, and to what extent does it work?" (Kiecolt-Glaser, Cacioppo, Malarkey, & Glaser, 1992).

Recalling the original rationale for the use of the technique, starting from James Pennebaker's earlier studies (e.g., Pennebaker, Kiecolt-Glaser, & Glaser, 1988; Pennebaker & Francis, 1996), yields the following:

a. Individuals often undergo traumatic events (or more prolonged traumatic situations) that are not sufficiently mentally worked through (due to inhibition or to the effect of trauma on mental functioning) and that are not shared with other people.
b. This causes the memory to remain in a raw form, often very partially verbal, disconnected from other areas of the mind. In addition, it prevents regulation of

[4] As regards the writing technique, in particular, the need for this kind of approach is very clearly emphasized in a paper by Norman et al. (2004).

related emotions and dilution of the experience with all other experiences in the person's life (many of which are presumably of a more positive quality).

c. This "capsule of distress" exerts a negative effect on people's mental and physical health, and on their capacities to thrive.
d. Writing about the event or situation helps modify this situation by bringing the mind to focus on the memory and so creating connections, dilution, and possibly the definite "filing" of the event (something that is referred to as "working through," "processing," or "assimilation").

A second set of considerations concerns the *type* of participants involved and the setting adopted:

a. Writing was offered to a specific segment of the general population (most often, college students), not to individuals showing any kind of psychological or physical distress.
b. Writing was offered without any request on the part of the participants in a nonclinical setting.

In our view, the latter aspects are both a strength and a possible limitation of the procedure. As to the former one, the writing technique appears to be an effective, fast, and low-cost way to make a psychological tool available to virtually anyone, without the need to portray oneself as ill or needing help (the request comes from outside), which is still one of the main reasons leading people to utilize psychological help only when problems are inveterate (this is the situation in Italy, but we believe it to be true elsewhere as well). In this sense, the writing technique appears useful as one of the few tools for true *health promotion*, rather than for treatment of disease or distress.

These very same features, on the other hand, feed the need for evidence that the technique is equally useful in specific distressed populations. Samples of college students can certainly contain highly distressed individuals, but not in high percentages, and it is possible that the technique failed in just these latter individuals: the results are average results. If severe distress can be dealt with in most cases by writing for just a few hours, then all of us who have been working once or more times a week with a patient for years would be wasting their time. Moreover, whereas most healthy individuals generally find the idea to write about any past trauma of their choice stimulating, intriguing, and fruitful, both clinical intuition and common sense suggest that a person currently going through deep distress should be respected in his or her time and pace regarding when to mentally address his or her condition, in order for writing to be useful. The high percentage of refusals and dropouts in bereavement studies (see below) supports this contention.

Although we agree with Pennebaker (personal communication, 2003) that no a priori limits should be posed on the study of the writing technique, we nevertheless would like to stress that any application departing substantially from the initial framework should be considered experimental, and that possible negative findings should not be taken as evidence of general ineffectiveness, and certainly not put in a meta-analysis together with more traditional applications. On the other hand, positive results in new situations, when repeatedly found, may serve to enrich the paradigm. New proposals in this sense include, for instance, the idea that the beneficial effects of writing might be connected to improved self-regulation and enhanced identity construction (King, 2002). Improvement of relationships between self and internal object representations (Costantini, 2005), increased working memory (Klein, 2002), and enhancement of nonverbal to verbal translation (Pennebaker & Chung, 2007) are some examples.

We would consider outside the original rationale all work dealing with traumatic situations that subjects are currently experiencing or which are so recent that it is difficult to assume the subject is not thinking about them. These situations are not only very different from the initial applications on healthy, non–help-requesting populations, but also may show thorough differences with each other. We shall now attempt to classify these applications—which we may broadly call clinical—together with the results obtained so far.

(1) *The recent loss of loved ones, or severe trauma, where the subject is asked to write about these actual events.* The results are consistently negative (Gidron, Peri, Connolly, & Shalev, 1996; Kovac & Range, 2000; Range, Kovac, & Marion, 2000; Segal, Bogards, Becker, & Chatman, 1999; Stroebe, Stroebe, Schut, Zech, & Van den Bout, 2002), with negligible exceptions. As Stroebe et al. (2002) conclude, after reviewing these studies, it is highly probable that "in the case of bereavement, the writing task is superimposed on the normal process of change and recovery expected for the recently bereaved" (p. 176); this is very different from writing about past trauma that individuals have not been thinking about for a long time, and which the writing task brings to recall. Referring to Horowitz's (1986) theory on the different phases of response to stress, we postulate that writing may interfere with moments of adaptive avoidance. "Taken together, these findings suggest that in cases of uncomplicated bereavement, the bereaved have to cope with their loss in their own time and their own way" (Stroebe et al., 2002, p. 177). The inappropriateness of this kind of intervention is also illustrated by the considerable reluctance of potential participants to take part, unseen in standard situations, as expressed by the percentages of refusals or dropouts (66% and 70%, respectively, in the two studies reported by Stroebe et al., 2002). In addition to the severity of the traumas considered, their being recent and the absence of a clinical request, we may notice that writing in this case cannot lead to any possibility for the subject to modify external reality.

Based on these data and those derived from research on crisis interventions (e.g., McNally, Byrant, & Ehlers, 2003), Pennebaker and Chung (2007) arrive at the conclusion that defenses such as denial, detachment, distraction, and distancing may in fact be quite healthy in the hours and days after an upheaval and they also conclude that a technique such as expressive writing may be inappropriate until several weeks or months later. These authors additionally encourage clinicians to delay their use of expressive writing until at least 1–2 months after an upheaval or as long as the patient is (obsessively) thinking too much about the event.

(2) *Chronic disease in a life-threatening phase, where the subject is asked to write about the disease itself.* De Moor et al. (2002, p. 616) asked patients with metastatic renal cancer to write about "their deepest thoughts and feelings about

their cancer." No effects were found. The considerations are similar to the preceding point. Here, too, the patients are in a situation that they are very probably already thinking about, and any further invitation or incitement to dwell on the subject, without offering professional help, seems most inappropriate. Also, in view of the negative results, we feel that this kind of intervention is not only scientifically but also ethically questionable.

(3) *Moderately severe or well-treated chronic disease, where the subject is asked to write about events other than the disease.* For these kinds of study participants, the results have been rather consistently positive. Improvements in physical and/or psychological conditions were obtained in rheumatoid arthritis (Kelley, Lumley, & Leisen, 1997; Smyth, Stone, Hurewitz, & Kaell, 1999), asthma (Smyth et al., 1999), HIV infection (Petrie, Fontanilla, Thomas, Booth, & Pennebaker, 2004), and cystic fibrosis (Taylor, Wallander, Anderson, Beasley, & Brown, 2003). These results suggest that patients with chronic, nonimmediately life-threatening diseases respond to the standard procedure equally well as the normal population. HIV infection might be seen as a somewhat more severe condition, but its high level of treatability makes it a definitely chronic, nonimmediately life-threatening disease. Moreover, the patients had a very straightforward possibility of exerting control on their clinical situation by improving adherence to treatment, which is possibly one of the reasons for the $CD4^+$ increase found in this study.

(4) *Moderately severe disease or moderately stressful life situations, where study participants are asked to write about the situation itself,* but where, unlike the previous two points, positive outcomes may be expected, in most cases through the participant's active participation.

Increased capacity to find new employment after job loss (Spera, Buhrfeind, & Pennebaker, 1994), a shorter hospital stay and increased well-being after minor surgery (Solano, Donati, Pecci, Persichetti, & Colaci, 2003), considerable improvement in the control of diabetes (Tabasso et al., 2004), decreased physical symptoms after effective treatment for breast cancer (Stanton et al., 2002), and a lower incidence of postpartum depression (Bucci, Donati, & Solano, 2004) were found after asking study participants to focus their writing on the difficulties of their ongoing situation (unemployment, hospital stay, diabetes, and pregnancy).

It goes without saying that neither the expectation of a positive outcome nor the belief in influencing the outcome are present after the loss of a loved one, whereas these factors may be more likely present in other conditions and stressful events, which may explain the more positive results in studies on the impact of writing after having been exposed to such experiences.

The different results obtained in these situations[5] support our contention that the effects of the writing technique should be considered in relation to the context it is employed in and therefore should not be lumped altogether.

[5] The idea of making these distinctions (or similar ones) is based on scientific findings (such as the importance for health of mastery over situations and the inverted U-shaped relationship between arousal and performance) but also on ordinary common sense. We believe that when common sense is put aside, this should be carefully motivated and explained.

An interesting line of research that emerges is the assessment of differential effects of the writing technique in participants experiencing different levels of distress (in the same study). An effort in this direction was made by our group (Solano, Pepe, Donati, Persichetti, Laudani, & Colaci, 2007) by measuring the effects of writing in hospital patients awaiting prostate resection: positive effects (in terms of length of postoperative stay in hospital and of subjective well-being) were obtained only in participants with low preoperative risk, therefore presumably less distressed, whereas high-risk patients who wrote were (non-significantly) worse off than non-writing high-risk controls.

Alexithymia as Moderator of the Effects of the Writing Technique

Another possible area of exploration concerns the role of individual differences as moderating the responses to the writing technique. One clear example is alexithymia, or a reduced emotional expression in general. This topic was thoroughly considered by Lumley, Tojek, and Macklem (2002) and Lumley (2003). The results of different studies seem rather contradictory; whereas some authors find writing to have more effect in alexithymic subjects, others demonstrate the intervention to be useless, or even detrimental, for alexithymic participants.

Here, too, we feel that we should drop the hope of arriving at a final, universal answer such as "alexithymics are the ones who benefit mostly (or hardly) from the writing technique." More humbly, but also more realistically, we can hope to define, for a well-defined group in a specific situation (e.g., people suffering from chronic disease of moderate severity; people looking for employment), ranges of scores to a specified test that may appear predictive of the effects of writing. Our position is based on the following.

a. *Alexithymia is not an all-or-nothing phenomenon.* The qualification "alexithymic" and "non-alexithymic" largely depends on the idiosyncratic definition of investigators. Results may therefore be very different and thus be hardly comparable if subgroups are formed by taking participants scoring above and below one standard deviation (as in Lumley, Naoum, & Kelley, 2001) or above and below the median (Paez, Velasco, & Gonzales, 1999; Solano et al., 2003), or the 12 + 12 extremely scoring individuals out of a sample of 554 (De Propris, Buttiglione, & De Gennaro, 2002).[6]

---

[6] This sampling, which was designed to obtain "true alexithymics" and "true non-alexithymics," led to the result that the two groups did not differ on the variables that were the object of the study. Whereas participants with extremely high TAS-20 scores appeared, in fact, to be alexithymic, those with very low scores produced verbal reports that were not so different from those of the control group. It may be that, as the population consisted of psychology students, a form of denial and/or self-idealization was involved.

b. *Different samples may have different mean alexithymia scores.* It is obviously different if a subject is in the upper quartile of a sample averaging 50 on the TAS-20 or if it is derived from a sample averaging 65. Therefore, results may only be combined when not only the operational definitions of "high" or "low" alexithymia are similar, but the average scores of the samples are comparable as well.
c. *Alexithymia scores may have different meanings in different samples and subsamples.* It is possible that, in addition to the actual score obtained, being in the "high" alexithymia group in a clinical sample (which is supposedly highly alexithymic as a whole) is different (that is, more extreme) than being in the "high" alexithymia group from a healthy sample. On the other hand, high scores in a sample of people requesting psychological help could have the more "benign" meaning of stressing the help request, rather than reflect true incapacity in handling emotions. The different meaning of high or low alexithymia scores in different cultural contexts should also be taken into account.

   Moreover, we should bear in mind that, in theory and in most of the literature (Taylor, Bagby, & Parker, 1997), high alexithymia scores are associated with a higher number of physical and mental symptoms. When this is not the case, we believe we should be very careful in drawing conclusions about the moderating effects of alexithymia scores on writing. In studies considered by Lumley et al. (2001), in which more alexithymic participants show a negative effect of writing, control groups showed *high alexithymia* scores to be associated with *less* physical symptoms; it may be that in these samples, the TAS-20 alexithymia scores are representing something different from what we generally mean with alexithymia, and this dimension appears to interact negatively with writing.

   In recent work by our group (Rago & Solano, 2004), we investigated the effects of group emotional disclosure on longitudinal changes of TAS-20 scores in the inmates of a therapeutic community for drug-dependent subjects. The baseline scores of a certain subgroup of these patients appeared surprisingly low (M = 34), which seems in contrast with the theory of alexithymia, which considers drug abuse as a substitute for ineffective emotional regulation. We therefore decided to devote specific attention to this subgroup: its L scores on the Minnesota Multiphasic Personality Inventory (MMPI) were significantly higher than that of the rest of the sample, confirming a trend toward denial and, whereas the latter group progressively decreased its TAS-20 scores in response to treatment, the scores of this subgroup progressively *increased* with treatment. This finding was interpreted as evidence for an increased authenticity and contact with actual difficulties in handling emotions. In this subgroup, too, therefore, TAS-20 scores apparently reflected a particular meaning.

When a sufficient number of studies has been conducted, it is possible that some general conclusions might be drawn, though not as general as might be expected following a naive main-effect approach. Our hypothesis is that writing should work better in individuals who are not as alexithymic as to have difficulty in performing the task, but who are also not as much in contact with their emotions that writing may add very little further benefit (ceiling effect). We also believe that clearer and somewhat general differentiations will emerge in the meaning and effects of alexithymia scores on writing in different groups, such as normal population samples, distressed individuals addressed by researchers, and distressed individuals requesting psychological help.

Conclusion

It is our belief that the effects of writing, emotional disclosure, or any other kind of psychological intervention[7] should always be evaluated in relation to the specific characteristics of the study participants and context of the application. The aspects we feel essential to consider, and which showed an influence on results, are (1) the presence of distress at the moment of intervention, (2) the degree of distress, (3) the possibility of different actual outcomes of the distressful situation, (4) the possibility of individuals to exert an influence on this outcome, (5) the presence or absence of a help request, and (6) alexithymia scores in relation to the specific group considered.

This approach is very different from the main-effect approach most commonly used in sciences of the inanimate world and also in biological and medical research (sometimes inappropriately in the latter case, in our view). The search for general answers, which may superficially appear more rigorous and scientific, is, in our opinion, a shortcut that is inadequate to the object of our study.

Acknowledgment

We wish to thank Prof. Mario Bertini, Director of the Postgraduate School in Health Psychology, University of Rome "La Sapienza," for his thoughtful comments and advice on this manuscript.

References

Bucci, F., Donati, V., & Solano, L. (2004). Elaborazione scritta dell'esperienza della gravidanza e salute pre e post-partum in 39 gestanti primipare. *VI Congresso Nazionale della Società Italiana di Psicologia della Salute*, Napoli.

Costantini, M. V. (2005). La Rivista come un diario. *Rivista di Psicoanalisi, 51*, 91–95.

De Propris, F., Buttiglione, D., & De Gennaro, L. (2002). Alessitimia e aspetti quantitativi e qualitativi del ricordo dei sogni. *Psicologia della Salute, 5,* 33–50.

De Moor, C., Sterner, J., Hall, M., Warneke, C., Gilani, Z., Amato, R., & Cohen, L.(2002). A pilot study of the effects of expressive writing on psychological and behavioral adjustment in patients enrolled in a phase II trial of vaccine therapy for metastatic renal cell carcinoma. *Health Psychology, 21*, 615–619.

[7] The same may be said for the effect of any psychosocial variable on health. This point was clearly made on several occasions by Lydia Temoshok (see, for instance, the discussion on this topic in Solano et al. [2002]).

Frisina, P. G., Borod, J. C., & Lepore, S. J. (2004). A meta-analysis of the effects of written emotional disclosure on the health outcomes of clinical populations. *Journal of Nervous & Mental Disease, 192,* 629–634.

Frisina, P. G., Lepore, S. J., & Borod, J. C. (2005).Written emotional disclosure and clinical populations: confirming and updating our meta-analytic findings. *Journal of Nervous & Mental Disease, 193,* 425–426.

Gidron, Y., Peri, T., Connolly J. F., & Shalev, A. Y. (1996). Written disclosure in posttraumatic stress disorder: Is it beneficial for the patient? *Journal of Nervous and Mental Disease, 184,* 505–507.

Horowitz, M. J. (1986). *Stress response syndromes* (2nd ed.). Northvale, NJ: Jason Aronson.

Hrobjartsson, A., & Gøtzche P. C.(2001). Is the placebo powerless? An analysis of clinical trials comparing placebo with no treatment. *New England Journal of Medicine, 344,* 1594–1602.

Kelley, J. E., Lumley, M. A., & Leisen, J. C. C. (1997). Health effects of emotional disclosure in rheumatoid arthritis patients. *Health Psychology, 16,* 331–340.

Kiecolt-Glaser, J. K., Cacioppo J. T., Malarkey, W. B., & Glaser, R. (1992). Acute psychological stressors and short-term immune changes: what, why, for whom, and to what extent? *Psychosomatic Medicine, 54,* 680–685.

King, L. A. (2002). Gain without pain? Expressive writing and self-regulation. In S. Lepore & J. M. Smyth (Eds.), *The writing cure* (pp. 119–134). Washington, DC: American Psychological Association.

Kovac, S. H., & Range, L. M.(2000). Writing projects: lessening undergraduates' unique suicidal bereavement. *Suicide and Life-Threatening Behavior, 30,* 50–60.

Lumley, M. A.(2003). Does alexithymia cause health problems? A critical examination of various pathways. In J. Denollet, I. Nyklicek, A.J.J.M. Vingerhoets (Eds.), *Third International Conference on the (Non) Expression of Emotions in Health and Disease* (p. 10). Tilburg, The Netherlands.

Lumley, M. A., Naoum, L., & Kelley, J. (2001). Alexithymia as a moderator of the effects of written and verbal emotional disclosure. Poster presented at the *Annual Meeting of the American Psychosomatic Society*, Monterey, CA.

Lumley, M. A., Tojek, T. M., & Macklem D. J. (2002). Effects of written emotional disclosure among repressive and alexithymic people. In: M S. Lepore & J. M. Smyth (Eds.), *The writing cure* (pp. 75–96). Washington, DC: American Psychological Association.

Meads, C. (2003). How effective are emotional disclosure interventions? A systematic review with meta-analyses. In J. Denollet, I. Nyklicek, A.J.J.M. Vingerhoets (Eds.), *Third International Conference on The (Non) Expression of Emotions in Health and Disease* (p. 97). Tilburg, The Netherlands.

Neisser, U. (1989). The ecological approach to cognitive psychology: II. Imagery and memory. *Comunicazioni Scientifiche di Psicologia Generale, 1,* 55–66.

Norman, S. A., Lumley, M. A., Dooley, J. A., & Diamond M. P. (2004). For whom does it work? Moderators of the effects of written emotional disclosure in a randomized trial among women with chronic pelvic pain. *Psychosomatic Medicine, 66,* 174–183.

Paez, D., Velasco, C., & Gonzales, J. L. (1999). Expressive writing and the role of alexithymia as a dispositional deficit in self-disclosure and psychological health. *Journal of Personality and Social Psychology, 77,* 630, 641.

Pennebaker, J. W., & Francis, M. (1996). Cognitive, emotional, and language processes in disclosure. *Cognition and Emotion, 10,* 601–626.

Pennebaker, J. W., & Chung, C. K. (2007). Expressive writing, emotional upheavals, and health. In H. Friedman & R. Silver (Eds.) *Handbook of health psychology*. New York: Oxford University Press.

Pennebaker, J. W., Kiecolt-Glaser, J. K., & Glaser, R. (1988). Disclosure of traumas and immune function: health implications for psychotherapy. *Journal of Consulting and Clinical Psychology, 56,* 239–245.

Petrie, K. J., Fontanilla, I., Thomas, M. G., Booth, R. J., & Pennebaker, J. W. (2004). Effects of written emotional expression on immune function in patients with human immunodeficiency virus infection: a randomized trial. *Psychosomatic Medicine, 66,* 272–275.

Rago, N., & Solano, L. (2004). Lo psicologo della salute in una comunità terapeutica per tossicodipendenti. *VI Congresso Nazionale della Società Italiana di Psicologia della Salute*, Napoli.

Range, L. M., Kovac, S. H.., & Marion, M. S. (2000). Does writing about bereavement lessen grief following sudden, unintentional death? *Death Studies, 24*, 115–134.

Segal, D. L., Bogards, J. A., Becker, L. A., & Chatman, C. (1999). Effects of emotional expression on adjustment to spousal loss among older adults. *Journal of Mental Health and Aging, 5*, 297–310.

Smyth, J. M., Stone, A. A., Hurewitz, A., & Kaell, A. (1999). Effects of writing about stressful experiences on symptom reduction in patients with asthma or rheumatoid arthritis. *JAMA, 281*, 1304–1309.

Solano, L., Donati, V., Pecci, F., Persichetti, S., & Colaci, A. (2003). Post-operative course after papilloma resection: effects of written disclosure of the experience in subjects with different alexithymia levels. *Psychosomatic Medicine, 65*, 477–484.

Solano, L., Pepe L., Donati, V., Persichetti, S., Laudani, G., & Colaci, A. (2007). Differential health effects of written processing of the experience of a surgical operation in high and low risk conditions. *Journal of Clinical Psychology 63,* 357–369.

Spera, S. P., Buhrfeind, E. D., & Pennebaker, J. W. (1994). Expressive writing and coping with job loss. *Academy of Management Journal, 37*, 722–733.

Stanton, A. L., Danoff-Burg, S., Sworowski, L. A., Collins, C. A., Branstetter, A. D., Rodriguez-Hanley, A., Kirk, S .B., & Austenfeld, J. L. (2002). Randomized, controlled trial of writen emotional expression and benefit finding in breast cancer patients. *Journal of Clinical Oncology, 20*, 4160–4168.

Stroebe, M. S., Stroebe, W., Schut, H., Zech, E., & Van den Bout, J. (2002). Does disclosure of emotions facilitate recovery from bereavement? Evidence from two prospective studies. *Journal of Consulting and Clinical Psychology, 70*, 169–178.

Tabasso, C., Pastena, R., Cirillo, D., Pepe, L., D'Alterio, G., Maida, P., Tatavitto, A., & Solano, L. (2004). Effetti sulla salute dell'elaborazione scritta delle emozioni: studio empirico su 32 soggetti con diabete di Tipo 2. *VI Congresso Nazionale della Società Italiana di Psicologia della Salute*, Napoli.

Taylor, G. J., Bagby, R. M., & Parker, J. D. A. (1997). *Disorders of affect regulation: alexithymia in medical and psychiatric illness*. New York: Cambridge University Press.

Taylor L. A., Wallander J. L., Anderson D., Beasley P., & Brown R. T. (2003). Improving health care utilization, health status, and adjustment in adolescents and young adults with cystic fibrosis: a preliminary report. *Journal of Clinical Psychology in Medical Settings, 10*, 9–16.

MIX
Papier aus verantwortungsvollen Quellen
Paper from responsible sources
FSC® C105338

If you have any concerns about our products,
you can contact us on
ProductSafety@springernature.com

In case Publisher is established outside the EU,
the EU authorized representative is:
Springer Nature Customer Service Center GmbH
Europaplatz 3, 69115 Heidelberg, Germany

Printed by Libri Plureos GmbH
in Hamburg, Germany